Catastrophic
Neurologic
Disorders
in the
Emergency
Department

CATASTROPHIC NEUROLOGIC DISORDERS IN THE EMERGENCY DEPARTMENT

Second Edition

EELCO F.M. WIJDICKS, M.D., Ph.D., FACP

Professor of Neurology, Mayo Clinic College of Medicine; Chair, Division of Critical Care Neurology, Department of Neurology, Mayo Clinic; Consultant, Neurologic-Neurosurgical Intensive Care Unit, Saint Marys Hospital and Mayo Medical Center, Rochester, Minnesota

OXFORD
UNIVERSITY PRESS
2004

SOUTH UNIVERSITY LIBRARY
COLUMBIA, SC 29203

OXFORD
UNIVERSITY PRESS

Oxford   New York
Auckland   Bangkok   Buenos Aires   Cape Town   Chennai
Dar es Salaam   Delhi   Hong Kong   Istanbul   Karachi   Kolkata
Kuala Lumpur   Madrid   Melbourne   Mexico City   Mumbai
Nairobi   São Paulo   Shanghai   Taipei   Tokyo   Toronto

Copyright © 2004, 2000 Mayo Foundation for Medical Education and Research.

First Edition published by Butterworth-Heinemann under the title
Neurologic Catastrophes in the Emergency Department.
Butterworth-Heinemann is a member of the Reed Elsevier group.

Published by Oxford University Press, Inc.
198 Madison Avenue, New York, New York 10016
http://www.oup.com

Oxford is a registered trademark of Oxford University Press

Library of Congress Cataloging-in-Publication Data
Wijdicks, Eelco F. M., 1954–
Catastrophic neurologic disorders in the emergency department /
Eelco F.M. Wijdicks.—2nd ed.   p. ; cm.
Rev. ed. of: Neurologic catastrophes in the emergency department / Eelco F.M. Wijdicks. c2000.
Includes bibliographical references and index.
ISBN 0-19-516880-1
1. Neurological emergencies. I. Wijdicks, Eelco F. M. 1954–
Neurologic catastrophes in the emergency department. II. Title.
[DNLM: 1. Nervous System Diseases—diagnosis.
2. Emergency Treatment. 3. Nervous System Diseases—therapy
WL 140 W662n 2004]   RC350.7.W556 2004   616.8′0425—dc21   2003053092

Nothing in this publication implies that Mayo Foundation endorses any of the products mentioned in this book. Care has been taken to confirm the accuracy of the information presented and to describe generally accepted practices. However, the authors, editors, and publisher are not responsible for errors or omissions or for any consequences from application of the information in this book and make no warranty, express or implied, with respect to the contents of the publication.

The authors, editors, and publisher have exerted every effort to ensure that drug selection and dosage set forth in this text are in accordance with current recommendations and practice at the time of publication. However, in view of ongoing research, changes in government regulations, and the constant flow of information relating to drug therapy and drug reactions, the reader is urged to check the package insert for each drug for any change in indications and dosage and for added warnings and precautions. This is particularly important when the recommended agent is a new or infrequently employed drug.

Some drugs and medical devices presented in this publication have Food and Drug Administration (FDA) clearance for limited use in restricted research settings. It is the responsibility of health care providers to ascertain the FDA status of each drug or device planned for use in their clinical practice.

9 8 7 6 5 4 3 2 1
Printed in the United States of America
on acid-free paper

To Barbara-Jane,
Coen, and Marilou,
for the best part of my day

Preface to the Second Edition

This book is part of a trilogy on critical care neurology published by Oxford University Press. Although some overlap is unavoidable, it stands separately from the others. I have always considered this monograph a serious attempt to fuse a neuroradiology text—adapted to acute neurologic conditions—with an emergency neurology manual, but without compromising academic rigor.

The second edition of *Catastrophic Neurologic Disorders in the Emergency Department* retains its unique organization with multiple examples of neuroimaging, algorithms, and inserts with background information (boxes). The title changed somewhat because several reviewers in the United Kingdom felt the title *Neurologic Catastrophes in the Emergency Department* implied a medicolegal book. (Not so!)

A neurologic catastrophe is a major interruption of an otherwise coordinated and functioning central or peripheral nervous system. However, the damage of an evolving catastrophe can be lessened if it can be predicted. Therefore, this new edition has an additional focus on urgent neurologic conditions that could rapidly progress into a catastrophic neurologic disorder.

The second edition has a wider scope, with eight additional chapters. Seven of these chapters form a new section on the evaluation of presenting symptoms, and their conversational titles echo common requests for urgent consultation. As one would expect, the differential diagnosis of these symptoms is very broad. However, the chapters emphasize the "red flags" that set the priorities and direction of the clinical approach. The chapters are intentionally brief and convey the initial overlapping of thoughts and action. They are intended only to orient readers, and they are directly clinical. The neurologic disorders considered are then discussed in more detail in Parts II and III, to which a chapter on forensic neurology has been added. The rest of the book has the same layout as the first edition, but I have added figures and updated the text wherever necessary. In some areas, due to new observations, I have changed my mind.

I hope the book will continue to serve as a practical guide for neurologists, neurosurgeons, and other physicians who are called upon to manage or evaluate deteriorating patients in the emergency department. I hope it will also benefit emergency physicians who are stationed there.

Rochester, Minnesota E.F.M.W.

Preface to the First Edition

The first 60 minutes ("golden hour") in acute neurologic emergencies remain critical, and failure to intervene immediately may result in poor outcome.

Currently available books on neurologic emergencies in the emergency department do not reach beyond the basics of neurologic examination and interpretation of the findings. This book tries to fill the need for a resource for neurologists, emergency room physicians, and neurosurgeons who evaluate, treat, and transfer patients with catastrophic neurologic disorders. Critical care neurology is often interdependent with other clinical disciplines, and the book should also be useful for any physician in the emergency department who interacts with neurologists. The material is written from a neurologist's perspective, but the approach by emergency department physicians is reflected as well.

This monograph completes my three-part book project on critical care neurology. The third book not only offers a practical approach to major neurologic disorders but also links early management in the emergency department with more prolonged care in the intensive care unit. It focuses on rapid but accurate neurologic assessment, on the most useful bedside tests, and particularly on interpretation of neuroradiologic images. The organization of the book is standardized, with a major focus on priorities of initial stabilization. I have placed great emphasis on the predictive value of diagnostic tests when they are available. The chapters are interspersed with flow diagrams to facilitate decision making and boxed capsules covering major topics in the subject under discussion. The text is brief to facilitate reading. Its aim is to quickly explain, not to fully discuss, complex topics. It is intended to reflect the train of thought and action in the emergency department.

This book draws on new material on evaluation and management of major neurologic disorders, but at the risk of presumption I feel compelled to state that it is also the result of years of contemplation of these problems and all I could find to read on the subject. However, in a discipline in its formative years, the "whats" are plentiful and the "whys" fewer. I hope this book is an informative guide to the recognition and management of acute neurologic catastrophes at their early stage of presentation and finds its way to neurologists, neurosurgeons, neuroradiologists, emergency physicians, residents, and fellows in these specialties.

E.F.M.W.

Acknowledgments

I owe a debt of gratitude to the Section of Scientific Publications and Media Support Services at Mayo Clinic. I am particularly grateful to David Factor for adding superb new drawings to this edition and Paul Honerman for his creative digital formatting of all the figures and tables. I thank my research secretary, Raquel J.S. Nelson, for her enthusiasm in keeping this project on track and her meticulous work ethic. I am fortunate to be associated with Oxford University Press, and I thank Fiona Stevens for bringing my "neurocritical care" books under Oxford's patronage.

Contents

Part I
Evaluation of Presenting Symptoms Indicating Urgency

Chapter 1
Short of Breath

A breathless patient with a suspected underlying neurologic disorder is alarming and requires a swift response. The patient feels that respiratory function is changing and, due to the increased work of breathing, may use descriptions such as "chest tightness."[1] Respiratory distress may not be apparent, noticeable only when provoked by change in position or with testing of respiratory mechanics. It may be the first defining sign of neuromuscular disease.[2–4] In other circumstances patients may present in coma, catching breaths or are even ceasing to breathe.

Neurologic disease can impair respiration at multiple levels (Fig. 1.1). The interconnections between cerebral hemispheres, respiratory centers in the brain stem and axons, motor neurons, phrenic nerves, and the respiratory muscles provide a functional system that moves air in and out of the lungs. If the system fails, hypercapnia results. The alveoli and pulmonary capillaries subsequently permit efficient gas exchange by diffusion through a foil-thin barrier; if that fails, hypoxemia results. Both conditions may occur simultaneously or one disorder may lead to the other when reduced airflow leads to poor alveolar recruitment and collapse.

There are a number of steps one could take to narrow down the diagnostic possibilities. In the initial evaluation, it is logical to ask three major questions (Table 1.1): Does the patient generate breaths? Is air getting to where it needs to go? Is the pulmonary apparatus intact?[5]

Clinical Assessment

Acute lesions of the hemisphere or brain stem impact on automatic or voluntary respiratory control. The automatic control of the respiratory drive is generated in the primary ventilatory nuclei in the brain stem (Box 1.1). Loss of automatic control (Ondine's curse) has been reported with neuroblastoma and syringobulbia but is extremely rare.

The voluntary control originates in the cortex and connects to spinal cord levels with motor neurons sending connecting fibers to the diaphragm, intercostal muscles, and abdominal muscles. Impaired voluntary breathing involves a gamut of respiratory disorders and is not discussed further. All of these breathing patterns result in hypoxemia and can rarely be observed well because patients have already been placed on a mechanical ventilator. Some of these patterns are apneustic breathing or cluster breathing, both common with acute lesions in the brain stem. *Cheyne-Stokes breathing* (an oscillating cycle of 2–3 minutes of hyperpnea separated by apnea) is very frequent and could lead to brief periods of oxygen desaturation.

Failure to maintain a patent airway may have originated directly from acute neurologic disease. Breathing may be obstructed at the pharyngeal or laryngeal level due to tongue displacement, vomit, or tooth fragments. Breathing may also be labored from stridor, recognized by a high-pitched noise

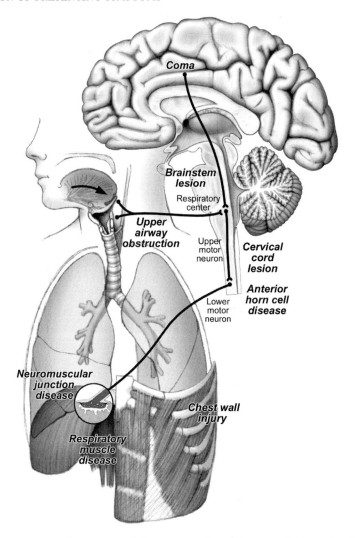

Figure 1.1 Causes of respiratory failure in neurologic disease at different levels of the nervous system.

at inspiration. It is not infrequent after extubation from subglottic edema or traumatic epithelial injury[6] but may be due to laryngeal dystonia (see Chapter 5) or vocal cord paralysis. Failure of gas exchange could be due to profound aspiration or, less commonly, neurogenic pulmonary edema. Frothy sputum and tachypnea often accompany hypoxemia and increased alveolar-arterial oxygen gradient.

Respiratory mechanics can become impaired due to lesions of the lower motor neuron (Box 1.2). However, disorders of the central nervous system may also impact on mechanics of the rib cage. Restricted muscle movements in advanced stages of Parkinson's disease are also reflected by

respiratory muscles causing incoordinated respiratory muscle pump function. Acute spinal cord lesions affecting higher cervical regions (C3–C5) result in ventilator dependence. Lesions below the level of C5 spare the nerve connections to the diaphragm, but expiratory effort is markedly reduced due to involvement of the abdominal and intercostal muscles. Placing the patient in a supine position improves expiration due to pressure of abdominal contents to the chest; breathing becomes labored when the patient is placed in a chair. Other lesions of the spinal cord (particularly multiple sclerosis) may cause diaphragmatic dysfunction, particularly when localized in the upper cervical cord.

Table 1.1. Three Major Causes of Respiratory Failure in Acute Neurologic Disease

Abnormal respiratory drive
    Sedatives (e.g., opioids, barbiturates, benzodiazepines, propofol)
    (Ponto)medullary lesion (hemorrhage, infarct, trauma)
    Hypercarbia
Abnormal respiratory conduit
    Upper airway obstruction
    Massive aspiration
    Neurogenic pulmonary edema
    Pneumothorax (e.g., after subclavian catheterization)
Abnormal respiratory mechanics
    Spinal cord lesion (e.g., trauma, demyelination, amyotrophic lateral sclerosis)
    Phrenic nerve lesion (e.g., Guillain-Barré syndrome)
    Absent or decreased neuromuscular junction traffic (e.g., organophosphates, botulism, tick paralysis, myasthenia gravis, Lambert-Eaton syndrome)
    Diaphragm weakness (e.g., myopathies) or associated trauma

The phrenic nerve may be injured, and unilateral damage could cause marked breathlessness during any form of exercise and prevent lying flat. Many cases are unexplained or due to neuralgic amyotrophy (associated with intense pain in shoulder muscles), stretch injury, or traumatic brachial plexus injury.[8] It is known to occur in compression of the brachial plexus due to tumor (commonly squamous cell lung carcinoma) or aneurysm (thoracic aorta), prior chest surgery or cannulation of subclavian or internal jugular vein, herpes zoster infection, or chiropractic manipulation.[9–11]

The focus of examination in patients with breathlessness due to neuromuscular disease should be on bulbar dysfunction, paradoxical breathing, and impaired coughing. Careful inspection and testing of the oropharyngeal muscles may point to a diagnosis. Longstanding dysfunction, such as in amyotrophic lateral sclerosis, is often evident by the presence of a wrinkled, fasciculating, slowly moving tongue and a hyperactive jaw reflex. In myasthenia gravis, next to ptosis and ophthalmoparesis, muscle weakness is prominent in the masseter muscles, and repetitive forceful biting on a tongue depressor is soon followed by inability to close the teeth. Passage of air through the nose when asked to blow up the cheek against counterpressure by the examiner's thumb and index finger reveals additional oropharyngeal weakness. The assessment of oropharyngeal weakness hints not only of involvement of the respiratory mechanics but also that ineffective swallowing could lead to aspiration. In a study on predictors of respiratory decline in Guillain-Barré syndrome, bulbar dysfunction predicted later requirement of mechanical ventilation.[12]

The symptoms and signs of acute neuromuscular respiratory failure are often very subtle. An initial cursory observation of breathing, blood gas, and chest X-ray could indicate no danger to the patient at all. However, after striking up a conversation, it becomes obvious that the patient frequently pauses in sentences to take a breath,

---

Box 1.1. The Anatomy of Central Control of Breathing

Two centers in the brain stem generate a respiratory oscillating pattern: the medulla oblongata central pattern generator and the pontine respiratory group. The medulla oblongata center consists of two major respiratory neuron groups with separate tasks. The dorsal respiratory group times inspiration and the respiratory cycle, and the ventral respiratory group is involved with expiration and includes the expiratory neurons of the Bötzinger complex. Within this ventral population is also the nucleus ambiguus, for dilator function of the upper airway during inspiration, and the nucleus paraambigualis, for inspiratory force. When these respiratory neurons in the medulla oblongata fire, specific patterns of the respiratory cycle are identified, suggesting architectural organization. The pontine center has a connecting link to the medulla center and functions as a time-tuning controller (e.g., setting lung volumes). Input to these centers comes from nonchemical reflexes (pharyngeal and pulmonary receptors and vagus nerve) and chemoreceptors (hydrogen ion). Stimulation is by decreased partial pressure of oxygen (PaO_2) (not content such as anemia) and increased partial pressure of arterial carbon dioxide ($PaCO_2$). The cortex can override these control centers, allowing speech, singing, coughing, and breath holding.

Box 1.2. The Anatomy of Pulmonary Mechanics

The activation of muscles in the upper airway, particularly the pharyngeal constrictor muscles and genioglossus, maintains a patent pharynx. The diaphragm is the major contributor to the respiratory pump. Using the abdomen as a bearing, its descent displaces the abdominal contents in a caudal and outward direction. The intercostal muscles run obliquely caudad and backward from the rib above to the rib below and thus provide, with contraction, an additional function. The muscles involved with respiration are not all active, and the inspiratory and expiratory muscles cycle during quiet breathing, the diaphragm contracts synchronously with the intercostal and scalene muscles (inspiration), and abdominal muscles barely assist with passive recoil of the rib cage (expiration).

The diaphragm controls most of the inspiration,

and dyspnea is expected with its dysfunction. When it contracts, the rib cage lifts due to its cephalocaudal fiber orientation. When it is not sufficient to lever it, accessory muscles such as sternocleidomastoid, pectoralis, trapezius, and latissimus dorsi, which harness the rib cage, are recruited. Expiration is assisted by contraction of the abdominal muscles. Coughing requires closure of the glottis and contraction of the diaphragm and abdominal muscles. The abdominal muscles can become severely affected in any neuromuscular disorder, reducing the effectiveness of coughing and atelectasis. Conversely, a patient with a forceful cough rarely has significant neuromuscular respiratory failure. Drugs (particularly opioids) and sleep can have an additional detrimental effect on respiratory drive and load.[7]

displays sweat accumulations at the hairline, demonstrates a mild tachycardia, and, when asked, confirms a sense of discomfort and increased work of breathing. The arterial blood gas can be entirely normal because the patient, due to an increase in frequency, is still able to compensate for a threatening hypoxemia. (The typical response in other medical disorders is increased tidal volume, but this is actually reduced because of respiratory muscle fatigue.) The tachypnea may be subtle, and respiratory rate is often increased to 20 breaths per minute and quickly rises. A useful bedside test is to have the patient count to 20 in one breath after maximal inhalation. If the patient can count, advancing one per second, the vital capacity is probably still within normal range. The classic clinical features of inspiratory paradox are characterized by inward movement of the abdomen during inspiration. With normal inspiration, lungs fill with positive pressure after the chest expands during diaphragm contraction, moving the abdominal contents out. When the diaphragm stops contracting, the positive pressure is replaced by a negative pressure, which causes the inward sucking movement of the abdomen. However, inspiratory paradox due to diaphragm weakness reveals itself late in the illness. Particularly when observed in a patient with an acute neuromuscular disorder, it more than likely indi-

cates that an early opportunity for endotracheal intubation has been missed. These patients are on the verge of apnea, often in the middle of the night.[13] It is important to note here that hypoxemia and hypercarbia are additional late phenomena, even in patients who are marginally compensated. Hypoxemia occurs due to significant shunting associated with collapse of multiple alveoli that are not recruited from breathing.

Bedside Respiratory and Laboratory Equipment

Pulmonary function tests provide quite useful values and are easy to obtain using non-electrical bedside devices. Commonly used peak flow devices (e.g., for asthma) are unreliable because expiratory peak flow rates can be normal. In neuromuscular respiratory failure, the airway is patent and lung recoil is actually increased. The simplest tests are assessment of vital capacity (VC), maximal inspiratory pressure (PImax), and maximal expiratory pressure (PEmax). The patient's position when these values are obtained is rather critical because clinically relevant diaphragmatic fatigue may become obvious in the supine position.

The technique of obtaining respiratory muscle function values is important, and scuba diving mouthpieces may reduce leakage, particularly when bilateral facial palsy is present. After the patient is connected to this apparatus, a nose clip is placed and the airway is occluded by blocking a port in the valve or by closing a shutter. VC is the volume of gas measured from a slow, complete forced expiration after maximal inspiration. VC can be reduced by additional airway and pulmonary disorders, certainly in patients with prior restricted pulmonary disease. PImax is recorded when a patient forcefully inspires against an occluded device. Typically, PImax is measured near residual volume at the end of maximal expiration and has a negative value as a result of the inspiratory effort in the presence of an occluded airway. PEmax measured near total lung capacity is the maximal pressure that can be generated by the patient making a forceful expiratory effort in an occluded airway. The manometer is able to record from 10 to 200 cm H_2O. The coaching of the patient is very important. Many patients have a tendency to produce a Valsalva maneuver, after which the required pressure is not generated and leads to falsely low values. Lack of understanding by the patient on how to perform this test remains a major problem in obtaining these spirometric values.

Normal adults can generate at least −60 cm H_2O of inspiratory pressures, and these are decreased in patients who have weakness of the mechanical function of the rib cage. PImax is largely a function of the abdominal and accessory muscles of respiration and some elastic recoil of the lungs. However, PImax can also be decreased in patients with hyperinflation disorders, such as emphysema. This condition in advanced stages makes the diaphragm flat due to trapped gas in the lungs.

There is little, if any, evidence of its usefulness in clinical assessment except in Guillain-Barré syndrome. A retrospective analysis of 114 patients with Guillain-Barré syndrome noted possible critical values of vital capacity of less than 20 mL/kg, PImax less than 30 cm H_2O, PEmax less than 40 cm H_2O (the so-called 20/30/40 rule) but also any reduction in vital capacity of more than 30% from baseline.[12]

Another study found VC 60% of the predictive value already a warning sign.[14]

An important correlation, or lack thereof, is reduction of respiratory muscle strength with PaO_2 or increased $PaCO_2$. Only when pulmonary function tests are markedly reduced is some rise in $PaCO_2$ expected; however, low-flow (0.5–2 L/min) O_2 administration may worsen hypercarbia substantially.[15] In these patients, measures to increase alveolar ventilation do not exist. In those patients with long-standing neuromuscular respiratory dysfunction and carbon dioxide retention, there is a dependence on a "hypoxemia drive." The additional administration of oxygen may cause apnea and hypercarbic coma.

The chest X-ray remains important in assessing pulmonary abnormalities. In neurogenic pulmonary edema it may show hazy opacities and airspace shadowing indistinguishable from cardiogenic pulmonary edema or aspiration pneumonitis (Fig. 1.2). Both acute lung injury and cardiac dysfunction may be present as a result of an adrenergic surge in acute hemispheric lesions or subarachnoid hemorrhage.[16] Suppression of cough reflex by sedatives or antiepileptic agents (e.g.,

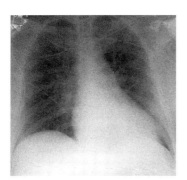 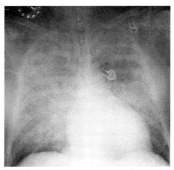 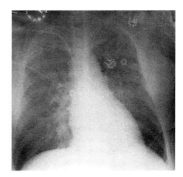

Figure 1.2 Serial chest X-ray in a patient with subarachnoid hemorrhage showing acute development of pulmonary edema. *Left*, Chest X-ray on admission. *Middle*, Acute development of pulmonary infiltrates and enlargement of the heart shadow, indicating pulmonary edema due to cardiac dysfunction. *Right*, After improvement in cardiac function with use of inotropes, infiltrates remain, suggesting dual injury to lungs and heart.[16]

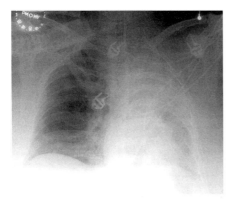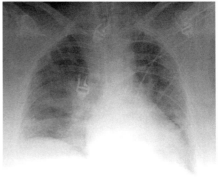

Figure 1.3 Acute bronchial occlusion from mucus plug (*left*), with reexpansion of the lung after bronchoscopic removal (*right*).

barbiturates) may cause mucus plugging of a main bronchus (Fig. 1.3). The chest X-ray may also show indirect signs of phrenic nerve injury (Fig. 1.4). Phrenic nerve conduction tests may document absent responses.[8]

Line of Action

Upper airway obstruction should be relieved, and in stridor laryngoscopy should be performed to view vocal cord erosion or epithelial damage. Elective endotracheal intubation must be per-

formed in any patient with persistent decrease in responsiveness and marginal oxygenation. Patients who have a mild tachycardia, display evidence of hypoxemia on a pulse oximeter, have evidence of increased work of breathing with change in posture,[17] or display the appearance of sweat beads need to be intubated preemptively.

In comatose patients, obstruction of the airway occurs for several reasons. First, muscles of the floor of the mouth and tongue become reduced in tone, and this changes the anatomic relationships. The tongue is repositioned to the back wall of the oropharynx and obstructs the airway. This

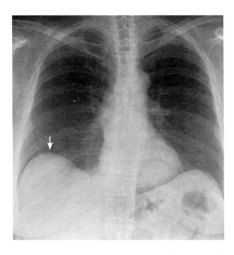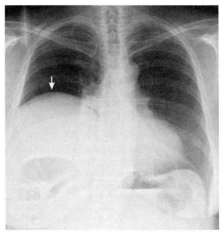

Figure 1.4 Serial chest X-rays showing development of hemidiaphragm elevation due to phrenic nerve injury on the right. (*Left*, normal; *right*, abnormal.)

position is even more exaggerated when the head is flexed. Therefore, with a simple technique the airway can be reopened. This so-called head-tilt/chin-lift (Fig. 1.5) tilts the head backward to what is often called the "sniffing position." In this position, the trachea and pharynx angulation is minimal, allowing for air transport. Also, the index and middle fingers of the examiner's hand lift the mandible and bring the tongue forward.

Another technique is the so-called jaw-thrust/head-tilt. The examiner places the ring, middle, and little fingers underneath the patient's jaw and lifts the chin forward. The examiner's index finger and thumb are free to fit a mask snugly to the face, with the other hand free to operate a resuscitation bag.

When the airway appears blocked by foreign material or dentures, this technique is modified by placing the thumb in the mouth, grasping the chin, and pulling it upward, leaving the other hand to clear any obstructing material from the airway (Fig. 1.5).

An oropharyngeal airway should be placed and is essential in patients who recently had a seizure because it prevents further tongue biting. The placement of this oral airway device is simple. The mouth is opened, a wooden tongue depressor is placed at the base of the tongue, and downward pressure is applied to displace the tongue from the posterior pharyngeal wall. The oropharyngeal tube is then placed close to the posterior wall of the oropharynx and is moved toward the tongue until the teeth are at the bite-block section. Alternatively, the jaw is thrust forward and the device is placed concave toward the palate and then rotated.[18] Dental injury, most commonly in patients who have significant dental or periodontal disease, rarely occurs.

Jaw thrust and mask ventilation securely maintain an open airway but must be followed by endotracheal intubation done by an experienced physician. Endotracheal intubation may be complicated in a traumatized patient with possible cervical spine injury. The ideal solution in these patients is to use fiberoptic bronchoscopy because with this procedure the risk of further neck trauma from neck movement is very low. Immediate endotracheal intubation is required in patients with penetrating neck trauma or significant intraoral bleeding. Temporarily, a cricothyrotomy can be made. A 14-gauge needle is inserted through the cricothyroid membrane, followed by insertion of a cannula. (The cricothyroid membrane is located just under the thyroid.) A formal tracheostomy should follow because ventilation through this small, highly flow-resistant tube is compromised.

Hypoxemia is often encountered, and oxygen administration has a high priority in patients with impaired consciousness. Nasal prongs are inefficient because they provide only 30% oxygen concentrations and often dislodge. Nasopharyngeal catheters provide 60% oxygen concentrations (but

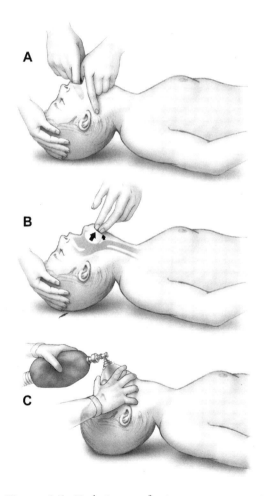

Figure 1.5 Techniques of airway management. *A*, Tongue jaw lift/finger sweep. *B*, Head tilt/chin lift. *C*, Jaw thrust/mask ventilation. From Wijdicks EFM, Borel CO.[18] By permission of Mayo Foundation.

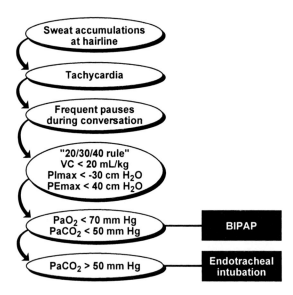

Figure 1.6 Critical steps in imminent neuromuscular respiratory failure. VC, vital capacity; PImax, maximal inspiratory pressure; PEmax, maximal expiratory pressure; PaO_2/$PaCO_2$, partial pressure of arterial oxygen/carbon dioxide; BIPAP, bilevel positive airway pressure ventilation.

only when the tip of the catheter is visible above the soft palate or face mask) and are a better alternative. Resuscitation bags are an optimal source of oxygen, and they can deliver a fraction of inspiratory O_2 (FiO_2) above 0.9 when the oxygen flow in the bag is 10 mL/minute. Oxygenation should be monitored with a pulse oximeter (O_2 saturation should exceed 90%) or measurement of an arterial blood gas sample (PaO_2 >100 mm Hg).

The indications for intubation in patients with acute neuromuscular failure are shown in Figure 1.6. Noninvasive bilevel positive airway pressure (BiPAP) ventilation in acute myasthenic crises, amyotrophic lateral sclerosis, and likely other chronic neuromuscular disorders should be tried first and may prevent mechanical ventilator dependence, tracheostomy, and volume-controlled, ventilator-associated pulmonary injury. BiPAP may avert intubation in acute myasthenic crises and amyotrophic lateral sclerosis.[19–22] However, presence of hypercapnia predicts failure of BiPAP, and volume-controlled mechanical ventilation is preferred.[21] Our initial experience in

Guillain-Barré syndrome is disappointing and we have seen respiratory distress persisting or emerging suddenly with BiPAP. Respiratory failure is commonly anticipated in patients with chronic neuromuscular disorders. This option ideally is addressed before intubation is undertaken.[23] In some patients (albeit very few), marked atelectasis, intervening pneumonia, or aspiration may have substantially contributed to respiratory failure. Thus, it should be emphasized that ventilatory dependence is not an incontrovertible outcome, and a period of rest with ventilatory support may lead to marked improvement.

After endotracheal intubation, virtually all patients are well served with an initial ventilator order that includes intermittent mandatory ventilation mode. The positive pressure breaths that are delivered by the mechanical ventilator are triggered by the patient, who has to generate only small pressure differences. The patient is able to breathe in between ventilator breaths and has entirely unsupported breaths. This ventilator order is particularly useful in neurologic patients because it allows for spontaneous breathing, and it can deliver hyperventilation if needed. A typical ventilator order for neurologically stable patients is a synchronized intermittent mandatory ventilation mode with an FiO_2 of 0.4–1.0, respiratory rate at 8–12 breaths/minute, tidal volume of 10–15 mL/kg, positive end-expiratory pressure of 2–5 cm H_2O, and an inspiration/expiration ratio of 1–3.[24,25]

REFERENCES

1. Sivak ED, Shefner JM, Sexton J: Neuromuscular disease and hypoventilation. *Curr Opin Pulm Med* 5:355, 1999.
2. Braun NMT, Arora NS, Rochester DF: Respiratory muscle and pulmonary function in polymyositis and other proximal myopathies. *Thorax* 38:616, 1983.
3. De Carvalho M, Matias T, Coelho F, et al.: Motor neuron disease presenting with respiratory failure. *J Neurol Sci* 139:117, 1996.
4. Kelly BJ, Luce JM: The diagnosis and management of neuromuscular diseases causing respiratory failure. *Chest* 99:1485, 1991.
5. Wijdicks EFM: Short of breath, short of air, short of mechanics. *Pract Neurol* 2:208, 2002.
6. Jaber S, Chanques G, Matecki S, et al: Post-extubation stridor in intensive care unit patients: risk factors evaluation and importance of the cuff-leak test. *Intensive Care Med* 29:69, 2003.

7. Ragette R, Mellies U, Schwake C, et al.: Patterns and predictors of sleep disordered breathing in primary myopathies. *Thorax* 57:724, 2002.

8. Chen YZ, Zu JG, Shen LJ, et al.: Phrenic nerve conduction study in patients with traumatic brachial plexus palsy. *Muscle Nerve* 24:1388, 2001.

9. Pandit A, Kalra S, Woodcock A: An unusual cause of bilateral diaphragmatic paralysis. *Thorax* 47:201, 1992.

10. Soler JJ, Perpiña M, Alfaro A: Hemidiaphragmatic paralysis caused by cervical herpes zoster. *Respiration* 63:403, 1996.

11. Piehler JM, Pairolero PC, Gracey DR, et al.: Unexplained diaphragmatic paralysis: harbinger of malignant disease? *J Thorac Cardiovasc Surg* 84:861, 1982.

12. Lawn ND, Fletcher DD, Henderson RD, et al.: Anticipating mechanical ventilation in Guillain-Barré syndrome. *Arch Neurol* 58:893, 2001.

13. Wijdicks EFM, Henderson RD, McClelland RL: Emergency intubation for respiratory failure in Guillain-Barré syndrome. *Arch Neurol* 60:947, 2003.

14. Sharshar T, Cheveret S, Bourdain F, et al.: Early predictors of mechanical ventilation in Guillain-Barré syndrome. *Crit Care Med* 31:278, 2003.

15. Gay PC, Edmonds JC: Severe hypercapnia after low-flow oxygen therapy in patients with neuromuscular disease and diaphragmatic dysfunction. *Mayo Clin Proc* 70:327, 1995.

16. De Chazal IR, Liopyris P, Wijdicks EFM: Cardiogenic shock and acute lung injury after aneurysmal subarachnoid hemorrhage (submitted for publication).

17. Allen SM, Hunt B, Green M: Fall in vital capacity with posture. *Br J Dis Chest* 79:267, 1985.

18. Wijdicks EFM, Borel CD: Respiratory management in acute neurologic illness. *Neurology* 50:11, 1998.

19. Lyall RA, Donaldson N, Fleming T, et al.: A prospective study of quality of life in ALS patients treated with non-invasive ventilation. *Neurology* 57:153, 2001.

20. Miller RG, Rosenberg JA, Gelinas DF, et al.: Practice parameter: the care of the patient with amyotrophic lateral sclerosis (an evidence-based review): report of the Quality Standards Subcommittee of the American Academy of Neurology: ALS Practice Parameter Task Force. *Neurology* 52:1311, 1999.

21. Rabinstein AA, Wijdicks EFM: BiPAP in acute respiratory failure due to myasthenic crisis may prevent intubation. *Neurology* 59:1647, 2002.

22. Sivak ED, Shefner JM, Mitsumoto H, et al.: The use of non-invasive positive pressure ventilation (NIPPV) in ALS patients. A need for improved determination of intervention timing. *Amyotroph Lateral Scler Other Motor Neuron Disord* 2:139, 2001.

23. Rumbak MJ, Walker RM: Should patients with neuromuscular disease be denied the choice of the treatment of mechanical ventilation? *Chest* 119:683, 2001.

24. Slutsky AS: Mechanical ventilation. American College of Chest Physicians' Consensus Conference. *Chest* 104:1833, 1993.

25. Wijdicks EFM, Borel CO: Respiratory management in acute neurologic illness. *Neurology* 50:11, 1998.

Chapter 2
Can't Walk or Stand

Acute impairment of the normal walking pattern is a comparatively common sign in patients arriving in the emergency department. Many patients present their symptom of inability to walk with sufficient explanation, and quite often it is due to an inability to support one's own weight from leg weakness or to maintain balance. Differentiating muscle weakness, lack of balance, or even inability to initiate a walk requires careful assessment and most of the time emergent neuroimaging. Examination of strength, sensation, and coordination should elicit a localization, severity of illness, and further determination of the specific diagnosis. Statistically, the most serious acute disorders associated with leg weakness are those due to acute spinal cord compression, acute spinal cord ischemia, and Guillain-Barré syndrome. To preserve the notion that acute leg weakness may be due to spinal cord compression, a separate chapter (Chapter 12) details recognition and management. Disorders with acute ataxia in adults (viral illness predominates in children) are invariably due to acute cerebellar or pontine (vestibular nuclei) lesions (see Chapter 15). Acute ataxic hemiparesis may be due to a pontine or capsular lesion (see Chapter 15).

Clinical Assessment

If the patient walks into the emergency department, balance and gait can be examined by following a simple set of tests. Proprioception after standing is tested by assessing vertical posture with eyes closed. Ability to maintain vertical stance with eyes closed could be impaired, with patients veering to one side. (One should note that keeling over consistently toward the examiner is psychogenic.) Walking is assessed next. Failure to initiate walking, "freezing" of gait during walking through a door, stepping and stride, and arm swing (including turns) are noted. Tandem gait and side-to-side pushes are finally added to assess gait.

Failure to initiate gait and lifting the feet off the floor ("as if glued to the floor, magnetic") may be due to acute frontal brain lesions or a more diffuse motor control failure, seen in patients with profound white matter lesions. Parkinsonian gait is usually suspected with small steps, audible shuffle, en bloc turns, and flexed posture. Freezing is common in parkinsonian syndromes and more a result of progression of the disease than an acute, first prominent manifestation.[1,2] Freezing may occur in a third of patients with hemiparetic stroke.[3] Unilateral thalamus lesions with sensory loss but no motor weakness could result in falls from falling backward or sideways.[4] The thalamofrontal connections and input from the cerebellum and spinal long tracts are responsible for this gait difficulty.

Gait apraxia is diagnosed when steps are inappropriate. Mayer and Barron[5] defined it as "loss of ability to properly use the lower limbs in the act of walking." Gait is counterproductive with perseverative leg movements, crossing legs while attempting to walk, and inability to mime march on the spot or wipe feet on an imagined mat.

Normally, during walking or running the feet slide very close to each other with minimal distance (less than 1 inch) between them. In cerebellar ataxia, the base widens and patients have instability of the trunk, poorly directed foot landing, and less specific inability to perform a tandem gait and sway and fall in all directions. Visual correction may reduce these manifestations. However, flocculonodular localizations do produce more sweep to one side with eyes closed.[6] Inability to even sit without falling over indicates a midline cerebellar vermis lesion.

Spastic gait with its typical scissoring and increased tone (rapid stretching causes increased resistance) proportionally involves the extensor muscles in the legs. Its presentation implies a much longer process, but patients may more or less acutely notice their symptoms becoming severe.

Loss of proprioception is a result of a disorder involving dorsal root ganglia cells and large fiber afferents in the posterior columns. These are usually known as "subacute" conditions due to prior use of chemotherapeutic agents such as cisplatin (dose >500 mg/m^2), nitrous oxide (abuse by dentists), and overdose with pyridoxine, or due to paraneoplastic destruction (Box 2.1). Pseudo-athetosis, areflexia, and absent position and vibration sense are hallmarks of this entity. When seen with spastic paraparesis and Lhermitte's sign, a cervical myelopathy (e.g., cervical spondylosis or multiple sclerosis) should be considered. Patients may have useless, numb, clumsy hands and may be unable to identify simple objects (e.g., coins) in their hands.

Inability to support one's own weight due to leg weakness and inability to get up from a sitting position, climb stairs, or walk uphill without taking countermeasures may eventually evolve into full paraplegia. These symptoms are so prominent that they may obscure equally important complaints of tingling and numbness. Progression may be in the ascending direction or suddenly complete.

The first principle is to determine a pattern of weakness. Proximal involvement favors muscle disease, myasthenia gravis, or myasthenic syndromes but also spinal cord disease. Purely distal weakness is more typical of peripheral nerve disease. Periodic paralysis is a rare disorder, but this channelopathy should be considered if the symptoms are repetitive.[10] Improving strength with repetitive testing argues for a presynaptic defect of the neuromuscular junction (Lambert-Eaton syndrome). Worsening strength with repetitive testing argues for a postsynaptic disorder of neuromuscular traffic (myasthenia gravis).[11] Tendon reflexes are lost early in acute polyradiculopathy and in spinal shock (see Chapter 12) and reduced in Lambert-Eaton syndrome and severe muscle disorders. Fasciculations and atrophy should be noted and indicate rapid worsening of a chronic neurologic disorder, mostly disorders involving the anterior horn cell or peripheral nerve. Muscle

---

Box 2.1. Paraneoplastic Syndromes Affecting Gait

Disabling ataxia, leg weakness, pains, and paresthesias may be presenting manifestations of cancer. Key syndromes are paraneoplastic cerebellar degeneration, opsoclonus, myoclonus and ataxia syndrome, sensory or motor polyneuropathy, and Lambert-Eaton syndrome. These manifestations are probably a result of a rapidly evolving immunologic mechanism and may become dramatically apparent in a matter of weeks. Paraneoplastic cerebellar degeneration associated with anti-Purkinje cell antibodies (PCA-1 or anti-Yo) increases suspicion of breast, ovarian, or genital tract cancer; when associated with ANNA (antineuronal nuclear autoantibody), anti-Ri, or anti-Hu, it predicts small cell lung cancer. In some patients, anti-Tr antibodies predict Hodgkin's lymphoma. Sensory neuropathies are associated with ANNA-1 or anti-Hu antibodies, which are rarely found in motor neuropathy. Voltage-gated calcium channel antibodies are almost always present in Lambert-Eaton syndrome. Positive antibodies should prompt more aggressive search using bronchoscopy, bone marrow aspiration, laparoscopy, or positron emission tomography. The serum antibodies that are found vary in type and detection and do not predict response to therapy, if any.[7–9]

tone is flaccid in acute Guillain-Barré syndrome, spinal shock, or cauda equina lesion.

Neurologic examination proceeds with sensory examination of the dermatomes and bladder assessment. The methods are discussed in Chapter 12 regarding spinal cord compression, where it is most relevant.

The differential diagnosis of acute or worsening paraplegia is quite broad but here is tailored toward disorders that, when not met with immediate attention, may result in permanent disability, bladder dysfunction, or even imperil respiration (Table 2.1). Acute paraplegia may be an immediate consequence of aortic dissection. Acute pain may be associated with widening mediastinum on chest X-ray. An emergent echocardiogram or magnetic resonance angiogram can confirm the diagnosis. Ischemic myelopathy may be due to reduced spinal blood flow, which in turn is due to increased intraspinal cerebrospinal fluid (CSF) pressure (Box 2.2).

Many other neurologic disorders can mimic spinal cord compression. Essential facts in the medical history include recent viral illness, vaccinations, illicit drug use, fever, weight loss, myalgia, severe back pain with radiation, recent tick bite, and skin rash, which may indicate acute myelitis or polyradiculopathy. It is very important to determine whether the patient is immunocompromised (e.g., cyclosporine, non-Hodgkin's lymphoma), has clinical evidence of human immunodeficiency virus (HIV) infection, or has risk factors for the acquired immunodeficiency syndrome (AIDS) virus, including previous blood or blood-product transfusions (the

Table 2.1. Acute Paraplegia

Disorder	History of	Suggests
Myelitis	Vaccination	Postvaccination myelopathy
	Febrile illness	Postinfectious transverse myelitis
	Optic neuritis	Multiple sclerosis or Devic's disease
	Travel	Schistosomiasis, cysticercosis
	Tick bite	Lyme disease
	Immunosuppression, AIDS	Tuberculosis, aspergillosis, coccidioidomycosis, syphilis
Myelopathy	Cancer	Acute necrotic myelopathy
	Aortic aneurysms or recent catheterization, low back pain	Infarction of the cord (thromboemboli, fibrocartilaginous emboli)
	Connective tissue disease (Sjögren's syndrome, SLE)	Vasculitis
	Cancer	Radiation myelopathy
		Paraneoplastic myelopathy
	Anticoagulation	Epidural hematoma
		Intramedullary hemorrhage
	Progressive symptoms with occasional exacerbation, profound muscle wasting	Spinal AVM
		Dural AV fistula
Polyradiculopathy	Diarrhea, URI, CMV, HS, EBV, diabetes mellitus, leukemia, sarcoidosis	Guillain-Barré syndrome
		Acute diabetic polyradiculopathy
		Infiltrative or inflammatory polyradiculopathy
Neoplastic meningitis	Carcinoma, lymphoma, or other hematologic–oncologic disease	Leptomeningeal spread
Neuromuscular dysfunction	Dysphagia, diplopia, ptosis, fatigability	Myasthenia gravis
	Small cell lung cancer	Lambert-Eaton syndrome
	Dry mouth; sixth nerve palsy; fixed, dilated pupils	Botulism
Myopathy	Autoimmune disorder	Polymyositis
	Malar, perioral skin rash	Dermatomyositis
	Exercise intolerance and myoglobinuria	Metabolic myopathy
	Periodic attacks (minutes to hours)	Hyperkalemic or hypokalemic paralysis

AIDS, acquired immunodeficiency syndrome; AV, arteriovenous; AVM, arteriovenous malformation; CMV, cytomegalovirus; EBV, Epstein-Barr virus; HS, herpes simplex; SLE, systemic lupus erythematosus; URI, upper respiratory infection.

Box 2.2. Paraplegia in Aortic Dissection

Immediate- or delayed-onset paraplegia from spinal cord ischemia can be a consequence of aortic dissection. It is often inappropriately considered permanent at onset. An acute lumbar puncture may lead to rapid recovery, and a high opening pressure is evident. Aortic occlusion of the descending aorta and cardiac outflow obstruction increase volume in the intracranial sinuses, translating into increased intraspinal volume and increased CSF pressure. Early spinal cord edema may cause the CSF pressure to rise also. Spinal cord perfusion is reduced and equal to spinal arterial pressure minus CSF pressure. Removal of 20 to 30 mL of CSF followed by continuous CSF drainage at a rate of 5 to 10 mL per hour can be dramatically effective, with resolution of symptoms within hours.[12,13]

risks were higher before 1985, when regular HIV screening was not available in blood banks). Recent travel may be relevant and may suggest a myelopathy from *Schistosoma* species (endemic in Brazil) or cysticercosis (any country in Latin America).

Acute transverse myelitis should be considered in patients between age 10 and 20 or 30 and 40 years but is highly uncommon. Criteria include development of sensorimotor or autonomic dysfunction from a cord lesion, defined sensory level; bilateral signs that can be asymmetric; and progression to maximal deficit within hours or 3 weeks.

Line of Action

It is imperative to admit any patient with acute severe impairment of gait or balance and to expedite evaluation.

With so many possible levels of involvement in the nervous system, the laboratory tests should focus on the most probable localization (Fig. 2.1). Magnetic resonance imaging (MRI) is mandatory because compression of the thoracic or lumbar spinal cord or meningeal pathology is common in acute or rapidly worsening weakness (if no further localization can be made). It is not unreasonable to proceed with an MRI of the entire neuraxis to visualize all structures involved in gait initiation. If no structural lesions are found, cerebrospinal fluid examination is warranted.

CSF examination should follow and may be immediately therapeutic in patients with ischemic myelopathy associated with aortic dissection. Failure to recognize this option of removing CSF under high pressure may lead to permanent deficit.[12]

Infectious myelitis is the most common alternative diagnosis in acute spinal cord syndromes and often involves viral infections. Viruses affecting spinal gray matter usually include herpes zoster, but other herpes viruses (cytomegalovirus, herpes simplex) may attack nerve roots. CSF in herpes zoster myelitis shows pleocytosis, increased protein levels, and normal glucose values. Viruses with a proclivity for white matter include HIV and human T-cell lymphotropic virus (type I). A viral serologic panel should be obtained in the emergency department in appropriate cases (HSV-1, HSV-2, HHV-6, VZV, CMV, EBV, HIV, and enteroviruses). Increased white cell count should suggest an acute transverse myelitis. In appropriate circumstances such as in concurrent TB infection, CSF and fast bacilli smear and culture should be obtained. A moderate lymphocytic pleocytosis is common in acute transverse myelitis and may be accompanied by increased IgG and oligoclonal

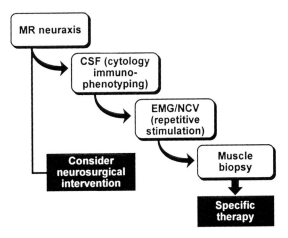

Figure 2.1 Critical steps in the evaluation of gait abnormalities or paraparesis. MR, magnetic resonance; CSF, cerebrospinal fluid; EMG/NCV, electromyography/nerve conduction velocity.

bands. Cytologic examination of CSF should focus on malignant cells (only 50% positive yield), and flow cytometry is indicated if atypical lymphocytes are found. Flow-cytometric immunophenotyping consists of antibodies against several antigens such as CD19, CD45, and κ and λ immunoglobulin light chains to characterize a possible blast population or monoclonal B-cell population.

Oligoclonal bands in CSF suggest multiple sclerosis, particularly if other white matter lesions are found (up to 80% positive predictive value). Visual evoked potentials can be useful to document optic neuritis, as in Devic's disease or multiple sclerosis. Systemic inflammatory disease may be complicated by myelitis, and autoantibodies (ANA [antinuclear antibodies], double-stranded DNA, SS-A [RO], SS-B [La], Sm [Smith], and RNP [ribonucleoprotein]) are useful.

More peripherally, other important rapid discriminating tests in the emergency department are creatine kinase and nerve conduction studies with repetitive stimulation (presynaptic rapid stimulation results in incremental amplitude, postsynaptic decremental amplitude at low stimulation rate).[14–17] Serum antibodies are tested for paraneoplastic syndromes, which can be quite rapid in presentation (Box 2.1).[7–9] Muscle and nerve biopsy is needed to document inflammatory myopathy.

REFERENCES

1. Giladi N: Freezing of gait. Clinical overview. *Adv Neurol* 87:191, 2001.
2. Giladi N, Kao R, Fahn S: Freezing phenomenon in patients with parkinsonian syndromes. *Mov Disord* 12:302, 1997.
3. Bussin JL, Abedin H, Tallis RC: Freezing episodes in hemiparetic stroke: results of a pilot survey. *Clin Rehabil* 13:207, 1999.
4. Masdeu JC, Gorelick PB: Thalamic astasia: inability to stand after unilateral thalamic lesions. *Ann Neurol* 23:596, 1988.
5. Mayer YS, Barron DW: Apraxia of gait: clinico-physiological study. *Brain* 83:261, 1960.
6. Masdeu JC: Neuroimaging and gait. *Adv Neurol* 87:83, 2001.
7. Moll JW, Antoine JC, Brashear HR, et al.: Guidelines on the detection of paraneoplastic and neuronal-specific antibodies. *Neurology* 45:1937, 1995.
8. Pittock SJ, Lucchinetti CF, Lennon VA: Anti-neuronal nuclear autoantibody type 2: paraneoplastic accompaniments. *Ann Neurol* 53:580, 2003.
9. Posner JB, Dalmau JO: Paraneoplastic syndromes of the nervous system. *Clin Chem Lab Med* 38:117, 2000.
10. Lehmann-Horn F, Jurkat-Rott K, Rudel R: Periodic paralysis: understanding channelopathies. *Curr Neurol Neurosci* 2:61, 2002.
11. Celesia GG: Disorders of membrane channels or channelopathies. *Clin Neurophysiol* 112:2, 2001.
12. Blacker DJ, Wijdicks EFM, Ramakrishna G: Resolution of severe paraplegia due to aortic dissection after CSF drainage. *Neurology* 61:142, 2003.
13. Killen D, Weinstein C, Reed W. Reversal of spinal cord ischemia resulting from aortic dissection. *J Thorac Cardiovasc Surg* 119:1049, 2000.
14. Pascuzzi RM: Pearls and pitfalls in the diagnosis and management of neuromuscular junction disorders. *Semin Neurol* 21:425, 2001.
15. Sanders DB: The Lambert-Eaton myasthenic syndrome. *Adv Neurol* 88:189, 2002.
16. Takamori M, Komai K, Iwasa K: Antibodies to calcium channel and synaptotagmin in Lambert-Eaton myasthenic syndrome. *Am J Med Sci* 319:204, 2000.
17. Moxley RT III: Channelopathies. *Curr Treat Options Neurol* 2:31, 2000.

Chapter 3
See Nothing, See Double, See Shapes and Images

Much like acute focal signs, sudden loss of visual acuity, clarity, or newly formed images may herald the rapid development of a major neurologic condition. A certain appearance (e.g., third nerve palsy) may indicate that immediate magnetic resonance imaging (MRI) or cerebral angiography is required. Some patients may need urgent neurosurgical intervention or a consultation by an ophthalmologist, particularly when a glaring contradiction between findings on examination and neuroimaging exists. Skill, knowledge, and additional investigations are required to diagnose acute neuro-ophthalmologic conditions. Many enigmatic presentations of monocular blindness are due to acute retinal or optic nerve disorders. Monocular visual loss may suggest a lesion involving the anterior cerebral circulation. Acute transient binocular visual loss may point to occlusion in the territory of the posterior cerebral circulation.

The emergency department may not be the place to commit oneself to definitively resolving the differential diagnosis of any of these conditions, and these patients may need admission. This chapter is included for the purpose of describing common urgent neuro-ophthalmologic disorders associated with decreased vision and positive visual phenomena.

Clinical Assessment

The testing methods in the emergency department are limited, but certain tests should be performed on every patient presenting with major symptoms of a defective visual system. Blindness is usually referred to as "vision of less than 20/200 with correction or a field not subtending an angle greater than 20 degrees" (legal blindness). It is simpler to describe it by a diagram (Box 3.1). Poor vision due to a refractive error is easily discovered by having the patient look through a pinhole punched in a piece of paper. (Vision will improve if decreased from a refractive cause.) The first test in a patient with marked reduction in vision is to assess "blink to threat." This is preferably performed in patients with reduced level of consciousness or those who claim no vision. The best technique is to approach both eyes from the lateral visual field with a closed fist and then open up the fist to a hand with spread-out fingers several inches before the eyes. (Blinking to bright light is not a reliable test.) Absence of blinking to threat often is noticed in hemianopic fields. Confrontation field testing is useful to delineate hemianopic and altitudinal defects, but it requires quiet cooperation of the patient and is not very sensitive. The best technique is to present two fingers in each visual field quadrant of both eyes,

Box 3.1. Degree of Visual Loss	
20/200	Legal blindness
20/800	Finger counting
2/1000	Arm movements
20/∞	Light perception
0	No light perception

typically midway between the patient and the examiner. Movement or finger counting can be used to indicate vision. Testing is followed by examination of the pupillary size and pupillary reaction to light. Pupillary abnormalities are important telltale signs, but the interpretation is much more difficult than appreciated. A common mnemonic, *PERRLA*, reminds the investigator of the different components of pupil assessment (*p*upil *e*qual, *r*ound, *r*eactive, *l*ight response, *a*ccommodation response); to further localize the anisocoria requires neuro-ophthalmologic examination with 10% cocaine or diluted pilocarpine. Anisocoria without any change in dim or bright light is physiologic and greater in dim light, possibly due to Horner's syndrome or structural pupillary abnormalities such as prior synechia or uveitis. In Horner's syndrome, interruption of the oculosympathetic pathway also produces ptosis or reduced upper lid folding. The face is warm, the skin is dry,

and conjunctival vessels may be dilated. Enophthalmos is an optical illusion due to a narrowed interpalpebral fissure. In carotid dissection, distention of the injured arterial wall damages the sympathetic fibers. Anhidrosis is typically absent in Horner's syndrome in lesions above the bifurcation (the fibers supplying the face accompany the external carotid below the carotid bifurcation). Anisocoria increasing in bright light is virtually always caused by mydriasis due to pharmacologic effects but could be due to a third nerve palsy if the reaction to diluted pilocarpine (0.1%) is negative and constriction occurs with 1.0% pilocarpine.

Dilating the pupils with phenylephrine, which stimulates the iris dilator, generally should be discouraged in acutely progressive neuro-ophthalmologic disorders because it may take several hours for the pupil to regain its response to light. Pupillary abnormalities are shown in Chapter 8 for further reference.

Funduscopy is necessarily limited to the optic disk and retinal vasculature, and specific note should be made of the caliber of the arteries, flame-like hemorrhages, edema, or change in color of the retinal pigment. Examination is followed by testing of ocular eye movements in the horizontal and vertical directions with the intent of detecting misalignment. Voluntary gaze in all fields includes up, down, left, and right, but it is useful to use figure-of-eight tracking (Fig. 3.1).

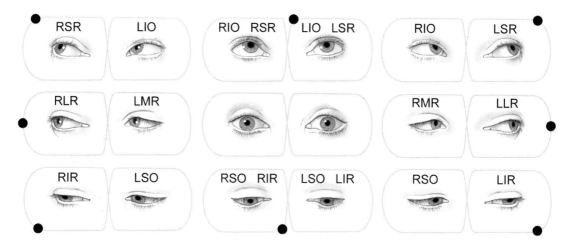

Figure 3.1 Baseline examination of eye movements and responsible muscles using standard figure-of-eight tracking. RSR, right superior rectus; LIO, left inferior oblique; RIO, right inferior oblique; LSR, left superior rectus; RLR, right lateral rectus; LLR, left lateral rectus; LMR, left medial rectus; RMR, right medial rectus; RIR, right inferior rectus; LIR, left inferior rectus; LSO, left superior oblique; RSO, right superior oblique.

Blindness

Monocular blindness is more common than acute loss of entire vision. In addition, transient monocular visual loss is more commonly encountered in the emergency department than persistent monocular defect. Transient monocular visual loss often includes embolization due to lesions of the aortic arch, heart valves, or carotid artery but may also include abnormalities associated with increased viscosity or hypercoagulability. It is not further considered here because many patients would need admission for further evaluation of its mechanism. Visual loss (uni- or bilateral) may result from lesions of the cornea and at any topographic location of the afferent visual system ending in the occipital poles. Monocular visual loss often indicates an ophthalmologic disorder, and these are shown in Table 3.1. A neurologic cause for monocular visual loss is most likely optic neuropathy. It typically manifests with markedly reduced visual acuity (20/200), inability to recognize color or its brightness (particularly red), and often no obvious findings on neurologic examination except an afferent pupil defect. The optic disk may take time to become abnormal but may show pallor or elevation. An afferent pupillary defect (Marcus Gunn) is traditionally examined, using the swinging flashlight test. The patient is asked to fixate on a distant target to eliminate the miotic effect of accommodation. A bright light is moved from one eye to the other. The response may vary from minimal asymmetry to pupils failing to constrict or dilate when the penlight moves to the affected eye. In its most pronounced form, pupils dilate immediately when the light shines into the diseased eye. Afferent pupillary defect is linked to optic neuropathy, but a retinal lesion or massive intravitreous hemorrhage (Terson's syndrome) may produce similar findings (see Chapter 13).

Optic neuritis is associated with periocular pain and pain on eye movement in 90% of cases.[1] The causes of optic neuritis are manyfold and can typically be divided into inflammatory causes and the first manifestations of multiple sclerosis (5-year probability of 30%).[2,3] Inflammatory causes may include common bacterial infections, such as streptococcus and staphylococcus, but also more exotic infections, such as toxoplasmosis, cryptococcosis, aspergillosis, and mucormycosis in susceptible immunosuppressed patients. In other patients, optic neuritis may occur after a vaccination or viral illness or in the setting of connective tissue disease or sarcoidosis. Hereditary optic neuropathy may also present with acute monocular visual loss; and in approximately 50% of patients, family history can be elicited. Certain toxic optic neuropathies have been described; they include methanol, ethambutol, isoniazid, thiamine (B_1) and folate deficiency.[4]

Acute blindness may involve both eyes and, excluding ophthalmologic disorders, points to bilateral involvement of the occipital lobes. Differential diagnosis involves acute basilar artery occlusive disease, sagittal sinus thrombosis, posterior reversible encephalopathy syndrome, and many drug-induced encephalopathies that include vincristine, methotrexate, cyclosporine, and tacrolimus (see Chapter 18).

Diplopia

Acute diplopia is complex to analyze, and the underlying deficit may remain ambiguous. Monocular diplopia, almost always due to abnormalities in the refractive media, precludes further neurologic work-up. Binocular diplopia is difficult to assess because in some patients multiple cranial nerve involvement is present. Questions that could clarify the chief complaint in acute diplopia should in-

Table 3.1. Ophthalmologic Disorders

Diagnosis	Findings
Central retinal artery occlusion	• Afferent pupil defect • Retinal edema • Optic disk pallor and cherry-red spots
Retinal vein occlusion	• "Blood and thunder" fundus (extensive intraretinal hemorrhages)
Retinal detachment	• Translucent gray wrinkled retina
Ischemic optic neuropathy	• Pale optic nerve • Milky, edematous • Scalp tenderness and absent temporal artery pulsation (giant cell arteritis)
Optic neuritis	• Normal findings ("patient sees nothing, doctor sees nothing") • Early pallor
Vitreous hemorrhage	• Diabetes, hypertension, or subarachnoid hemorrhage

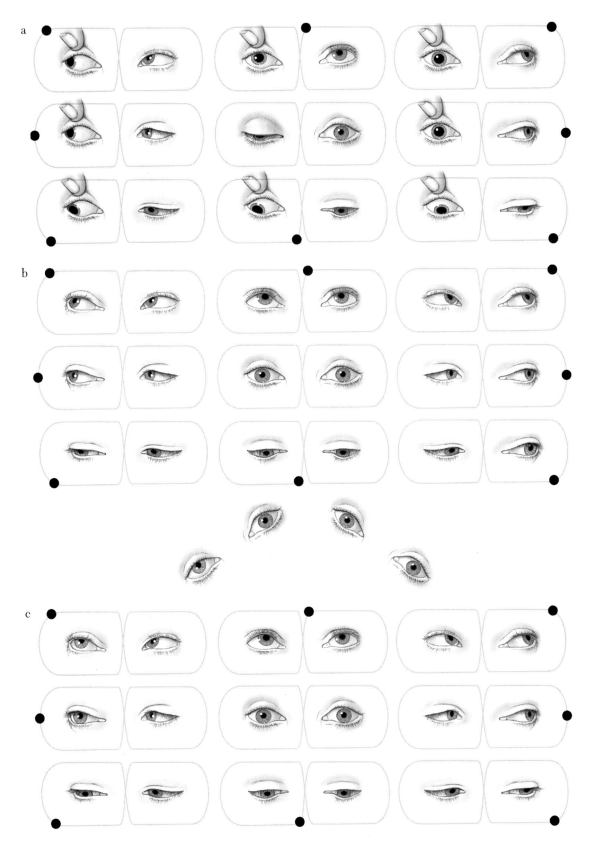

Figure 3.2 Nine gaze positions in (*a*) III nerve palsy, (*b*) IV nerve palsy, and (*c*) VI nerve palsy.

clude mode of onset, diplopia disappearing after one eye is closed, whether vertically or horizontally oriented, whether always present or fluctuating, and whether more pronounced in a certain gaze.

Figure 3.2 shows nine cardinal positions of gaze in oculomotor palsies, each providing fairly characteristic deviations of the globe. In addition, Table 3.2 provides an oversimplification of, but is useful in sorting out, the different cranial nerve palsies associated with diplopia. Table 3.3 lists disorders that indicate the need for urgent evaluation. Skew deviation may be associated with diplopia and indicates an internuclear lesion. It is a result of abnormalities in fibers ascending vertically from vestibular nuclei with the medial longitudinal fasciculus. Not infrequently, it is due to a pontine stroke in elderly patients and multiple sclerosis in younger patients (Fig. 3.3).

The cause of acute diplopia, however, may also include other factors, such as difficulty with movement of the globe due to mass effect in the orbit (thyrotoxicosis), diplopia caused by an acute manifestation of myasthenia gravis, and chronic progressive external ophthalmoplegia, particularly if ptosis is bilateral. A cavernous sinus lesion should be considered when an abducens lesion is associated with Horner's syndrome.

Acute oculomotor palsy with preceding retroorbital pain may be a sign of unruptured posterior communicating aneurysm, and two-thirds may be smaller than 6 mm (Fig. 3.4). It may herald rupture and indicate rapid aneurysm growth.[5] Development of pupil involvement, albeit uncommon, may be particularly worrisome for pending rupture.[6] A very urgent condition is carotid cavernous fistula. Trauma to the orbit may be remote (e.g., hit windshield) or comparatively early, such as after transsphenoidal pituitary surgery, carotid endarterectomy, or ethmoidal surgery.[7–9] Associations with Ehlers-Danlos syndrome and pregnancy have been noted. It may occur spontaneously. Lid swelling and orbital pain with characteristic pul-

Table 3.3. Urgent Disorders in Acute Diplopia

Acute III nerve palsy	• Basilar artery aneurysm, posterior communicating artery aneurysm° • Pituitary apoplexy • Acute midbrain infarct or hemorrhage • Mucormycosis° • Carotid cavernous fistula • Granulomatous inflammation (Tolosa-Hunt) • Diabetic microvascular disease†
Acute VI nerve palsy	• Carotid aneurysm • Cavernous sinus thrombosis° • Nasopharyngeal carcinoma • Increased intracranial pressure
Acute IV nerve palsy	• Trauma • Meningitis, infectious or neoplastic° • Herpes zoster ophthalmicus°

°Also known as the painful ophthalmoplegias.
†More often pupil-sparing.

sating exophthalmos and tortuous conjunctival vessels point to its diagnosis *(see Color Fig. 3.5 in separate color insert).* Funduscopy may demonstrate pulsating venous dilation and, in more extreme forms, disk edema and ophthalmoplegia. Ophthalmoplegia may be due to restricted excursions or cranial nerve injury in the segments traversing the cavernous or petrosal sinus. Visual loss is a consequence of increased intraocular pressure and reversal of flow or thrombus in the superior ophthalmic vein. There is a need for full angiographic documentation. Immediate opacification of the cavernous sinus is seen after carotid injection.

Complete Ptosis

A curious phenomenon is apraxia of eyelid opening when the patient is unable to open the eyes.[10,11] The orbicularis oculi does not contract, and the frontalis muscles are used to try to perform this act, though the eyes may remain completely closed. This disorder has been linked to acute nondominant hemispheric lesions (e.g.,

Table 3.2. Diplopia Due to Cranial Nerve Palsy

Cranial Nerve	Position of Eye	Diplopia	Additional Features
III	Down and out	Crossed	Ptosis, dilated fixed pupil
IV	Higher	Vertical	Head tilted away from affected side, chin down
VI	Inward	Uncrossed	Head turned to affected side

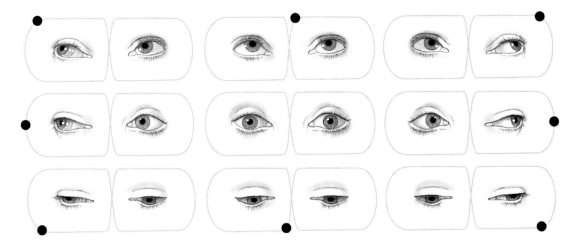

Figure 3.3 Internuclear ophthalmoplegia.

putaminal hemorrhage and large hemispheric in-farcts).[12–14] The pathways are unknown but involve supranuclear connections in the nondominant hemisphere (Fig. 3.6). It may be at brain-stem level and is more common when herniation occurs.[14]

Visual Illusions

Positive visual phenomena may need careful attention and evaluation. Images perceived as false may indicate an acute hemispheric lesion or significant neurotoxicity. Visual hallucinations may take many forms, from dots, geometric shapes, and lines to dream-like descriptions of figures, animals (often frightening), and detailed movie-like scenes (midbrain peduncular hallucinations). First, neurotoxicity should be excluded by history. Drugs to treat Parkinson's disease (e.g., levodopa, lisuride, mesulergine, pergolide) or depression (e.g., amitriptyline, imipramine, lithium carbonate), stimulants (amphetamine, cocaine), and immunosuppressive agents (cyclosporine, tacrolimus) should be considered. Hallucinations with migrainous components, such as fortifications (zigzag lines in parallel) that are constantly in the same visual field, could point to an arteriovenous malformation.[15] Visual hallucinations could be due to seizures—albeit rare—certainly when isolated, not accompanied by head or eye deviation or rapid blinking, or associated with a transient hemianopic field defect. However, it is not always appreciated that colored comma shapes or white

streaks flashing in a vertical direction may be due to vitreous detachment.

Palinopsia involves an image that persists after looking at a subject, rapidly fades or returns hours later, and is superimposed on certain objects. It has been noted with encephalitis, fulminant multiple sclerosis, and brain tumors; but illicit drugs (lysergic acid diethylamide) and major psychiatric pathology are equally common.[16–19]

Micropsia (objects appear smaller) is rarely caused by cerebral lesions and is more typically seen with retinal lesions. Unilateral *metamorphopsia* (illusion that objects are distorted) (also common in macular degeneration) may indicate a parietal lobe lesion and may be limited to facial images. It probably only occurs as an ictal phenomenon.[20]

Line of Action

There are many conditions associated with diplopia or visual loss. Some acute neuro-ophthalmologic conditions may point to an acute neurologic condition that needs immediate evaluation. The critical steps in gathering key features of the patient with the most urgent concerns are shown in Figure 3.7. This most likely involves immediate MRI or cerebral angiography. A neurosurgical consult is mandated in any patient with a painful ophthalmoplegia, due to its correlation with lesions that may require skull base surgery or endovascular procedures. A compressive or in-

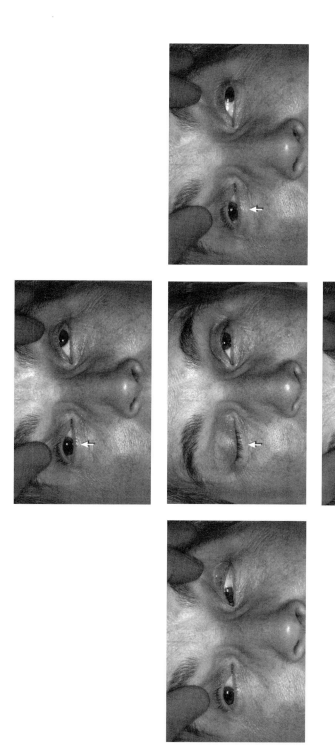

Figure 3.4 III nerve palsy due to posterior communicating artery aneurysm.

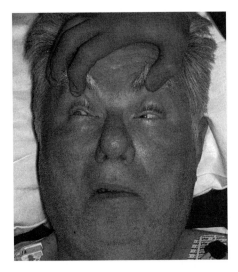
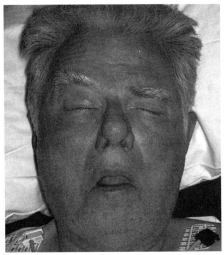

Figure 3.6 Complete ptosis in hemispheric stroke in non-dominant hemisphere. Note gaze preference.

filtrative lesion that affects the optic nerve should be excluded by an MRI scan. An MR angiogram to exclude an intracranial aneurysm should be considered when appropriate because an anterior cerebral aneurysm can leak into the optic sheath and be responsible for acute monocular blindness.[21] Balloon or coil occlusion in carotid-cavernous fistula has been successful but not without worsening of symptoms. However, reversibility of blindness has been reported.[22]

Unexpected loss of vision may have many causes and can be further delineated by an emergent ophthalmology examination. A particularly worrisome condition is anterior ischemic optic neuropathy. When considered, and when the erythrocyte sedimentation rate is elevated (normal age plus 12 in males and normal age plus 10 to 12 in females), immediate administration of methylprednisolone 250 mg IV qid for 3 days should be done to prevent involvement of the opposite eye.

REFERENCES

1. Hickman SJ, Dalton CM, Miller DH, et al.: Management of acute optic neuritis. *Lancet* 360:1953, 2002.
2. Kaufman DT, Beck R, ONTT Study Group: The 5-year risk of MS after optic neuritis: experience of the Optic Neuritis Treatment Trial. *Neurology* 49:1404, 1997.
3. Soderstrom M, Ya-Ping J, Hillert J, et al.: Optic neuritis: prognosis for multiple sclerosis from MRI, CSF, and HLA findings. *Neurology* 50:708, 1998.
4. Glaser JS: *Neurophthalmology*, 3rd ed. Philadelphia: Lippincott Williams & Wilkins, 1999.
5. Yanaka K, Matsumaru Y, Mashiko R, et al. Small unruptured cerebral aneurysms presenting with oculomotor nerve palsy. *Neurosurgery* 52(3):553, 2003.
6. Lee AG, Hayman LA, Brazis PW. The evaluation of isolated third nerve palsy revisited: an update on the evolving role of magnetic resonance, computed tomography, and catheter angiography. *Surv Ophthalmol* 47(2):137, 2002.
7. Kushner FM: Carotid-cavernous fistula as a complication of carotid endarterectomy. *Ann Ophthalmol* 13:979, 1981.
8. Paullus WS, Norwood CW, Morgan CW: False aneurysms

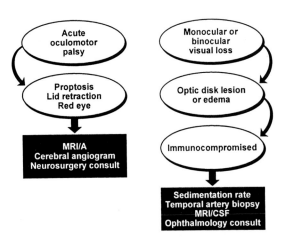

Figure 3.7 Critical steps in acute neurophthalmology. MRI/A, magnetic resonance imaging/angiography; CSF, cerebrospinal fluid.

of the cavernous carotid artery and progressive external ophthalmoplegia after transsphenoidal hypophysectomy. *J Neurosurg* 51:707, 1979.

9. Pederson RA, Troost BT, Schramm VL: Carotid-cavernous sinus fistula after external ethmoid-sphenoid surgery. Clinical course and management. *Arch Otolaryngol* 107:307, 1981.

10. Defazio G, Livrea P, Lamberti R, et al.: Isolated so-called apraxia of eyelid opening: report of 10 cases and a review of the literature. *Eur Neurol* 39:201, 1998.

11. Schmidtke K, Buttner-Ennever JA: Nervous control of eyelid function: a review of clinical, experimental, and pathological data. *Brain* 115:227, 1992.

12. Averbuch-Heller L, Leigh RJ, Mermelstein V, et al.: Ptosis in patients with hemispheric strokes. *Neurology* 58:620, 2002.

13. Verghese J, Milling C, Rosenbaum DM: Ptosis, blepharospasm, and apraxia of eyelid opening secondary to putaminal hemorrhage. *Neurology* 53:652, 1999.

14. Blacker DJ, Wijdicks EF: Delayed complete bilateral ptosis associated with massive infarction of the right hemisphere. *Mayo Clin Proc* 78:836, 2003.

15. Kupersmith MJ, Vargas ME, Yashar A, et al.: Occipital arteriovenous malformations: visual disturbances and presentation. *Neurology* 46:953, 1996

16. Bender MB, Feldman M, Sobin AJ: Palinopsia. *Brain* 91:321, 1968.

17. Kawasaki A, Purvin V: Persistent palinopsia following ingestion of lysergic acid diethylamide (LSD). *Arch Ophthalmol* 114:47, 1996.

18. Lefebre C, Kolmel HW: Palinopsia as an epileptic phenomenon. *Eur Neurol* 29:323, 1989.

19. Young WB, Heros DO, Ehrenberg BL, et al.: Metamorphopsia and palinopsia. Association with periodic lateralized epileptiform discharges in a patient with malignant astrocytoma. *Arch Neurol* 46:820, 1989.

20. Nass R, Sinha S, Solomon G: Epileptic facial metamorphopsia. *Brain Dev* 7:50, 1985.

21. Chan JW, Hoyt WF, Ellis WG, et al.: Pathogenesis of acute monocular blindness from leaking anterior communicating artery aneurysms: report of six cases. *Neurology* 48:680, 1997.

22. Albuquerque FC, Heinz GW, McDougall CG: Reversal of blindness after transvenous embolization of a carotid-cavernous fistula: case report. *Neurosurgery* 52: 233, 2003.

Chapter 4
Spinning

Akin to other equally less precise descriptions, spinning (or the perception of movement) may have different meanings. The sensation of spinning in a patient acutely admitted to the emergency department frequently is due to near fainting, hyperventilation, acute peripheral vestibular disease,[1–4] anxiety, or other disorders outside the purview of acute neurology (Box 4.1). Naturally, it is essential to extrapolate urgent disorders from patients reporting signs such as acute floating, giddiness, wooziness, drunkenness, tilting, and imbalance. Some of these disorders are discussed in more detail in the third section of this book and include vertigo as presenting signs of cerebellar hematoma, acute embolus to the basilar artery, and dissection of the vertebral artery. Other key neurologic signs and neuroimaging features usually point to the diagnosis. The main task is to find convincing arguments for a lesion in the central nervous system as a cause of spinning and certain elements in the history that should point to a lesion of the central vestibular system or cerebellum. When present, they justify an urgent magnetic resonance imaging (MRI) study for which the patient may be transferred to a tertiary center. There are both otologic and neurologic emergencies that need to be considered. Otologic emergencies should be considered because emergent antibiotic or antiviral therapy could minimize longstanding sequelae (*see Color Fig. 4.1 in separate color insert*). These disorders are summarized in Table 4.1.[7]

Clinical Assessment

When acute spinning represents vertigo, the history may provide additional clues. Autonomic symptoms such as vomiting, nausea, pallor, and sweating are less pronounced in central lesions but are so common and come in different degrees of severity that they cannot be used as major discriminating factors. Vertigo due to positional change, coughing, sneezing, fluctuating hearing loss, nonpulsatile tinnitus, and hearing loss is more typical of peripheral vestibular disease.[8]

Oscillopsia is another important sign, in which patients feel images are moving or bouncing. When combined with spontaneous nystagmus and transient vertigo, a peripheral source is likely. Central causes may be strongly considered when oscillopsia is induced by head movement. Lesions in the cerebellum produce a spinning sensation, but more often severe scanning speech and impaired finger-to-nose and heel-knee-shin testing predominate in the clinical picture. Ipsilateral hearing loss points to an occlusion of the anterior inferior cerebellar artery.[9] Ipsifacial numbness, hypophonia, and Horner's syndrome localize in the lateral medulla oblongata. Details of these disorders and other cerebrovascular-related occlusions are found in Chapter 15.

Several neurologic signs need careful documentation. The characterization of nystagmus is necessary and an important determinant.[10,11] Central nystagmus has a characteristic direction

Box 4.1. Systemic Illness and Drug-Induced Dizziness

Certain metabolic derangements could produce a profound (and sometimes permanent) effect on the vestibular system. Longstanding juvenile diabetes mellitus, fat emboli, and hyperviscosity syndromes may acutely occlude the common cochlear artery.[5] Less clear mechanisms known for acute vertigo are dialysis, acute anemia, and hypothyroidism; and many of the vasculitic syndromes such as polyarteritis no-

dosa, Wegener's granulomatosis, Behçet's disease, connective tissue disorders. Vertigo can be a paraneoplastic manifestation. Drugs known to damage the auditory system are aminoglycosides, anti-epileptic drugs, loop diuretics, and *cis*-platin. Exposure to these drugs may be only brief, and toxic levels are not always required to produce permanent destruction of auditory and vestibular systems.[6]

dependence. When present, gaze to where the fast component of nystagmus beats increases the frequency and amplitude in any type of nystagmus. In central causes of nystagmus, gaze away from the direction of the fast component will achieve the opposite effect and may abolish or, in extremes of gaze, reverse the direction of nystagmus. A vertical nystagmus (up- or downbeat) is almost always central but can be drug-induced (particularly opioids).[12] Gaze-evoked nystagmus with similar amplitudes in both directions is due to drugs but has been reported in myasthenia gravis, multiple sclerosis, and cerebellar atrophy.[10] Periodic alternating nystagmus (nystagmus changing in direction) has typically been considered in disease of craniocervical function but can be due to phenytoin intoxication or lithium.[13] Common central types of nystagmus are shown in Table 4.2.

Peripheral vestibular and congenital nystagmus can be markedly muted by visual fixation of the patient.[14] Nystagmus can be observed with eye closure, but it is easier to examine the eye with the ophthalmoscope covering the opposite eye. This maneuver eliminates fixation and brings on

alternating drift and correcting jerks of the retina as a manifestation of the nystagmus. Frenzel glasses (30 plus lenses) also eliminate fixation, and both eyes can be observed due to the great magnification (Frenzel glasses are rarely available in emergency rooms and require ear, nose, and throat consultation). Positional nystagmus can be documented after a rapid change from sitting to head hanging over the examination table, turning the head sideways. A torsional and vertical nystagmus appears after 10 seconds' delay and produces a vertiginous sensation that fades away with repeated testing. Both delay and fatigability are characteristic of this positional nystagmus. This maneuver (Dix-Hallpike) is helpful to bring on a vestibular lesion mostly due to canalithiasis. Its absence may suggest a central cause.

Vestibulospinal reflexes (i.e., neuronal connections from labyrinths and vestibular neurons to anterior horn cells) are tested by past-pointing, the Romberg test, and tandem walking. Past-pointing is tested by having the patient touch the hand of the examiner with an extended arm, close his or her eyes, point up, and try to touch the examiner's

Table 4.1. Vertigo and Otologic Emergencies

Diagnosis	Clues	Therapy
Herpes zoster oticus	Ear lobe vesicles, hearing loss, facial palsy	Acyclovir 1 g/day for 10 days
Bacterial labyrinthitis	Acute deafness, prior cholesteatoma, meningitis	Surgical management or specific antibiotics
Malignant external otitis (*Pseudomonas aeruginosa*)	Extreme ear pain, facial palsy (may be multiple cranial nerves)	Ciprofloxacin or gentamicin
Perilymph fistula	Tinnitus, hearing loss, position vertigo, prior strain or Valsalva or barotrauma	Conservative first, then surgery
Labyrinth hemorrhage	Nausea, vomiting, hearing loss, trauma	Correct underlying coagulopathy

Data from Cummings et al.[7]

Table 4.2. Nystagmus in Acute Lesions of the Central Vestibular System

Type	Features	Lesion
Downbeat	Increasing amplitude with downgaze	Cervicomedullary junction
Upbeat	Increasing amplitude with upgaze	Dorsal medulla oblongata
Rebound	With continuous lateral position, reversal or disappearance	Cerebellum
Dissociated	Disconjugate	Brain stem
Ocular bobbing	Downward jerk with slow return to midposition	Pons

hand again in a repeated to and fro movement but with eyes closed. Past-pointing occurs toward the damaged side. Abnormalities of the past-pointing test may not be replicated by the more traditional finger-to-nose test because joint and muscle proprioception during this coordinated movement may compensate. Another technique is vertical writing with eyes closed. This test identifies unilateral vestibular dysfunction, but this may occur in both peripheral and central causes.[15]

Static posture is tested by Romberg's test. Standing with feet close together and eyes closed can be maintained for 30 seconds in normal individuals less than 70 years old.[7] Crossing the arms against the chest adds a touch of difficulty and may bring on more subtle swaying. Tandem gait walking (10 steps) evaluates vestibular function when done with eyes closed and cerebellar function with eyes opened. Dysbalance due to acute vermian or cerebellar hemisphere lesion can be dramatic because patients are unable to sit steady or unable to stand unassisted.

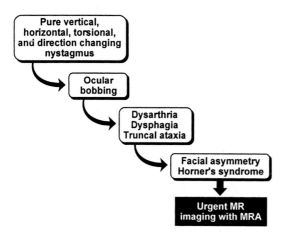

Figure 4.2 Critical steps in vertigo evaluation due to central nervous system cause. MRA, magnetic resonance angiography.

Line of Action

A few patients presenting with spinning will have an emergent neurologic disorder. In many, an acute nonviral labyrinthitis can be diagnosed or drug toxicity has emerged.[5,6] As mentioned before, a full-scale neurologic evaluation should proceed only after otologic emergencies have been considered and rejected as possible explanations. The signs and symptoms that point to a central cause of vertigo and warrant urgent MRI and magnetic resonance angiography are summarized in Figure 4.2. This will image the posterior fossa structures and flow interruptions in the vertebrobasilar circulation. Cerebrospinal fluid examination could document elevated immunoglobulin G synthesis and oligoclonal bands supporting a first bout of multiple sclerosis or pleocytosis with a wide range of diagnostic possibilities, including meningeal carcinomatosis and major central nervous system infections (see Chapter 18).

REFERENCES

1. Friedland DR, Wackym PA: A critical appraisal of spontaneous perilymphatic fistulas of the inner ear. *Am J Otol* 20:261, 1999.
2. McShane D, Chapnik JS, Noyek AM, et al.: Malignant external otitis. *J Otolaryngol* 15:108, 1986.
3. Robillard RB, Hilsinger RL Jr, Adour KK: Ramsay Hunt facial paralysis: clinical analyses of 185 patients. *Otolaryngol Head Neck Surg* 95:292, 1986.
4. Baloh RW. Vestibular neuritis. *N Engl J Med* 348:1027, 2003.
5. Tay HL, Ray N, Ohri R, et al.: Diabetes mellitus and hearing loss. *Clin Otolaryngol* 20:130, 1995.
6. Schacht J: Aminoglycoside ototoxicity: prevention in sight? *Otolaryngol Head Neck Surg* 118:674, 1998.
7. Cummings CW, Fredrickson JM, Harker LA, et al.: *Otolaryngology*, 3rd ed. St. Louis: Mosby, 1998.
8. Magnusson M, Karlberg M: Peripheral vestibular disorders with acute onset of vertigo. *Curr Opin Neurol* 15:5, 2002.

9. Lee H, Sohn SI, Jung DK, et al.: Sudden deafness and anterior inferior cerebellar artery infarction. *Stroke* 33:2807, 2002.

10. Baloh RW, Honrubia V: *Clinical Neurophysiology of the Vestibular System*, 3rd ed. New York: Oxford University Press, 2001.

11. Serra A, Leigh RJ: Diagnostic value of nystagmus: spontaneous and induced ocular oscillations. *J Neurol Neurosurg Psychiatry* 73:615, 2002.

12. Henderson RD, Wijdicks EFM: Downbeat nystagmus associated with intravenous patient-controlled administration of morphine. *Anesth Analg* 91:691, 2000.

13. Lee MS, Lessell S: Lithium-induced periodic alternating nystagmus. *Neurology* 60:344, 2003.

14. Leigh RJ, Zee DS: *The Neurology of Eye Movements,* 3rd ed. New York: Oxford University Press, 1999.

15. Fukuda T: Vertical writing with eyes covered: a new test of vestibulospinal reaction. *Acta Otolaryngol* 50:26, 1959.

Chapter 5
Twitching and Spasms

The presentation of abnormal movements may doubtlessly have many causes, not to mention parallel systemic illness. Many emergency room physicians ask neurologists to classify, resolve, and treat the cause. Movement disorders may indicate a new lesion to the brain, may be due to drug effect, endocrine pathology, or connective tissue disease, or may even be factitious.[1,2] Of patients with new movement disorders, the similarities between certain acute movement disorders would make recognition elusive, and particularly, naming the abnormal movement remains difficult when it presents as a mixture of things. (Even a proverbial neurologist may say "I have no idea what this is.")

This chapter attempts to clarify the commonly observed acute movement disorders in the emergency department but concentrates on the more serious and those that are drug-induced.

Clinical Assessment

In plain terms, involuntary movements are described using the following characteristics: rhythm, regularity, displacement by movement, generalized or same muscle group, presence or absence with relaxation, and whether the movement is fast, slow, flowing, or resembling spasm.[3] Movement disorder can be very difficult to differentiate from a focal seizure or epileptic partialis continua. Staring, automatisms, and lip smacking may be absent, and the abnormality may just be a continuous repetitive jerk in one limb. Clonic jerks can be felt or seen and may evolve into a generalized seizure. (An electroencephalogram may be the only option to differentiate it from another movement disorder.)

Myoclonus is applied to muscle contractions that are brief, of small amplitude, and shock-like. The movements may be random or rhythmic, generalized or limited to one or multiple groups of muscles. Usually they are chaotic and arrhythmic but, when rhythmic, have been denoted as myorhythmias. Myoclonus due to lesions in the cortex is touch- and sound-sensitive and in awake patients caused by attempted motion (action myoclonus) or muscle stretch.[4] Myoclonus can originate from the cortex, basal ganglia, brain stem, or spinal cord.[5] In severe anoxic–ischemic brain injury, all of these locations may be involved. Myoclonus status epilepticus in a comatose patient after cardiac resuscitation is a result of devastating multilayer cortical damage and an indicator of poor prognosis (see Chapter 10).[6]

Drug-induced myoclonus may involve manifestations of first exposure or appear in toxic doses (Table 5.1).[3,7–11] Generalized myoclonus is common in acute metabolic derangements but usually at end-stage organ failure such as hepatic and renal disease. It has been observed in hypernatremia, hypomagnesemia, and nonketotic hyperglycemia. Unusual causes are heat stroke, decompression injury, and pesticide exposure. The toxic exposure may have caused permanent

Table 5.1. Drugs Causing Myoclonus

Drug Type	Drug
Antidepressants	Monoamine oxidase inhibitors
	Tricyclic antidepressants
	Lithium
	Fluoxetine
Antimicrobials	Penicillin
	Ticarcillin
	Carbenicillin
	Cephalosporins
	Acyclovir
	Isoniazid
Anesthetics	Etomidate
	Enflurane
	Isoflurane
	Fentanyl
Anticonvulsants	Valproic acid
	Carbamazepine
	Clozapine
	Vigabatrin
Calcium channel–blocking drugs	Verapamil
	Nifedipine
	Diltiazem
Opiate derivatives	Meperidine
	Methadone
	Morphine
	Oxycodone
Other drugs	Bismuth
	Chlorambucil
Overdoses or poisonings	Antihistamine overdose
	Methyl bromide fumes
	Organic mercury poisoning
	Gasoline sniffing
	Dichloromethane ingestion
	Strychnine poisoning
	Chloralose (rodenticide)

Source: Adapted from Vadlamudi L, Wijdicks EFM: Multifocal myoclonus due to verapamil overdose. *Neurology* 58:984, 2002. By permission of Lippincott Williams & Wilkins.

damage to the cortex and basal ganglia (see Chapter 8).

Segmental myoclonus affecting the arm or leg may be due to acute spinal cord injury including trauma. Segmental myoclonus may closely mimic epilepsia partialis continua, in which the jerking movements are more regular and at a repetitive fast rate.

Dystonia is reserved for movements characterized by a persistent posture in one extremity. There is sustained patterned spasm but normal tone in between. The positions may be bizarre in the limbs and trunk.[12] In the emergency department, it is use-

ful to distinguish between a generalized or focal dystonia and whether dystonia occurs at rest. Sensory tricks (touching limb to reduce spasm), also known as *geste antagoniste,* are characteristic in dystonia. A form of dystonia is ocular deviation (oculogyric crises). Oculogyric crises may be associated with backward or lateral flexion of the neck, and the tongue may protrude. The deviation of the eyes upward, sideways, or downward is held for several minutes and can only for a brief moment be corrected by effort. This eye movement is commonly drug-induced, and discontinuation of the drug is rapidly successful. Oculogyric crises do occur in serious neurologic conditions such as bilateral paramedian thalamic infarction, multiple sclerosis, head injury, and tumors in the ventricles. Drugs causing oculogyric crises and oromandibular dyskinesis include phenothiazines and many of the antipsychotic drugs but also carbamazepine, gabapentin, lithium, ondansetron, and, perhaps best known, metoclopramide (Fig. 5.1). However, they may be seen as a manifestation of schizophrenia alone. Acute drug-induced dystonia is not prevalent along with antipsychotic drug use, but other well-established associations have been reported (Table 5.2).[7,9,13]

Dystonia is a common symptom in Parkinson's disease and neurodegenerative disorders associated with extrapyramidal signs, such as progressive supranuclear palsy, multisystem atrophy, corticobasal ganglia degeneration, and inherited movement disorders.[14] Any physician seeing patients with acute dystonia should consider Wilson's disease, particularly when patients are 20–30 years old. Additional findings are artificial grin (retracted lips) and brown iris in previously blue-eyed persons. Diagnostic tests include reduced serum ceruloplasmin level (in 5% of patients it is normal), Kayser-Fleischer rings under slit lamp, and increased signal in basal ganglia and cortex on magnetic resonance imaging (MRI).

Chorea and athetosis are movements that are often combined and overlapping. Chorea is arrhythmic, with a jerky, thrusting component that is always purposeless but often incorporated into a voluntary movement. It may include grimacing, respiratory muscles producing grunts, or "dance-like" walk. Athetosis involves slow, undulating movements seen with the attempt to sustain a posture. Fairly typical movement patterns are known, such as alteration between extension–pronation

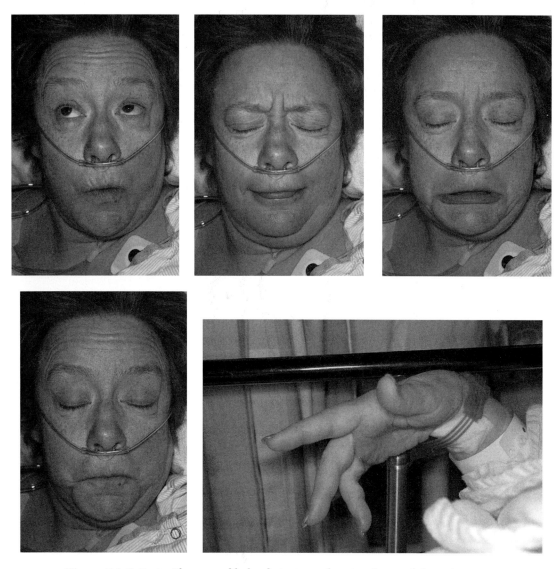

Figure 5.1 Patient with oromandibular dystonia, oculogyric crises, and dystonic posturing after ondansetron administration. The facial images were made within 90 seconds.[13]

and flexion–supination of arm, flexion–extension of fingers, and foot inversion. Pursing and parting of the lips or side-to-side movement of the neck is observed commonly.

Drug-induced chorea is shown in Table 5.3, with a well-established presentation of central nervous system (CNS) stimulants and oral contraceptives.

Chorea gravidarum and its association with birth control medication show an increased susceptibility in some patients but many patients had prior Sydenham's chorea and heart valve damage from streptococcal infection. Chorea is also associated with new-onset hyperthyroidism, polycythemia vera, and systemic lupus erythematosus. Structural CNS lesions commonly involve ischemic or hemorrhagic stroke in basal ganglia but usually are one-sided (hemichorea).

Finally, tremor is common and diagnosed by synchronous contractions of opposing muscles. Tremor produces rhythmic oscillations. Acute tremors may indicate damage to the red nucleus (Benedikt's syndrome, see Table 15.2) that may produce a rubral tremor and has a frequency of

Table 5.2. Drug-Induced Dystonia

Anesthetics
Antiepileptic drugs
Benzodiazepines
Calcium antagonists
Dextromethorphan
Dopamine agonists
Metoclopramide
Monoamine oxidase inhibitors
Ondansetron
Ranitidine
Selective serotonin reuptake inhibitors
Sumatriptan
Amitriptyline

Table 5.4. Drug-Induced Tremors

Antiepileptic drugs
Antidepressants
Antihyperglycemic drugs
Calcium channel blockers
Corticosteroids
Dopamine receptor–blocking agents
Lithium
Theophylline
Thyroxine

2–5 Hz. It is typically seen in action and with posture holding and not at rest.

Drug-induced tremors (Table 5.4) are usually postural and primarily enhanced physiologic tremors. Withdrawal of alcohol, barbiturates, benzodiazepines, β-blockers, and opioids may produce tremors.

Certain rare entities can be encountered in the emergency department and require prompt action. Acute parkinsonism may be induced by toxins such as MPTP (1-methyl-4-phenyl-1,2,3,6-tetrahydropyridine), organophosphates, carbon monoxide, carbon disulfide, cyanide, and methanol. It may also be particularly severe in acute withdrawal from dopaminergic drugs in patients with established Parkinson syndrome. Many chemotherapeutic agents have been implicated, including paclitaxel, vincristine, and CHOP (cyclophosphamide, hydroxydaunomycin, vincristine [Oncovin], and prednisone). Response to levodopa or prednisone is potentially present but not in toxic parkinsonism. Parkinsonism can be part of neuroleptic malignant syndrome, and fever, dysautonomia, and elevation of serum creatine

Table 5.3. Drug-Induced Chorea

Amphetamines
Cocaine
Pemoline
Tricyclic oral contraceptives
Tricyclic antidepressants
Selective serotonin reuptake inhibitors
Theophylline
Lithium
Antiepileptic drugs

kinase usually point in that direction (see Chapter 9).

In addition, there are reasonably well-delineated disorders that include lethal catatonia (due to a prior major lesion to the CNS) and serotonin syndrome (due to serotonin-specific reuptake inhibitors, "ecstasy," and a combination of monoamine oxidase inhibitors and meperidine).[15,16] Neuroleptic malignant syndrome should be rapidly considered when hyperthermia, rigidity, autonomic features, and increased creatine kinase are present. Acute serotonin syndrome has a profile similar to any of the acute dysautonomias, but profound myoclonus and shivering may be present (Box 5.1).

Acute laryngeal dystonia may occur after recent administration of phenothiazine or other neuroleptic agents.[17–19] Manji and coworkers[20] from Queens Square London coined the term *status dystonicus*. Life-threatening complications occurred in these patients with respiratory failure due to upper airway obstruction or decreased respiratory function. Myoclonus may affect the diaphragm, and generalized dystonic spasm may impair swallowing. A tracheostomy was needed in more than a third of patients, and rhabdomyolysis from persistent spasm did occur.

Line of Action

Acute movement disorders could point to a structural lesion and justify an MRI scan. Paroxysmal dyskinesias, whether dystonia, chorea, or athetosis, could be due to a secondary cause.

Toxicity from overdose is a common occurrence, and one should not be satisfied with other

Box 5.1. Akinetic Rigid Crises with Hyperthermia

The diagnostic spectra of these mostly poorly understood disorders overlap and include profuse perspiration, fluctuating pulse rate and blood pressure, and hyperthermia due to impaired thermoregulation. Untreated, the condition leads to rhabdomyolysis and dehydration and may become lethal due to myocardial stress or deep venous thrombosis and pulmonary emboli. This condition may be drug-induced (neuroleptic agents or serotonin syndrome—mostly due to recent use or increase in dose of selective serotonin reuptake inhibitors) or due to drug withdrawal (dopamine withdrawal in severe Parkinson's disease or as a result of a major brain injury, encephalitis, or anoxic–ischemic damage). The degree of increase in creatine kinase is variable but expected, with prolonged symptoms. Therapy is supportive, with oxygenation, rehydration, anticoagulation, and options include dantrolene (1–10 mg/kg), bromocriptine (5 mg), lisuride (0.02–0.25 mg/hour), or, certainly not as a last resort, electroconvulsive therapy.

explanations until they are carefully excluded. All drug-induced movement disorders are self-limiting, but failure to recognize their severity may lead to progression of the disorders, with hypotension and cardiac arrhythmias.

In patients with severe myoclonus, medication to enhance γ-aminobutyric acid (GABA) inhibition could be useful, including lorazepam and valproate. Propofol infusion (titrating to effect) is successful in myoclonus status epilepticus.[6,21]

Acute dystonic reactions are often successfully treated with intravenous or oral administration of anticholinergics (benztropine) or antihistaminic agents (diphenhydramine).[22] Benzodiazepines may be useful as well. In status dystonicus, neuromuscular paralysis and sedation may be needed for several days, followed by benzhexol, tetrabenazine, and pimozide or haloperidol. Intravenous diphenhydramine 25–75 mg dramatically resolved the status in acute laryngeal dystonia.

Dantrolene, bromocriptine, lisuride, or electroconvulsive therapy is effective in neuroleptic malignant syndrome or lethal catatonia (Box 5.1).[23] Cyproheptadine has shown promise in serotonin syndrome.[24] The management in movement disorders leading to major systemic involvement or airway involvement is summarized in Figure 5.2.

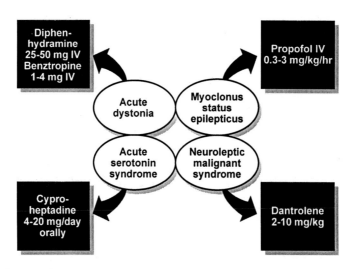

Figure 5.2 The four major acute movement disorders and initial therapy.

REFERENCES

1. Blakeley J, Jankovic J: Secondary causes of paroxysmal dyskinesia. *Adv Neurol* 89:401, 2002.

2. Calne DB, Lang AE: Secondary dystonia. *Adv Neurol* 50:9, 1988.

3. Watts R, Koller WC: *Movement Disorders*. New York: McGraw-Hill, 1997.

4. Lance JW, Adams RD: The syndrome of intention or action myoclonus as a sequel to hypoxic encephalopathy. *Brain* 86:111, 1963.

5. Caviness JN: Myoclonus. In CH Adler, JE Ahlskog (eds), *Parkinson's Disease and Movement Disorders: Diagnosis and Treatment Guidelines for the Practicing Physician*. Totowa, NJ: Humana Press, 2000, p. 339.

6. Wijdicks EFM, Parisi JE, Sharbrough FW: Prognostic value of myoclonus status survivors of cardiac arrest. *Ann Neurol* 35:239, 1994.

7. Hicks CB, Abraham K: Verapamil and myoclonic dystonia. *Ann Intern Med* 103:154, 1985.

8. Klawans HL, Carvey PM, Tanner CM, et al.: Drug-induced myoclonus. In: S Fahn, CD Marsden, MH Van Woert (eds), *Myoclonus*. New York: Raven Press, 1986, p. 251.

9. Lang A: Miscellaneous drug-induced movement disorders. In AE Lang, WJ Weiner (eds) *Drug-Induced Movement Disorders*. New York: Futura, 1992, p. 339.

10. Vadlamudi L, Wijdicks EFM: Multifocal myoclonus due to verapamil overdose. *Neurology* 58:984, 2002.

11. Savin S, Cartigny B, Azaroual N, et al. 1H NMR spectroscopy and GC-MS analysis of alpha-chloralos. Application to two poisoning cases. *J Anal Toxicol* 27:156, 2003.

12. Fahn S, Bressman S, Marsden CD: Classification of dystonia. *Mov Disord* 12(Suppl 3):1, 1997.

13. Ritter MJ, Goodman BP, Sprung J, et al. Ondansetron-induced multifocal encephalopathy. *Mayo Clin Proc* 78:1150, 2003.

14. Gasser T, Bressman S, Durr A, et al.: State of the art review: molecular diagnosis of inherited movement disorders. Movement Disorders Society Task Force on Molecular Diagnosis. *Mov Disord* 18:3, 2003.

15. Radomski JW, Dursun SM, Reveley MA, et al.: An exploratory approach to the serotonin syndrome: an update of clinical phenomenology and revised diagnostic criteria. *Med Hypotheses* 55:218, 2000.

16. Sternbach H: The serotonin syndrome. *Am J Psychiatry* 148:705, 1991.

17. Flaherty JA, Lahmeyer HW: Laryngeal–pharyngeal dystonia as a possible cause of asphyxia with haloperidol treatment. *Am J Psychiatry* 135:1414, 1978.

18. Koek RJ, Pi EH: Acute laryngeal dystonic reactions to neuroleptics. *Psychosomatics* 30:359, 1989.

19. Marion M, Klap P, Perrin A, et al.: Stridor and focal laryngeal dystonia. *Lancet* 339:457, 1992.

20. Manji H, Howard RS, Diller DH, et al.: Status dystonicus: the syndrome and its management. *Brain* 121:243, 1998.

21. Wijdicks EFM: Propofol in myoclonus status epilepticus in comatose patients following cardiac resuscitation. *J Neurol Neurosurg Psychiatry* 73:94, 2002.

22. Vaamonde J, Narbona J, Weiser R, et al.: Dystonic storms: a practical management problem. *Clin Neuropharmacol* 17:344, 1994.

23. Addonizio G, Susman VL: ECT as a treatment alternative for patients with symptoms of neuroleptic malignant syndrome. *J Clin Psychol* 48:102, 1987.

24. Graudins A, Stearman A, Chan B: Treatment of the serotonin syndrome with cyproheptadine. *J Emerg Med* 16:615, 1998.

Chapter 6
A Terrible Headache

Many times over, emergency departments are visited by patients with refractory severe headaches. Within this melee of patients traveling through the emergency department are some with a potentially life-threatening condition, uncommon in frequency but devastating if not recognized. The emergency department physician and neurologist are commonly held responsible for their triage.[1,2] The dilemma of improper "playing it safe" with a series of tests throwing up false-positives or running the risk of litigation due to incomplete investigations has become a major area of contention.[2,3] Not all patients require neuroimaging studies or cerebrospinal fluid (CSF) examination; in fact, most do not. However, a split-second onset of persistent severe ("terrible") headache typically indicates aneurysmal subarachnoid hemorrhage (see Chapter 13), and evaluation is urgently needed. In addition, this chapter considers other neurologic or nonneurologic disorders responsible for acute headache syndromes.

Clinical Assessment

Minute analysis of onset and character of the presenting headache is a skill, and most of the time the diagnosis is reached after exposing characteristic features. These warning signs are shown in Table 6.1. Most disorders are acute neurologic conditions; in addition, acute severe headache may indicate equally serious disorders, such as acute sphenoid sinusitis, a first manifestation of

malignant hypertension, or acute-angle glaucoma (Table 6.2). All of these disorders need different therapeutic approaches but should be considered by the neurologist.

A thunderclap headache should receive all attention. This headache refers to a split-second, extremely intense, totally unexpected headache that has not been experienced before and the patient feels as if struck by lightning (thunderclap) or as if the top of the head was blown off (like a volcano). When a loud handclap or finger snap is demonstrated, to indicate the sudden onset, patients will recognize that. Headache of this character may be short in maximal intensity but may persist for hours or be brief.[1]

Subarachnoid hemorrhage remains the main diagnostic consideration, and the diagnosis is established by computed tomography (CT) in 98 of 100 cases if seen within 12 hours of onset. The vast majority will be due to aneurysmal rupture.

Unfortunately, clinical signs, such as nuchal rigidity (rarely in the first hours), retinal or subhyaloid hemorrhage (predominantly patients in a very poor condition from a subarachnoid hemorrhage), or cranial nerve deficits (third nerve or sixth nerve palsy), are uncommon leads or absent in a ruptured aneurysm. Other infrequent conditions have been associated with thunderclap-like headaches, all very serious (Table 6.3).

Thunderclap headache may be without any objective abnormalities on neuroimaging (CT and all other magnetic resonance [MR] modalities) and CSF examination but this benign form is rather

Table 6.1. Warning Signs in Acute Headache

Signs and Symptoms	Diagnosis to Consider
Split-second onset, unexpected, worst and not previously encountered, loss of consciousness, vertigo, or vomiting	Aneurysmal subarachnoid hemorrhage, cerebellar hematoma
Acute cranial nerve deficit (particularly oculomotor palsy)	Carotid artery aneurysm
Carotid bruit in a young individual	Carotid artery dissection
Fever and skin rash	Meningitis
Shock, Addison's disease	Pituitary apoplexy
Immunosuppressed state	Cryptococcal meningitis, toxoplasma
Coagulopathy or anticoagulation	Subdural or intracerebral hematoma

Table 6.2. Acute Severe Headache Syndromes from Nonneurologic Causes

Disorder	Location or Type	Time Profile	Pathognomonic Features
Acute-angle glaucoma	Eye pain, frontal	Acute	Red eye, midrange pupil, decreased vision
Temporal arteritis	Sharp or dull	Rapidly built up	Temporal artery painful, sedimentation rate >55 mm/hour
Acute sinusitis	Frontal and maxilla	Hours	Fever, pressure pain on maxillary frontal sinus
Pheochromocytoma	Bilateral	Rapidly increasing intensity	Sweating, pallor, systolic blood pressure >200 mm Hg
Herpes zoster ophthalmicus	Eye pain, frontal	Hours-days	Vesicular rash may be delayed; visual loss; facial edema

Table 6.3. Symptomatic Thunderclap Headache Other than Subarachnoid Hemorrhage

Diagnosis	Clues in History	Clues in Examination	MR Features
Hypertensive encephalopathy	Poorly controlled hypertension	Systolic blood pressure more than 200 mm Hg	T2 abnormality predominantly in parieto-occipital lobes
Cerebral venous thrombosis	None	Increased CSF opening pressure	Transverse or sagittal sinus obstruction on MRV
Retroclival hematoma	None	CSF xanthochromia	Clot posteriorly and at level of clivus
Pituitary apoplexy	Cranial nerve deficit	Hypotension, hyponatremia	Pituitary tumor with hemorrhage
CSF hypovolemia syndrome	Marfan characteristics	Headache posture-related	Meningeal enhancement Subdural hematoma "Sagging brain"
Carotid or vertebral artery dissection	Trauma, chiropractic therapy	Horner's syndrome, dysarthria, carotid bruit	Recent cerebral infarcts; double lumen sign

MR, magnetic resonance; CSF, cerebrospinal fluid; MRV, magnetic resonance venography.

Table 6.4. "Benign" Acute Headache Syndromes

Disorder	Location	Time Profile	Quality	Pathognomonic Features
Cluster headache	Oculofrontal, temporal	30–90 minutes	Severe, stabbing	Rocking, restless, Horner's syndrome, rhinorrhea
Chronic paroxysmal hemicrania	Unilateral	2–30 minutes	Severe	Conjunctival injection, not restless, lacrimation on symptomatic side (common in females)
Acute migraine	Mostly unilateral	6–30 hours	Moderately severe	Nausea and photophobia in ~80%
Trigeminal neuralgia	Unilateral (face only)	Seconds	Severe, electrical	Provoked by chewing, cold wind, shaving, tooth brushing

uncommon. The term for this clinical entity was coined by Day and Raskin[4] but is also known as *crash* or *blitz migraine.*[5] Some patients may go on to develop common migraine but not invariably so, and the link with established types of migraine is uncertain. Onset associated with exertion or orgasm is relatively common in thunderclap headaches.[6] In a few patients, diffuse segmental vasospasm has been found by MR angiography (MRA) and angiogram.[7] The phenomenon is not explained well, but an increased sympathetic tone has been proposed.[7] Nifedipine may be helpful in some cases.[8] Recurrences do occur in 10%–15% of cases, mostly within the first 6 months, but outcome is very good.[9–12]

Status migrainous, refractory trigeminal neuralgia, and cluster headache are other causes for acute severe headache.[13] Severe-intensity, pulsating unilateral headache is aggravated by normal physical activity and associated with nausea and vomiting. Photophobia and sonophobia are common features in all of these disorders, but other differences of these more or less benign headaches are apparent (Table 6.4).

Refractory trigeminal neuralgia is characterized by episodic electrical sharp jabs of facial pain triggered by facial touch, chewing, talking, tooth brushing, and is commonly refractory to medication. Doses have been so high that intolerance has become a limiting factor.

Refractory cluster headache is fairly certain when patients present with excruciating retro-orbital forehead, jaw, or cheek pain following the first division of the trigeminal nerve, with lacrimation, nasal congestion, ptosis, and eyelid swelling. Attacks last approximately 1 hour and are commonly accompanied by restlessness and rocking motions.[13]

Line of Action

The critical steps in patients with a new thunderclap headache are shown in Figure 6.1.

Subtle subarachnoid hemorrhage can be very difficult to detect (Fig. 6.2). If the CT scan is negative, CSF would still be able to document xanthochromia up to 2 weeks.[14–16] However, CSF examination should be deferred until 4 hours have passed, to allow detection of xanthochromia from hemolysed erythrocytes freeing up oxyhemoglobin. CSF examination should include cell count, protein, and CSF pressure before sampling, as well as assessment of xanthochromia (*see Color Fig. 6.3 in separate color insert*).[17,18] Spectrophotometry would be a valuable method to prove xanthochromia that is due to bilirubin or oxyhemoglo-

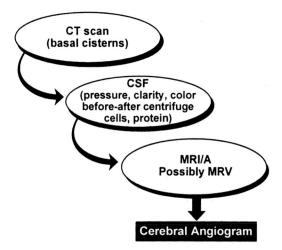

Figure 6.1 Critical steps in the evaluation of acute headache. CT, computed tomography; CSF, cerebrospinal fluid; MRI/A, magnetic resonance imaging/angiography; MRV, magnetic resonance venography.

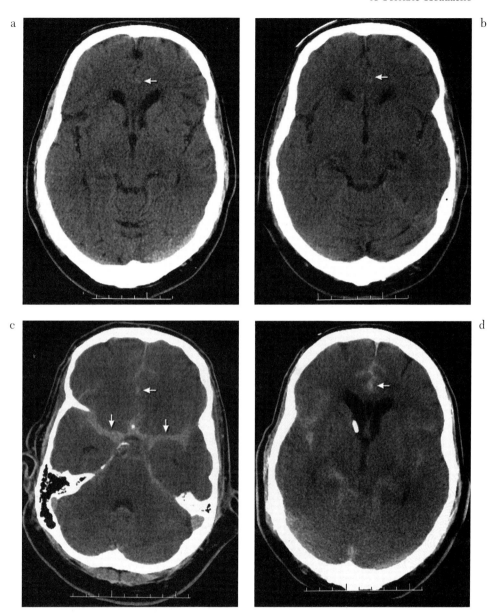

Figure 6.2 Serial computed tomographic scans of missed "warning leak." Very subtle hemorrhage in the interhemispheric fissure in a patient with thunderclap headache initially interpreted as normal (*a* and *b*). Follow-up 2 months later (*c* and *d*) documents more dramatic presentation of ruptured anterior communicating artery aneurysm after recurrent severe headache.

bin, but the technique is not used in the United States. Conditions other than aneurysmal subarachnoid hemorrhage have only been recognized after MRI and thus undermine the generally held tenet that CSF and CT should be sufficient to exclude underlying causes. No series of MRIs have been published on patients with thunderclap headaches; thus, categorical recommendations to proceed with MRI or MRA in all cases are not solidly based on data. MRI has documented thunderclap headache associated with hypertensive encephalopathy, pituitary apoplexia, signs of intracranial hypotension and meningeal enhancement, and retroclival hematoma.[19–22] MRA has

Box 6.1. The Triptans

It is postulated that triptans inhibit the peripheral trigeminal nerve terminals and central transmission within the medulla sensory nuclei. They have an additional potent vasoconstrictor effect on cerebral meningeal and dural arteries. These effects are mediated through binding and activation of specific 5-hydroxytryptamine receptors and thus are classified as serotonin agonists.

Major adverse effects involve facial flushing, tingling, and chest discomfort, which may be due to constriction of coronary arteries. Various triptans are available with different pharmacologic profiles, but comparison studies are scarce. Improvement of headache at 2 hours is approximately 60% with 100 mg of sumatriptan, with approximately 30% pain-free at 2 hours.[25,26]

documented carotid or vertebral artery dissection[23] but should include the entire region from the origin of the arch to the circle of Willis to scrutinize for arterial dissection. Magnetic resonance venography may discover cerebral venous thrombosis. However, in retrospect, each of these disorders had other clinical or laboratory clues suggesting the diagnosis.

In uncertain cases or in patients with ambiguous results, it is appropriate to proceed with a four-vessel cerebral angiogram. A cerebral angiogram may also seem appropriate in patients with a personal or family history of subarachnoid hemorrhage and disorders associated with cerebral aneurysms (e.g., polycystic kidney disease).[14] In all other patients, a cerebral angiogram is probably not recommended if neurologic examination, CT, and CSF are normal. There are very few data on patients with a thunderclap headache, a normal CT and CSF, and uncontrovertible evidence

of a recent rupture during visual inspection of the aneurysm by the neurosurgeon. Presence of an unruptured aneurysm can be coincidental, and the link between its discovery in patients with thunderclap headache may be a result of aggressive pursuit in evaluation of signs.[24]

Many patients with a migraine attack respond well to 900 mg of aspirin, 1000 mg of acetaminophen, or high doses of nonsteroidal antiinflammatory agents. However, triptans (Box 6.1) and droperidol have been used,[27] including in the emergency department. Contraindications include familial hemiplegic migraine, basilar migraine, ischemic stroke, ischemic heart disease, Prinzmetal's angina, uncontrolled hypertension, combination with monoamine oxidase inhibitors or ergot compounds, and pregnancy.[25,26] Abortive treatments for patients with "therapy-resistant, persistent" headache lasting for hours are shown in Table 6.5.[28–36] This designation of severity is

Table 6.5. Abortive Therapies in Unrelenting Head Pain

Disorder	Therapy Options
Migraine	• Sumatriptan (6 mg SC); repeat after 1 hour, if needed • Droperidol (2.75–8.25 mg IM) • Dexamethasone (20 mg IV) • Meperidine (100 mg IM) and hydroxyzine (50 mg IM) • Valproate sodium (500 mg IV [20 mg/minute drip]) • Dihydroergotamine (1–3 mg IV at hourly intervals) and metoclopramide (10 mg IM)
Cluster headache	• Oxygen therapy (7 L/minute facemask) • Metoclopramide (10 mg IM) • Sumatriptan (6 mg SC) • Nasal butorphanol (1 mg/1 puff) • Intranasal lidocaine 4% (4 sprays)
Trigeminal neuralgia	• Fosphenytoin IV loading (15–20 mg/kg IV) • Lamotrigine (50–100 mg per day) • Topiramate (50–100 mg per day)

very difficult to define, and the boundaries with rebound headache and analgesic-induced headache are not always that clear. The success of each of these pharmaceutical approaches in this more severe state comes more from anecdotal clinical experience than clinical trials.

A randomized trial of intravenous magnesium sulfate and metoclopramide in migraine showed a less favorable response than with metoclopramide alone.[37] The effect of dexamethasone may be much less than originally claimed.

Antiepileptic drugs, antispasticity drugs, and tricyclic antidepressants, often in combination, may not be successful in refractory trigeminal neuralgia. In these patients, a preliminary study has shown that fosphenytoin loading (15–20 mg/ kg) was rapidly successful.[38] Lamotrigine or topiramate may take weeks to exert a maximal effect. Other options are surgical, including ganglionic opioid analgesia, stereotactic radiosurgery, microvascular decompression, or percutaneous balloon compression.[28,39–41]

The response of cluster headache to subcutaneous sumatriptan or oxygen by nasal cannula is excellent, and refractory cases are quite uncommon.[42] The trigeminal nerve, at least its peripheral position, may not be of major importance in generating cluster headache, because cluster headaches have remained after section of the nerve, and response to sumatriptan remained.[43] Intranasal lidocaine or corticosteroids are good abortive second-line therapies.[44] The options for severe cluster headache are shown in Table 6.5.

REFERENCES

1. Perry JJ, Stiell IG, Wells GA, et al.: The value of history in the diagnosis of subarachnoid hemorrhage for emergency department patients with acute headache. *Acad Emerg Med* 10:553, 2003.
2. Jagoda AS, Dalsey WC, Fairweather PG, et al.: Clinical policy: critical issues in the evaluation and management of patients presenting to the emergency department with acute headache. *Ann Emerg Med* 39:108, 2002.
3. Saper JR: Medicolegal issues: headache. *Neurol Clin* 17:197, 1999.
4. Day JW, Raskin NH: Thunderclap headache: symptom of unruptured cerebral aneurysm. *Lancet* 2:1247, 1986.
5. Fisher CM: Painful states: a neurological commentary. *Clin Neurosurg* 31:32, 1984.
6. Green MW: A spectrum of exertional headaches. *Med Clin North Am* 85:1085, 2001.
7. Dodick DW, Brown RD, Britton JW, et al.: Non-aneurysmal thunderclap headache with diffuse, multifocal, segmental, and reversible vasospasm. *Cephalalgia* 19:1, 1999.
8. Jacome DE: Exploding head syndrome and idiopathic stabbing headache relieved by nifedipine. *Cephalalgia* 21:617, 2001.
9. Linn FHH, Rinkel GJE, Algra A: Follow-up of idiopathic thunderclap headache in general practice. *J Neurol* 246:946, 1999.
10. Linn FHH, Wijdicks EFM, van der Graaf Y: Prospective study of sentinel headache in aneurysmal subarachnoid haemorrhage. *Lancet* 344:590, 1994.
11. Markus HS: A prospective follow-up of thunderclap headache mimicking subarachnoid hemorrhage. *J Neurol Neurosurg Psychiatry* 53:1117, 1991.
12. Wijdicks EFM, Kerkhoff H, van Gijn J: Long-term follow-up of 71 patients with thunderclap headache mimicking subarachnoid haemorrhage. *Lancet* 11:68, 1988.
13. Olesen J, Goadsby PJ: *Cluster Headache and Related Conditions*. Oxford: Oxford University Press, 1999.
14. Edlow JA, Caplan LR: Avoiding pitfalls in the diagnosis of subarachnoid hemorrhage. *N Engl J Med* 342:29, 2000.
15. Edlow JA, Wyer PC: How good is a negative cranial computed tomographic scan result in excluding subarachnoid hemorrhage? *Ann Emerg Med* 36:507, 2000.
16. Hughes RL: Identification and treatment of cerebral aneurysms after sentinel headache. *Neurology* 42:1118, 1992.
17. Evans RW: Diagnostic testing for the evaluation of headaches. *Neurol Clin* 14:1, 1996.
18. Field AG, Wang E: Evaluation of the patient with nontraumatic headache: an evidence based approach. *Emerg Med Clin North Am* 17:127, 1999.
19. de Bruijn SF, Stam J, Kappelle LJ: Thunderclap headache as first symptom of cerebral venous sinus thrombosis. CVST Study Group. *Lancet* 348:1623, 1996.
20. Dodick DW: Thunderclap headache. *J Neurol Neurosurg Psychiatry* 72:6, 2002.
21. Schievink WI, Thompson RC, Loh CT: Spontaneous retroclival hematoma presenting as a thunderclap headache. Case report. *J Neurosurg* 95:522, 2001.
22. Schievink WI, Wijdicks EF, Meyer FB: Spontaneous intracranial hypotension mimicking aneurysmal subarachnoid hemorrhage. *Neurosurgery* 48:513, 2001.
23. Silbert PL, Mokri B, Schievink WI: Headache and neck pain in spontaneous internal carotid and vertebral artery dissections. *Neurology* 45:1517, 1995.
24. Witham TF, Kaufmann AM: Unruptured cerebral aneurysm producing a thunderclap headache. *Am J Emerg Med* 18:88, 2000.
25. Jamieson DG: The safety of triptans in the treatment of patients with migraine. *Am J Med* 112:135, 2002.
26. Loder E: Safety of sumatriptan in pregnancy: a review of the data so far. *CNS Drugs* 17:1, 2003.
27. Silberstein SD, Young WB, Mendizabal JE, et al.: Acute migraine treatment with droperidol: a randomized, double-blind, placebo-controlled trial. *Neurology* 60:315, 2003.

28. Spacek A, Bohm D, Kress HG: Ganglionic local opioid analgesia for refractory trigeminal neuralgia. *Lancet* 349: 1521, 1997.

29. Goadsby PJ, Lipton RB, Ferrari MD: Migraine—current understanding and treatment. *N Engl J Med* 346:257, 2002.

30. Potrebic S, Raskin NH: New abortive agents for the treatment of migraine. *Adv Intern Med* 46:1, 2001.

31. Robbins L: Intranasal lidocaine for cluster headache. *Headache* 35:83, 1995.

32. Wasiak J, Anderson JN: Is dexamethasone effective in treating acute migraine headache? *Med J Aust* 176:83, 2002.

33. Zakrzewska JM, Chaudhry Z, Nurmikko TJ: Lamotrigine (Lamictal) in refractory trigeminal neuralgia: results from a double-blind placebo controlled crossover trial. *Pain* 73:223, 1997.

34. Zvartau-Hind M, Din MU, Gilani A: Topiramate relieves refractory trigeminal neuralgia in MS patients. *Neurology* 55:1587, 2000.

35. Cady R, Dodick DW: Diagnosis and treatment of migraine. *Mayo Clin Proc* 77:255, 2002.

36. Vinson DR: Emergency department treatment of migraine headaches. *Arch Intern Med* 162:845, 2002.

37. Corbo J, Esses D, Bijur PE, et al.: Randomized clinical trial of intravenous magnesium sulfate as an adjunctive medication for emergency department treatment of migraine headache. *Ann Emerg Med* 38:621, 2001.

38. Cheshire WP: Fosphenytoin: an intravenous option for the management of acute trigeminal neuralgia crisis. *J Pain Symptom* 21:506, 2001.

39. Elias WJ, Burchiel KJ: Microvascular decompression. *Clin J Pain* 18:35, 2002.

40. Hasegawa T, Kondziolka D, Spiro R: Repeat radiosurgery for refractory trigeminal neuralgia. *Neurosurgery* 50:494, 2002.

41. Skirving DJ, Dan NG: A 20-year review of percutaneous balloon compression of the trigeminal ganglion. *J Neurosurg* 94:913, 2001.

42. Bahra A, May A, Goadsby PJ: Cluster headache: a prospective clinical study with diagnostic implications. *Neurology* 58:354, 2002.

43. Matharu MS, Goadsby PJ: Persistence of attacks of cluster headache after trigeminal nerve root section. *Brain* 125:976, 2002.

44. Couch JR, Ziegler DK: Prednisone therapy for cluster headache. *Headache* 18:219, 1978.

Chapter 7
Confused and Febrile

Fever and confusion are common presenting problems in the emergency department and thus are combined here. Fever in sick, dazed patients is often tied to an acute neurologic illness. It matters in which emergency department, in which place in the world the patient has recently traveled,[1] whether patients present in summer and fall, and whether the patient is immunocompromised.[2,3] Infection of the central nervous system (CNS) is readily considered, and decisions may have to be made quickly on a few clinical clues. The mortality and morbidity from the ravages of infection as a result of procrastination are very high. Also, evidence of an infection outside the CNS may not be immediately obvious and a great number of diagnostic possibilities are present. Fever and confusion can be caused by bacteremia, focal bacterial infection (upper respiratory tract, skin, and soft tissue infection), and nonbacterial illness such as viremia, drug fever, or malignant neuroleptic syndrome, malignancy, connective tissue disease, and thromboembolism. One should pity the physician (mostly the neurologist) who must make sense out of a perplexed, irritable, impulsive, desultory, markedly uncooperative febrile patient making smutty remarks. This chapter provides methodological diagnostic steps in organizing the evaluation of these patients. More specific disorders are discussed in Chapters 17 and 18.

Clinical Assessment

The diagnostic possibilities remain beyond measure if not narrowed down by additional distinctive symptoms. The most useful inquiries in the histories are shown in Table 7.1. For example, neurologic examination could indicate that confusion means aphasia, a postictal state, or nonconvulsive status epilepticus. Unusual signs may need attention and certainly could have a nonneurologic, infectious explanation. These are muscle rigidity (strychnine in illicit drugs, rabies, tetanus), myoclonus (*Salmonella typhi*), and trismus (tetanus). Fever and confusion can be associated with marked rigidity and tremors in the face and arms and should suggest an acute autonomic storm (neuroleptic malignant syndrome, lethal catatonia, or serotonin syndrome; see Chapter 5).[4]

The major domains of neurologic examination of a confused and febrile patient should include a serious attempt to assess demeanor and orientation, followed by thought content, attention, language, memory, and visuospatial skills. Each of these cognitive spheres may be judged in only a hurried cursory manner when agitation or delirium is prominent (Box 7.1).[5] First, it is important to observe the patient's poise. Uneasiness and restlessness may also indicate a medical disorder (e.g., hyperthyroidism, hypoglycemia, severe hypoxemia) or drug intoxication (e.g., theophylline, lidocaine). Impulsivity and emotional outburst and their opposite manifestation, abulia, are largely due to acute frontal lesions. Second, orientation is addressed and requires simple questions such as "How did you get here?" or "Where are you?" or "What is the month and year?" or "Why are you here?" However, the content of the answers may be disturbed with perseveration (continuation of thoughts) and intrusions (words

Table 7.1. Critical Observations and Clues in the Confused Febrile Patient

- Debilitated, wasted, underfed (drug abuse, alcoholism, cancer)
- Prior transplantation or AIDS (*Toxoplasma* encephalitis or aspergillus)
- Beginning of endemic encephalitis (arboviruses)
- Exposure to wilderness, tropics, animal bite (rabies)
- Exposure to excessive heat (heatstroke)
- Recent travel or immigration from developing country (neurocysticercosis, fungal meningitis)
- Recent vaccination (ADEM)

ADEM, acute demyelinating encephalomyelitis; AIDS, acquired immunodeficiency syndrome.

from prior context, often due to aphasia). Attention tests include spelling words backward, reciting the days of the week in reverse order, or other spelling tests. Language should at least include assessment of fluency, inflection and melody, rate, volume, articulation, and comprehension. Memory testing is challenging in confused febrile patients, but remote memory (significant life events in the family) or recent breaking news can be assessed. Visuospatial orientation may be briefly assessed by the patient localizing body parts or clock drawing and filling in the numbers. All of these manifestations may be stable, progressing, or fluctuating.

Confusional behavior may be due to mass lesions, which often produce language disorders. Masses in the frontal lobe that are located on the right (in right-handed persons) may enlarge to impressive tumors that may not be detected by even the most meticulous neurologic examination. A left frontal lobe mass, particularly if the lesion extends posteriorly, is manifested by Broca's aphasia. Its characteristics are distinct; the patient is constantly unable to repeat an exact sentence, speaks in short phrases and with revisions, and makes major grammatical errors together with loss of cohesion in lengthier narratives. Frontal lobe syndrome has been well recognized and appears in many guises, such as loss of vitality and notable slow thinking. It may be manifested by weird behavior, sexual harassment, cynically inappropriate remarks in an attempt to be humorous, or intense irritability. Any executive function requiring planning ahead or some type of organization and planning is disturbed but may be covered up by euphoria, platitudes in speech, or

"robot-like" behavior, in many with preservation of social graces.

Masses in the temporal lobe may also generate changes in behavior and therefore may remain unnoticed or be delayed in recognition. Left-sided masses may change a normal personality into one of depression and apathy. More posterior localization in the temporal lobe may produce Wernicke's aphasia. This classic type of aphasia is recognized by continuously "empty" speech, often with syllables, words, or phrases at the end of sentences and characteristically with incomprehensible content (e.g., one of our patients, asked to define *island,* responded "place where petos . . . no trees . . . united presip thing" and to define *motor,* responded "thing that makes the drive thing"). Involvement of the nondominant temporal lobe may be manifested by an upper quadrant hemianopia and nonverbal *auditory agnosia* (inability to recognize daily familiar sounds, such as a loud clap or tearing of paper).

Parietal lobe masses also produce effects that depend on localization. Right parietal lesions usually cause neglect of the paralyzed right limb up to entire unawareness but also cause marked inertia and aloofness. A dominant (left in right-handed persons) parietal lobe impairs normal arithmetical skills, ability to copy three-dimensional constructions (e.g., making interlocking rings with the index finger and thumb), recognition of fingers, and right–left orientation. A nonfluent aphasia may occur as well.

Occipital lobe masses produce hemianopia. When only the inferior occipital cortex is involved, *achromatopsia* (loss of color vision in a hemianopic field) or abnormal color naming ("What is the color of the sky, an apple, a tomato") may result. Extension into the subcortical area from edema might produce alexia without agraphia, but all in a left occipital lesion.

Systemic signs can provide a clue to the infectious agent. Obviously, an illness beginning with a cough suggests a primary respiratory infection, but there is a broad differential diagnosis. Community-acquired respiratory infections with a proclivity for systemic manifestations include influenza A and B, adenoviral infection, *Mycoplasma pneumoniae, Legionella pneumophila,* and reactivation of tuberculosis. All of these disorders could have neurologic manifestations. An illness with a prominent rash, fever, and confusion

---

Box 7.1. DSM-IV Diagnostic Criteria for Delirium due to Multiple Etiologies

A. Disturbance of consciousness (i.e., reduced clarity of awareness of the environment), with reduced ability to focus, sustain, or shift attention.
B. A change in cognition (e.g., memory deficit, disorientation, language disturbance) or the development of a perceptual disturbance that is not better accounted for by a prescription-existing, established, or evolving dementia.
C. The disturbance develops over a short period of time (usually hours to days) and tends to fluctuate during the course of the day.

D. There is evidence from the history, physical examination, or laboratory findings that the delirium has more than one etiology (e.g., more than one etiologic general medical condition, a general medical condition plus substance intoxication, or medication side effect).

Coding note: Use multiple codes reflecting specific delirium and specific etiologies (e.g., delirium due to viral encephalitis, alcohol withdrawal delirium).

With permission from American Psychiatric Association: *Diagnostic and Statistical Manual of Mental Disorders*, 4th ed. Washington DC: American Psychiatric Association, 1994.

---

could be due to viral, bacterial, and fungal agents with a possibility of seeding in the CNS (Table 7.2).

The multisystem involvement (myocarditis, pneumonia, lymphadenopathy, or hepatorenal dysfunction) associated with encephalopathy could indicate a certain infectious agent. Diagnostic considerations should include Q fever[6] (periventricular or focal edema on magnetic resonance imaging [MRI]), pneumonia, lymphocytic pleocytosis caused by zoonotic agent *Coxiella burnetii*, leptospirosis (meningitis, hepatic dysfunction, muscle pain, conjunctivitis), tularemia (ulceroglandular disease, conjunctivitis, and lymphadenopathy), *Mycoplasma pneumoniae* (pneumonia, transverse myelitis, conjunctivitis), and cat-scratch disease (lymphadenopathy, vasculitis caused by *Bartonella henselae*).[7]

In any patient, it is important to consider an immunocompromised state, which raises an entirely different set of possibilities.[2] Acute HIV infections can be present in a young adult with fever, confusion, lymphadenopathy, pharyngitis, and rash. One may consider questioning patients about sexual practice or intravenous drug abuse.

It would be inappropriate to have a too narrow scope in analyzing causes of febrile confusion, linking it only to meningoencephalitis. Specialization may in fact be a disadvantage when interpreting clinical signs in patients with such a broad presentation. Many systemic illnesses may produce a confusional state and agitation, and the major considerations are shown in Table 7.3.[6]

Febrile neutropenia is a common finding in patients with recently treated malignancies, particularly with aggressive myelosuppressive drugs. Infections become frequent and severe, with neutrophil counts less than 100 cells/mL. Remission induction therapy for acute leukemia is commonly followed by a prolonged period of virtually absent neutrophils. The most common pathogens in patients with neutropenia are *Staphylococcus*

Table 7.2. Clinical Signs Indicating Central Nervous System Disease in Confused Febrile Patients

Signs	Disorder
Skin rash	• Rickettsial diseases • Vasculitis • Aspergillosis
Petechiae	• Thrombocytopenic purpura • Meningococcemia • Endocarditis • Drug eruption from intoxication • Leukemia
Splenomegaly	• Toxoplasmosis • Tuberculosis • Sepsis • Human immunodeficiency virus infection • Lymphoma
Pulmonary infiltrates	• *Legionella* species • Fungi • Tuberculosis • Mycoplasma • Pneumonia • Q fever • Tick-borne diseases

Table 7.3. Systemic Illnesses Producing Fever and Confusion

- Septic shock
- Thyrotoxicosis
- Anticholinergic drug intoxication
- Streptococcal shock syndrome
- Heat stroke
- Lobar pneumonia
- Acute osteomyelitis
- Abdominal suppuration
- Endocarditis
- Erysipelas
- Measles
- Psittacosis
- Influenza
- Yellow fever
- Typhoid fever
- Cholera

epidermidis, Streptococcus spp., *Staphylococcus aureus, Escherichia coli,* and *Pseudomonas aeruginosa.* Many yeasts or fungi can be implicated. In hematologic malignancies, *Listeria monocytogenes, Cryptococcus neoformans, Toxoplasma gondii,* and *Nocardia* are common CNS infections when patients present with febrile neutropenia. When an Ommaya reservoir is in situ for chemotherapeutic delivery in leptomeningeal disease, coagulase-negative staphylococci and other skin inhabitants can be implicated. Patients seen in the emergency department with neutropenia, prior induction therapy or bone marrow transplant, pneumonia, or other documented infection as well as a major comorbid condition should be admitted using empirical broad-spectrum antibiotics and aggressive evaluation of its source.

Line of Action

It is virtually impossible to approach these patients from every conceivable angle. Clearly, primary disorders of the CNS need rapid assessment because therapeutic options are limited and time-locked. Encephalitis (particularly arboviruses),[8,9] meningitis, vasculitis, parainfectious encephalopathy, or a postictal state from epilepsy should be considered.

Studies with the highest yield and in the shortest period of time are needed and should be prioritized. To bring some clarity in patients who present with multiple converging problems, steps are shown in Figure 7.1. When the suspicion of intracranial disease is high, it is quite justifiable to temporarily sedate the patient (e.g., propofol), intubate, administer antibiotic agents and acyclovir, and obtain MRIs while obtaining cerebrospinal fluid (CSF).

The most reasonable sequence of evaluation is first to obtain laboratory data that could suggest a possible systemic infection. The chance of a bacterial infection increases with age (>50 years), erythrocyte sedimentation rate (>30), white blood cell count (>15,000), bands (>1500), and comorbid illness.[10,11] Laboratory tests should include a toxicology screen and drug levels, if needed, in addition to routine chemistry and hematology markers. Initially, an electroencephalogram should have some priority but may be artifactually abnormal or show a medication effect when sedative drugs are needed to control agitation. If no obvious or clearly defined abnormalities are present, one should proceed with a computed tomographic scan or MRI when encephalitis is present. MRI will, early in the disease, document

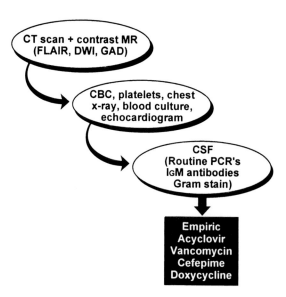

Figure 7.1 Critical steps in the evaluation of the febrile confused patient. CT, computed tomography; MR, magnetic resonance; FLAIR, fluid attenuation inversion recovery; GAD, glutamic acid decarboxylase; CBC, complete blood count; CSF, cerebrospinal fluid; PCR, polymerase chain reaction; IgM, immunoglobulin M; DWI, diffusion-weighted imaging.

Table 7.4. Etiologies of Central Nervous System Disease and Their Detection by Laboratory Methods

Disease	Etiology	Diagnostic Tests Recommended
Encephalitis Viral (with or without accompanying meningitis)	Herpes simplex virus-1	Polymerase chain reaction (PCR) and cell culture of cerebrospinal fluid (CSF) and tissue
	Varicella-zoster virus (VZV)	PCR and cell culture of CSF and tissue
	Cytomegalovirus	PCR and cell culture of CSF and tissue
	Epstein-Barr virus	Antibody (serum), PCR of tissue
	Arboviruses°	Immunoglobulin M (IgM) and IgG antibody (serum and CSF), antigen detection and PCR (brain tissue) available for some viruses
	West Nile virus	PCR testing of CSF, IgM antibody (CSF and serum)
	Colorado tick fever virus	Antibody (serum)
	Human immunodeficiency virus	Laboratory testing not specific for central nervous system (CNS) involvement
	JC polyoma virus (agent of progressive multifocal leukoencephalopathy)	PCR testing of CSF, PCR or in situ hybridization of brain tissue
	Rabies	Antigen testing of skin biopsy (hair follicles), conjunctival smear or brain tissue, PCR testing of tissue
	Herpes B virus	Cell culture or PCR of lesion (special biocontainment laboratory required)
	Postinfectious†	Document recent infection at primary site outside CNS
Nonviral Bacterial causes	Rickettsia rickettsii (Rocky Mountain spotted fever)	Antibody (serum)
	Borrelia burgdorferi	Antibody (serum and CSF), PCR testing of CSF
	Treponema pallidum	Antibody (serum and CSF)
	Mycoplasma pneumoniae	Antibody (serum), culture
Fungal causes		Fungal culture for all
	Blastomyces dermatitidis	Fungal stain of CSF recommended
	Coccidioides immitis	Antibody (serum and CSF)
	Cryptococcus neoformans	Cryptococcal antigen (CSF and serum)
Parasitic causes	Naegleria species	Histopathology, direct microscopic examination for ameba
	Plasmodium falciparum	Examination of thick and thin smears made with finger-stick blood
	Toxoplasma gondii	Histopathology, antibody (serum)
Meningitis Acute (neutrophilic pleocytosis)	Streptococcus pneumoniae	Gram stain and aerobic culture for all except amebas and anaerobes
	Neisseria meningitidis	Bacterial antigen testing rarely useful
	Listeria monocytogenes	Bacterial antigen testing rarely useful
	Streptococcus agalactiae	Bacterial antigen testing rarely useful
	Haemophilus influenzae	Bacterial antigen testing rarely useful
	Staphylococcus aureus	
	Gram-negative bacilli°	
	Anaerobic bacteria	Anaerobic transport and culture
	Ameba (Naegleria and Acanthamoeba species)	Microscopic examination of CSF and coculture with Escherichia coli or Stenotrophomonas maltophilia
Chronic (predominantly lymphocytic pleocytosis) Bacterial causes	Nocardia asteroides complex	Modified acid-fast stain, aerobic bacterial or fungal culture
	Brucella species	Aerobic bacterial cultures, hold agar plates 14 days, inoculate aerobic blood culture bottle with additional fluid

(continued)

Table 7.4. Etiologies of Central Nervous System Disease and Their Detection by Laboratory Methods (*Continued*)

Disease	Etiology	Diagnostic Tests Recommended
	Leptospira interrogans	CSF dark-field examination and culture, antibody tests (serum)
	Mycobacterium tuberculosis	CSF acid-fast culture and PCR where available
	Treponema pallidum	Antibody tests (serum and CSF)
	Borrelia burgdorferi	Antibody tests (serum and CSF)
	Fungal causes	CSF fungal culture for all
	Cryptococcus neoformans	Cryptococcal antigen test (CSF)
	Candida species	Gram stain for fungi (CSF) useful with shunt infections
	Coccidioides immitis	Antibody tests (CSF and serum)
	Histoplasma capsulatum	Histoplasma antigen testing (CSF and urine)
	Blastomyces dermatitidis	Gram stain for fungi (CSF) may be useful
	Other opportunistic filamentous fungi	Gram stain for fungi (CSF) may be useful
Parasitic causes	*Taenia soleum* (cysticercosis)	Microscopic examination of aspiration material or biopsy, antibody (serum by immunoblot)
	Echinococcus granulosis (echinococcosis)	Examination of removed cyst or cyst fluid for scolices
	Toxoplasma gondii	PCR testing of CSF
	Trichinella spiralis	Microscopic examination of muscle for larvae, antibody testing (serum)
	Angiostrongylus species	Eosinophilic meningitis
	Baylisascaris (raccoon ascarid)	Eosinophilic meningoencephalitis
Viral "aseptic" (initially neutrophilic, then mononuclear pleocytosis)		
	Enteroviruses	PCR testing of CSF, cell culture of lesion, antibody (serum) occasionally useful
	Mumps virus	CSF cell culture, IgM and IgG antibody (serum)
	Herpes simplex viruses 1 and 2	PCR testing of CSF
	Lymphocytic choriomeningitis virus	Antibody (serum)
	Varicella-zoster virus	PCR testing of CSF
	Cytomegalovirus	PCR testing of CSF
	Epstein-Barr virus	PCR testing of CSF

°Includes common arboviruses in North America, such as St. Louis encephalitis, LaCrosse encephalitis, and eastern and western equine encephalitis viruses.

†Postinfectious encephalitis caused by measles virus, VZV, influenza virus, and vaccinia (pox) virus.

Source: Thomson RB Jr, Bertram H: Laboratory diagnosis of central nervous system infections. *Infect Dis Clin North Am* 15 (no. 4):1047, 2001. By permission of Elsevier.

characteristic findings of herpes simplex (temporal lobe subinsular region), mosquito-borne encephalitis (cortical spotted lesions and basal ganglia), hyperintensities, or enhancing meninges (fungal or bacterial meningitis).[12] Almost simultaneously, CSF analysis should be sent for multiple polymerase chain reactions (PCRs), and failure to do so is a lost opportunity to diagnose the underlying organism.[13] PCRs are robust in documenting the presence of herpes simplex, Epstein-Barr virus, and varicella-zoster DNA and may detect organisms that do not grow in culture.[14] Fungal meningoencephalitis is very uncommon, but cryptococcosis, coccidioidomycosis, *Histoplasma capsulatum*, and *Blastomyces dermatitidis* are more endemic.[12] Detection by growth in CSF or of specific antibody is possible, but multiple CSF specimens are needed to detect a positive culture.

CSF in herpes simplex encephalitis will show a characteristic formula of normal or raised pressure at 10–200 cells (lymphocytes)/mm^3, normal glucose, and increased protein but can be normal in 5% of presenting cases.[15,16] CSF and serum antibodies (immunoglobulins M and G) should be obtained specific to any mosquito-borne viral encephalitis and repeated after 1 week. Indirect immunofluorescent assays are useful if Rocky Mountain spotted fever or ehrlichiosis is considered.[16,17]

When CSF is suggestive of an infection, it would be prudent to start with a multipronged approach directed against possible resistant bacteria (fourth-generation cephalosporin), herpes simplex (acyclovir and vancomycin), and ticks (doxycycline), while awaiting test results. The importance of dexamethasone is discussed in Chapter 17. The current laboratory methods assisting in diagnosis of meningitis or encephalitis are shown in Table 7.4. The interpretation of MRI and CSF is not considered further but is described in Chapters 16 and 17.

REFERENCES

1. Shlim DR, Solomon T: Japanese encephalitis vaccine for travelers: exploring the limits of risk. *Clin Infect Dis* 35:183, 2002.
2. Cunha BA: Central nervous system infections in the compromised host: a diagnostic approach. *Infect Dis Clin North Am* 15:423, 2000.
3. Frank LR, Jobe KA: *Admission and Discharge Decisions in Emergency Medicine*. Philadelphia: Hanley & Belfus, 2002.
4. Brendel DH, Bodkin JA, Yang JM: Massive sertraline overdose. *Ann Emerg Med* 36:524, 2000.
5. American Psychiatric Association: *Diagnostic and Statistical Manual of Mental Disorders*, 4th ed. Washington DC: American Psychiatric Association, 1994.
6. Bernit E, Pouget J, Janbon F, et al.: Neurological involvement in acute Q fever: a report of 29 cases and review of the literature. *Arch Intern Med* 162:693, 2002.
7. Libenson MH, Yang JM: Case 12-2001—A 16-year-old boy with an altered mental status and muscle rigidity. *N Engl J Med* 344:1232, 2001.
8. Deresiewicz RL, Thaler SJ, Hsu UL, et al.: Clinical and neuroradiographic manifestations of eastern equine encephalitis. *N Engl J Med* 336:1867, 1997.
9. McJunkin JE, De Los Reyes EC, Irazuzta JE, et al.: La Crosse encephalitis in children. *N Engl J Med* 344:1801, 2001.
10. Leibovici L, Cohen O, Wysenbeek AJ: Occult bacterial infection in adults with unexplained fever. Validation of a diagnostic index. *Arch Intern Med* 150:1270, 1990.
11. Mellors JW, Horwitz RI, Harvey MR, et al.: A simple index to identify occult bacteremia infection in adults with acute unexplained fever. *Arch Intern Med* 147:666, 1987.
12. Gottfredsson M, Perfect JR: Fungal meningitis. *Semin Neurol* 20:307, 2000.
13. Lambert AJ, Martin DA, Lanciotti RS: Detection of North American eastern and western equine encephalitis viruses by nucleic acid amplification assays. *J Clin Microbiol* 41:379, 2003.
14. Johnston RT: *Viral Infections of the Nervous System*, 2nd ed. Philadelphia: Lippincott-Raven, 1998.
15. Buringer JR: Herpes simplex virus encephalitis. In LE Davis, PGE Kennedy (eds), *Infectious Diseases of the Nervous System*. Oxford: Butterworth-Heinemann, 2000, p. 139.
16. Kennedy PGE, Chaudhuri A: Herpes simplex encephalitis. *J Neurol Neurosurg Psychiatry* 73:237, 2002.
17. Ratnasa MYN, Everett ED, Roland WE, et al.: Central nervous system manifestations of human ehrlichiosis. *Clin Infect Dis* 23:314, 1996.

Part II

Evaluation and Management
of Evolving Catastrophes
in the Neuraxis

Chapter 8
Altered Arousal and Coma

Catastrophic brain injury has widespread effects, among them coma. The assessment of comatose patients permeates the practice of all physicians. The causes of coma are many. Structural injury to the brain results in coma if it closely follows or directly affects the relay nuclei and connecting fibers that make up the ascending reticular activating system (ARAS). Its connections with the thalamus and both cortices make for a complex network (Box 8.1).

Elucidating the cause of coma cannot be compartmentalized into a simple algorithm, and novices may blanch and become unsure of themselves when a hastily ordered computed tomography (CT) scan and initial laboratory results are normal. The priorities in the evaluation of comatose patients have changed considerably with the arrival of magnetic resonance imaging (MRI). However, this may have encouraged a misconception that the cause of coma is easily established with neuroimaging. Relying solely on these tests can be counterproductive and potentially dangerous. Failure to recognize diabetic coma, thyroid storm, acute hypopituitarism, fulminant hepatic necrosis, nonconvulsive status epilepticus, or any type of poisoning while wasting time performing neuroimaging tests and waiting for cerebrospinal fluid (CSF) results may potentially lead to a rapidly developing neurologic fiasco.

The circumstances under which comatose patients are discovered can also be misleading. For example, a patient found next to an empty bottle of analgesic medication may have fulminant meningitis, traumatic head injury with skin lacerations may be a consequence of a fall from acute hemiplegia or brief loss of consciousness, and patients with massive intracerebral hematomas may be intoxicated. Comatose patients presenting with flexor posturing may have self-administered alkaloids as a recreational drug and, although suspected initially, may not have a primary structural lesion.[1] Another dramatic situation occurs when a patient with diabetes consumes a little alcohol but fails to have dinner and is brought in comatose and smelling of alcohol but also is profoundly hypoglycemic. All of these eventualities have the potential for misjudgment.

Evaluation of comatose patients requires a systematic approach, exploring five major categories: (1) unilateral hemispheric mass lesions that compress or displace the diencephalon and brain stem; (2) bilateral hemispheric lesions that damage or compress the reticular formation in the thalamus, interrupting the projecting fibers of the thalamus-cortex circuitry; (3) lesions in the posterior fossa below the tentorium that damage or compress the reticular formation; (4) diffuse brain lesions affecting the physiologic processes of the brain; and (5) less commonly, psychiatric unresponsiveness, mimicking a comatose state (Table 8.1). Accidental and self-inflicted poisoning and illicit drug overdose are common in the emergency department and thus receive proportionally more attention in this chapter.

Three major issues in the clinical approach to comatose patients are discussed. First, this chap-

Box 8.1. Ascending Reticular Activating System

The role of the ARAS is to arouse and maintain alertness. Despite identifiable structures, its definition remains conceptual. Coma is understood as a dysfunction of this anatomic neural network, which spans a large part of the rostral upper pons, mesencephalon, and thalamus and projects to the cerebral cortex of both hemispheres. Populations of neurons situated in the tegmentum of the pons and mesencephalon, intralaminar nuclei of the thalamus, and posterior hypothalamus are linked to the basal forebrain and associated cortex (Fig. 8.1). These networks communicate through neurotransmitters, such as acetylcholine, norepinephrine, serotonin, and dopamine and, through activation of the forebrain, produce wakefulness.

ter merges a thorough physical examination with a neurologic examination. Second, it emphasizes stabilization of the patient in a threatening state. Many stabilizing measures are simple, require virtually no specific skills, are easily mastered, and should be applied by physicians without delay. Third, it consolidates the priorities of diagnostic tests and provides recommendations for management and triage in each of the major categories.

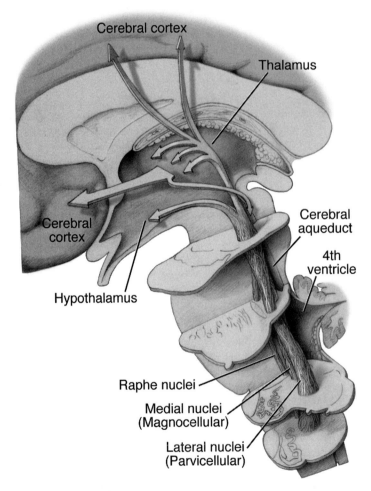

Figure 8.1 Ascending reticular activating system. By permission of Mayo Foundation.

Table 8.1. Classification and Major Causes of Coma

Structural Brain Injury	***Acute Metabolic-Endocrine Derangement***

Hemisphere
  Unilateral (with displacement)
    Intraparenchymal hematoma
    Middle cerebral artery occlusion
    Hemorrhagic contusion
    Cerebral abscess
    Brain tumor
  Bilateral
    Penetrating traumatic brain injury
    Multiple traumatic brain contusions
    Anoxic-ischemic encephalopathy
    Multiple cerebral infarcts
    Bilateral thalamic infarcts
    Lymphoma
    Encephalitis
    Gliomatosis
    Acute disseminated encephalomyelitis
    Cerebral edema
    Multiple brain metastases
    Acute hydrocephalus
    Acute leukoencephalopathy
Brain stem
  Pontine hemorrhage
  Basilar artery occlusion
  Central pontine myelinolysis
  Brain stem hemorrhagic contusion
Cerebellum (with displacement of brain stem)
  Cerebellar infarct
  Cerebellar hematoma
  Cerebellar abscess
  Cerebellar glioma

Acute Metabolic-Endocrine Derangement

Hypoglycemia
Hyperglycemia (nonketotic hyperosmolar)
Hyponatremia
Hypernatremia
Addison's disease
Hypercalcemia
Acute hypothyroidism
Acute panhypopituitarism
Acute uremia
Hyperbilirubinemia
Hypercapnia

Diffuse Physiologic Brain Dysfunction

Generalized tonic-clonic seizures
Poisoning, illicit drug use
Hypothermia
Gas inhalation
Basilar migraine
Idiopathic recurrent stupor

Psychogenic Unresponsiveness

Acute (lethal) catatonia, malignant neuroleptic syndrome
Hysterical coma
Malingering

Examination of the Comatose Patient

In assessing the nature of coma, an examination that sorts out representative localizing neurologic findings remains of great importance. Equally important is a reliable history. Relatives, bystanders, and police may all provide important information, including personal belongings and medical alerts.

The onset of coma may provide a clue. Acute onset in a previously healthy person points to aneurysmal subarachnoid hemorrhage, a generalized tonic-clonic seizure, traumatic brain injury, or self-induced drug poisoning. Gradual worsening of coma most often indicates an evolving intracranial mass, a diffuse infiltrative neoplasm, or a degenerative or inflammatory neurologic disorder.

A general physical examination is essential and may unpredictably provide a plausible explanation for altered awareness.

General Clinical Features

The general appearance of the patient may be deceptive, but extremely poor hygiene or anorexia may indicate alcohol or drug abuse. A foul breath in most instances means poor dental and periodontal hygiene or alcohol consumption. The classic types of foul breath should be recognized. These are "dirty restroom" (uremia), "fruity sweat" (ketoacidosis), "musty or fishy" (acute hepatic failure), "onion" (paraldehyde), and "garlic" (organophosphates, insecticides, thallium).

Fever and particularly hyperthermia (>40°C) in comatose patients may indicate an inflammatory cause, such as acute bacterial meningitis or encephalitis, but can occur in massive pontine hemorrhage, aneurysmal subarachnoid hemorrhage, and traumatic head injury. It may originate from direct compression, ischemia, or contusion of the hypothalamus. Hypothermia (<35°C) in-

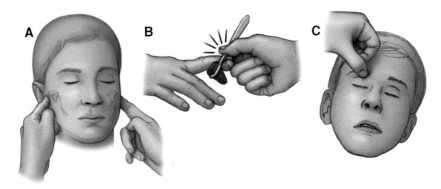

Figure 8.4 Methods of pain stimuli in coma. *A:* Compression of temporomandibular joints. *B:* Compression of nailbed with handle of reflex hammer. *C:* Supraorbital nerve compression. By permission of Mayo Foundation.

dicates exposure to a cold environmental temperature, a systemic illness, or intoxication. In patients with a devastating traumatic brain and spine injury, it may be a systemic sign of brain death or acute spinal cord transection.

Examination of the skin may provide important additional findings leading to the cause of coma. Bullae or excoriated blisters at compression points are nonspecific in most comatose patients but may indicate barbiturate overdose *(see Color Fig. 8.2 in separate color insert).* Carbon monoxide exposure, amitriptyline, theophylline, and diabetic ketoacidosis have also been linked to this curious skin manifestation.[2–4] In a patient with a long bone fracture, rapidly developing pulmonary edema, and acute unresponsiveness, petechiae in the axilla strongly indicate fat emboli *(see Color Fig. 8.3 in separate color insert).* Intravenous illicit drug use should be considered when appropriate, and the skin should

be carefully inspected for needle marks in multiple sites outside the cubital fossa. (However, scars in the cubital fossa alone often may indicate that the patient is a blood donor or receives regular blood transfusions.) Significant periorbital ecchymosis ("raccoon eyes") and retroauricular ecchymosis (Battle's sign) indicate midface or skull base fractures; they should be carefully looked for but often become apparent much later. The skin should be touched at different areas to assess its texture; both dry skin and skin drenched in sweat may point to certain intoxications (Table 8.2). Dry skin in a comatose patient (particularly in moist locations such as the feet, groin, and axilla) points to overdose of anticholinergic agents (common tricyclic antidepressant). Characteristically, these intoxications are associated with tachycardia, fever, and cardiac arrhythmias. As discussed in a later section, because electrocardiographic abnormalities can be

Table 8.2. Important Skin Abnormalities That May Have Discriminatory Value in Assessment of Coma

Sign or Symptom	Meaning
Acne	Long-term anticonvulsant use
Bullae	Barbiturates, sedative-hypnotic drugs
Butterfly eruption on face	Systemic lupus erythematosus
Cold, malar flush, yellow tinge, puffy face	Myxedema
Dark pigmentation	Addison's disease
Dryness	Barbiturate poisoning, anticholinergic agents
Edema	Acute renal failure
Purpura	Meningococcal meningitis, thrombocytopenic purpura vasculitis, disseminated intravascular coagulation, aspirin intoxication
Rash	*Streptococcus pneumoniae* (maculopapular) or *Staphylococcus aureus* (limited petechial) meningitis
Wetness	Cholinergic poisoning, hypoglycemia, sympathomimetics, malignant catatonia or sympathetic storm, thyroid storm

Table 8.3. Common Changes in Vital Signs in Coma from Poisoning

Toxin	Blood Pressure	Pulse	Respiration	Temperature	Additional Signs
Amphetamines	↑	↑	↑	↑	Mydriasis
Arsenic	↓	↑	~	~	Marked dehydration
Barbiturates	↓	~	↓	↓	Bullae, hypoglycemia
β-Adrenergic blockers	↓	↓	~	~	Seizures
Carbon monoxide	~	~	~	~	Seizures
Cocaine	↑	↑	~	↑	Mydriasis, seizures
Cyclic antidepressants	↓	↑	~	↑	Mydriasis
Ethylene glycol	~	↑	↑	~	Anion gap and osmol gap, metabolic acidosis
Lithium	↓	~	~	~	Seizures, myoclonus
Methanol	↓	~	↑	~	Anion gap and osmol gap, acidosis
Opioids	↓	↓	↓	↓	Miosis
Organophosphates	↓	↓ / ↑	↑ / ↓	~	Fasciculations, bronchospasm, hypersalivation, sweating, miosis
Phencyclidine	↑	↑	~	↑	Miosis, myoclonus
Phenothiazine	↓	↑	~	↓ / ↑	Dystonia
Salicylates	~	~	↑	↑	Anion gap, metabolic acidosis, respiratory alkalosis
Sedative-hypnotics	↓	~	↓	↓	Bullae

↑, increase; ↓, decrease; ~, no change.

entirely absent in tricyclic antidepressant overdose, its recognition may thus be extremely difficult. Profuse sweating should always point to organophosphate pesticide poisoning or severe hypoglycemia.

Hypertension is a common clinical feature in coma associated with acute structural CNS lesions and therefore has little predictive value. It usually subsides after the sympathetic outburst associated with the initial insult wanes, but unexplained surges of hypertension indicate poisoning from certain drugs, such as amphetamines, cocaine, phenylpropanolamine, hallucinogens, and sympathomimetic agents. Conversely, hypertension should be considered a cause of diffuse encephalopathy only in patients with profound hypertension (diastolic values ≥140 mm Hg), documented seizures, and papilledema, key signs that are often preceded by visual hallucinations.

Combinations of changes in vital signs may suggest certain poisonings. They are summarized in Table 8.3 and may be helpful in narrowing down the endless list of possible intoxications.

Neurologic Features

It should reflect the astuteness of a clinical neurologist to first evaluate whether the patient truly is comatose, in locked-in syndrome, or malingering. In locked-in syndrome, an acute structural lesion in the pons (which spares pathways to oculomotor nuclei of the mesencephalon and reticular formation) causes a nearly uncommunicative state. Before pain stimuli are applied, the patient should be asked to blink and look up and down. Grim accounts have been published of failure to appreciate this entity.[5]

The depth of coma should be documented, and many coma scales have been devised. Only the Glasgow Coma Scale (a combination of the best possible eye, motor, and verbal responses, as summarized in Table 8.4) has been tested for its

Table 8.4. Glasgow Coma Scale

Eye opening
  4 Spontaneous
  3 To speech
  2 To pain
  1 None
Best motor response (arm)
  6 Obeying
  5 Localizing pain
  4 Withdrawal
  3 Abnormal flexing
  2 Extensor response
  1 None
Best verbal response
  5 Oriented
  4 Confused conversation
  3 Inappropriate words
  2 Incomprehensible sounds
  1 None

reliability in daily clinical practice.[6,7] This scale remains unsurpassed. (The need for the scale arose when researchers in Glasgow realized that a standard language had to be used rather than vague statements such as "He seems a bit brighter today."[8]) The individual components of the Glasgow Coma Scale have been graded, at times summed to a score between 3 and 15. Grading coma by sum scores of the Glasgow Coma Scale alone is misleading because similar sum scores could represent different levels of decreased consciousness. A stimulus to elicit a response to pain, if needed, must be standardized: compression of the nailbed with the handle of the reflex hammer or pen, compression of the supraorbital nerve, or compression of the temporomandibular joint (Fig. 8.4).[9] Alter-

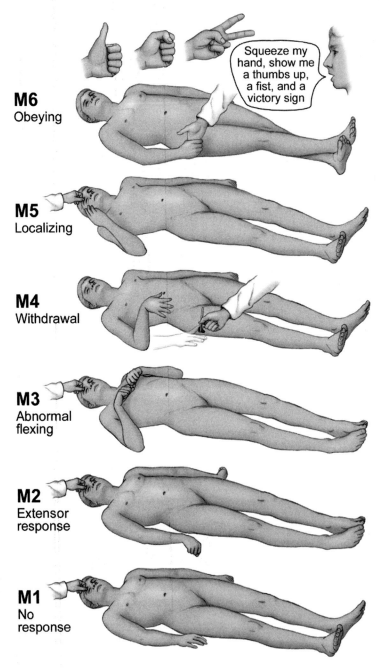

Figure 8.5 Glasgow coma score. By permission of Mayo Foundation.

native stimuli are sternal and axillary rubs or squeezing the trapezius muscle.

The components of the Glasgow Coma Scale (Fig. 8.5) are as follows:

1. *Eye opening.* By definition, patients in coma have their eyes closed. Spontaneous eye opening, however, does not portend awareness. Patients in a persistent vegetative state frequently have their eyes open, and they spontaneously blink. Eye opening can be produced by aural stimulus, such as a loud voice, or pain stimulus. Obviously, one should take care not to use both a loud voice and a pain or sternal rub stimulus at the same time. Eye opening is difficult to assess in patients with facial trauma or periorbital edema.

2. *Motor response.* By convention, the "best" motor response of the arm is noted, particularly when a different response between left and right exists. Responses in the legs are noted. They may vary from none to a triple-flexion response (flexion of hip, knee, and ankle) to following commands to wiggle the toes. In the fully alert patient, the legs can be crossed, mostly indicating a comfortable degree of relaxation (arguably this position is not seen in patients in acute distress).

The motor response is one of the most important elements in the neurologic examination of the comatose patient. Motor response is graded from "following commands or obeying" to "no response after a pain stimulus." It additionally is useful to ask the patient to follow simple commands rather than to squeeze a hand alone because reflex

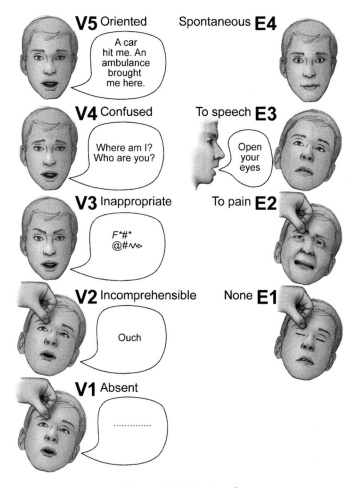

Figure 8.5 *Continued*

grasping may be misinterpreted as obedience. An example of a simple command is to ask the patient to show a thumbs-up, fist, or victory sign.[10] For localization of a pain response, the arms should either cross the midline toward a contralateral nail bed compression or reach above shoulder level toward a stimulus applied to the face. Withdrawal to pain is quick (snap-back response), usually involving only flexion and not arm or wrist flexion and adduction. Motor responses may include the so-called primitive responses. Both abnormal flexor responses (decorticate rigidity) and abnormal extensor responses (decerebrate rigidity) are nonlocalizing, indicating bilateral hemisphere diencephalic or brain stem lesions. Abnormal extensor responses imply a more severe lesion but not necessarily a worse prognosis. An abnormal flexion response in the arms (decorticate) is indicated by stereotyped, slow flexion of the elbow, wrist, and fingers, with adduction of the arms. An abnormal extensor response in the arms (decerebrate) consists of adduction and internal rotation of the shoulder and pronation of the hand with extension, internal rotation, and plantar flexion of the legs. Extreme extensor posturing may result in fist formation (thumb in palm) or wedging of the thumb between the index and middle fingers. Its presence is indicative of imminent demise (Fig. 8.6).

3. *Verbal response.* A normal verbal response is speech that implies awareness of self, environment, and circumstances. The patient knows who he or she is, where he or she is, and why he or she is there. Confused conversation is conversational speech with disorientation in content. Inappropriate speech is intelligible but consists of isolated words only and may include profanity and yelling. The term *incomprehensible speech* refers to the production of fragments of words, moaning, or groans alone. Lack of speech may denote mutism or anarthria and speech is obviously absent in endotracheally intubated patients.

Meningeal irritation should be assessed (Fig. 8.7 and 8.8) but becomes less apparent in patients with deeper stages of coma (e.g., no eye opening to pain, abnormal motor responses, and moaning only). Both the classic Kernig sign (inability to extend the leg with flexion at the hip) and the Brudzinski sign (flexing the neck causes flexion of the hips and knees) may be useful, but the diagnostic value for meningitis has been questioned by some.[11] Muscle tone can be flaccid (normal in coma but may indicate intoxication with benzodiazepine or tricyclic antidepressant poisoning) or rigid (e.g., neuroleptic agents, etomidate, strychnine, malignant catatonia, or malignant hyperthermia). Abnormal movements such as twitching in the eyelids (may indicate seizures), tremors, myoclonus (anoxic-ischemic encephalopathy, lithium intoxication, penicillin intoxication, pesticides), asterixis (acute renal, liver, or pulmonary failure), and shivering (sepsis, hypothermia) should be noted and integrated into the interpretation of the examination.

Neurologic examination proceeds with the cranial nerves. The size of the pupils and whether

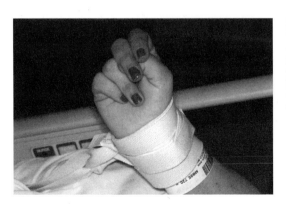
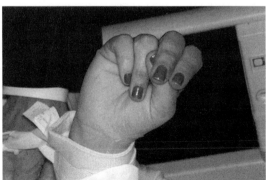

Figure 8.6 Extreme form posturing, poor prognostic sign (fist and thumb in fingers).

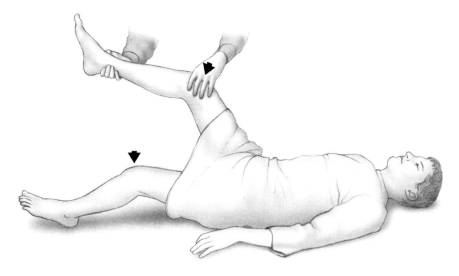

Figure 8.7 Kernig's sign.

they are equal, round, oval, or irregular should be noted. It is important to understand the meaning of a unilateral dilated, fixed pupil (frequently designates uncal herniation); bilateral fixed, midposition pupils (frequently designate diencephalic herniation, brain death, or intoxication with scopolamine, atropine, glutethimide, or methyl alcohol); and pinpoint pupils (frequently designate narcotic overdose, acute pontine lesion, or syphilis [Argyll Robertson pupils]). The pupillary reactions to an intense beam from a flashlight are studied for both eyes. A magnifying glass may be needed to evaluate questionable "sluggish" pupillary responses, particularly in patients with small

pupils. Pupillary abnormalities and their significance are shown in Figure 8.9.

Funduscopy may reveal diagnostic findings in comatose patients. Subhyaloid hemorrhage *(see Color Fig. 8.10A in separate color insert)* is seldom seen in coma but when present implies aneurysmal subarachnoid hemorrhage (see Chapter 13) or shaken-baby syndrome (see Chapter 20). Papilledema *(see Color Fig. 8.10B in separate color insert)* indicates acutely increased intracranial pressure but also is present in some patients with acute asphyxia.

Absence of spontaneous eye movement should be documented, along with lateral deviation to ei-

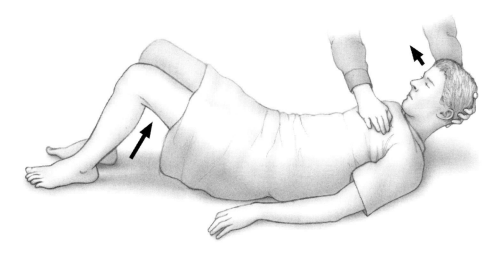

Figure 8.8 Brudzinski's sign.

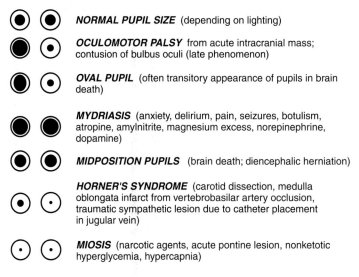

Figure 8.9 Pupil abnormalities in altered consciousness and coma.

ther side or disconjugate gaze at rest. Forced gaze deviation indicates a large hemispheric lesion at the site looked at. Spontaneous eye movements— periodic alternating gaze, ocular dipping, and retractory nystagmus—may be seen in coma but have no localization value other than indicating diffuse brain injury. (However, ocular bobbing— rapid downward, slow return to baseline—is typical for acute pontine lesions.) The oculocephalic responses are evaluated in conjunction with passive, brisk horizontal head turning, and, if appropriate, the response to vertical head movements can be tested. (In patients with any suspicion of head or spine injury, the oculocephalic responses should not be tested because movement may luxate the cervical spine if fractured and immediately cause spinal cord trauma.) Oculovestibular responses are tested by irrigating each external auditory canal with 50 mL of ice water with the head 30 degrees above the horizontal plane (an intact tympanum needs to be confirmed). Comatose patients exhibit tonic responses with conjugate deviation toward the ear irrigated with cold water. Bilateral testing can be done by rapidly squirting 50 mL of ice water in each ear, resulting in a forced downward eye movement. Abduction of the eye only on the side being irrigated with ad-

duction paralysis of the opposite eye implies a brain stem lesion (internuclear ophthalmoplegia) as a cause of coma (Fig. 8.11).

Finally, corneal responses are tested by drawing a cotton wisp fully across the cornea. Spontaneous coughing or coughing after tracheal suctioning is recorded (to-and-fro movement of the endotracheal tube is not an adequate stimulus). Absence of coughing may indicate either that the neurologic catastrophe has evolved into brain death or that sedative or anesthetic drugs or neuromuscular blocking agents for emergency intubation have markedly muted these responses.

Brain Death

The clinical diagnosis of brain death is strongly suspected when all brain stem reflexes are absent in a comatose patient, but the cause of the catastrophic event should be known and demonstrated to be irreversible.[12–14] It often is suggested when patients with fixed pupils stop bucking the ventilator and blood pressure suddenly decreases to low systolic values around 80–90 mm Hg. Brain death can be diagnosed in the emergency department but remains a presumptive diagnosis, and organ donation should not proceed directly from this lo-

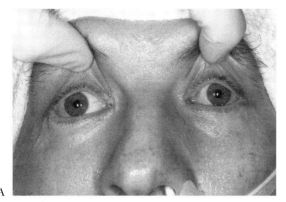

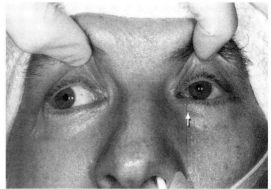

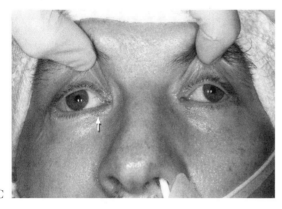

Figure 8.11 Internuclear ophthalmoplegia associated with acute pontine lesion. Eye position with eyelid opening *(A)*. Adduction paralysis *(arrow)* can be elicited by cold water irrigation of the right ear *(B)* or the left ear *(C)*.

cation. Any physician assessing a patient with brain death should be very sensitive to the possibility that confounding causes may be present, particularly in patients admitted directly to the emergency department. Even when a catastrophic brain lesion is demonstrated on neuroimaging, the circumstances should be considered ambiguous until the history is complete and, if appropriate, a toxicologic study has ruled out drug ingestion.

The accepted clinical criteria for brain death are shown in Figure 8.12. The technical procedure for the apnea test is shown in Table 8.5.

Assessment of Patients with Structural Causes of Coma

Structural lesions are often acute (hemorrhage, infarct, abscess) or may be a critical extension of an infiltrating tumor, abscess, or giant mass. The boundary in the vertical axis is the lower pons. Destructive lesions below this level may lead to acute dysfunction of autonomic nuclei, resulting in failure to drive respiration or vascular tone.

Coma or impaired consciousness in localized medulla oblongata lesions therefore is only an indirect consequence of hypercapnia or hypotension-induced global hemispheric injury. These lesions do not involve the ARAS structures and thus by themselves do not produce coma or hypersomnia.[15] These medullary structural lesions may involve hemorrhages (often arteriovenous malformation or cavernous hemangioma), metastasis, lateral or medially located medullary infarct, or an inflammatory lesion such as a bacterial or fungal abscess.

Tegmental pontine lesions interrupt the ARAS midway but result in impaired consciousness only with bilateral injury. The base of the pons does not participate in arousal; therefore, large lesions such as infarcts or central pontine myelinolysis do not impair consciousness but may interrupt all motor output except vertical eye movement and blinking initiated by centers in the mesencephalon. As alluded to earlier, this "locked-in syndrome" is often mistaken for coma until blinking and repeated up-and-down eye movements seem to coincide with questions posed to the pa-

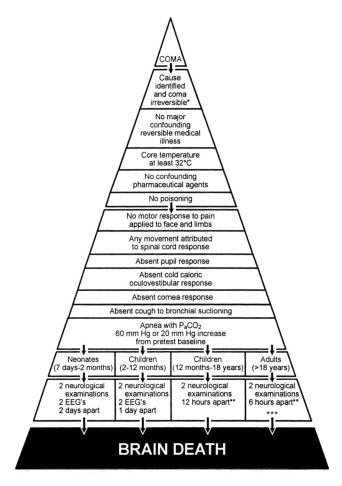

COMA

↓

Cause
identified
and coma
irreversible*

No major
confounding
reversible medical
illness

Core temperature
at least 32°C

No confounding
pharmaceutical agents

No poisoning

↓

No motor response to pain
applied to face and limbs

Any movement attributed
to spinal cord response

Absent pupil response

Absent cold caloric
oculovestibular response

Absent cornea response

Absent cough to bronchial suctioning

Apnea with P$_a$CO$_2$
60 mm Hg or 20 mm Hg increase
from pretest baseline

Neonates (7 days–2 months)	Children (2–12 months)	Children (12 months–18 years)	Adults (>18 years)
2 neurological examinations 2 EEG's 2 days apart	2 neurological examinations 2 EEG's 1 day apart	2 neurological examinations 12 hours apart**	2 neurological examinations 6 hours apart** ***

BRAIN DEATH

Figure 8.12 Brain death diagnosis and guidelines for confirmatory testing. °Evidence preferably based on computed tomographic scan or cerebrospinal fluid exam. °°Confirmatory test such as cerebral angiography, nuclear scan, or transcranial Doppler ultrasonography may obviate observation over time. °°°Criteria vary worldwide. P$_a$CO$_2$, partial pressure of arterial CO$_2$; EEG, electroencephalogram.

tient. Cognition is intact, and patients may communicate through code systems.

Mesencephalic damage usually is seldom seen in isolation and more commonly occurs from extension of a lesion in the thalamus (e.g., destructive intracranial hematoma) or as a result of occlusion of the tip of the basilar artery, producing simultaneous infarcts in both thalami and in the mesencephalic tegmentum.

Bilateral thalamic damage resulting in coma most often involves the paramedian nuclei, but damage to interlaminar, ventrolateral, or lateral posterior nuclei may impair consciousness by interrupting the thalamic cortex and thalamocortical projections. Infarcts in the distribution of the penetrating thalamogeniculate or anterior thala-

mic perforating arteries are the most common causes of bilateral thalamic damage, but an infiltrating thalamic tumor or infiltrative intraventricular masses in the third ventricle can produce sudden coma. Ganglionic hemorrhages may extend into the thalamus and compress the opposite thalamus.[16] Bithalamic hematoma is more commonly seen as an extension of pontine hematoma (see Chapter 14). Combined thalamic and mesencephalic damage may result in so-called slow syndrome, characterized by immobility, voicelessness, flat emotions, and somnolence most of the day.[15]

Bihemispheric structural damage may involve the white matter or cortex or both, and a diversity of disorders may produce damage severe

Table 8.5. The Apnea Test
(Apneic Diffusion Method)

Precautionary Measures

1. Core temperature $\geq36.5°C$ (4.5°C higher than the required 32°C for clinical diagnosis of brain death)
2. Systolic blood pressure ≥90 mm Hg
3. Euvolemia
4. Eucapnia
5. Normoxemia (preoxygenate)
   - Connect a pulse oximeter to the patient.
   - Disconnect the ventilator.
   - Deliver 100% O_2, 6 L/minute (place a cannula close to the level of the carina).

Assessing for Apnea

- Look closely for respiratory movements. Respiration is defined as abdominal or chest excursions that produce adequate tidal volumes.
- Measure arterial PO_2, PCO_2, and pH after approximately 8 minutes and reconnect the ventilator.
- If respiratory movements are absent and arterial PCO_2 is ≥60 mm Hg or there is an increase of 20 mm Hg in the PCO_2 over a baseline normal value, the apnea test result is positive (supports the clinical diagnosis of brain death).
- If respiratory movements are observed, the apnea test result is negative (does not support the clinical diagnosis of brain death), and the test should be repeated.

PO_2/PCO_2, partial pressure of O_2/CO_2.

enough to reduce arousal. The most notable disorders are anoxic-ischemic encephalopathy from cardiac standstill destroying most of the cortical lamina, multiple brain metastatic lesions, multifocal cerebral infarcts from isolated central nervous system (CNS) vasculitis, multiple emboli from a cardiac source, markedly reduced global cerebral blood flow from acute subarachnoid hemorrhage, cerebral edema, hydrocephalus, blunt head trauma causing extensive scattered lesions in white and gray matter structures, and encephalitis (see Table 8.1). Unusual structural causes for coma are bilateral internal carotid occlusions, very commonly leading to loss of all brain function from profound swelling within days.[17]

Assessment of Patients with Acute Unilateral Hemispheric or Cerebellar Mass

Two major clinical manifestations may be observed in patients with an acute hemispheric mass:

first, direct destruction of brain tissue leading to clinical features related to the involved lobe and, second, remote effects from herniation and buckling of essentially normal tissue.

The differential diagnosis in unilateral brain masses is extensive (Table 8.6).

The quintessential patterns of brain herniation from mass effect are (1) cingulate herniation, (2) central syndrome of rostrocaudal deterioration (herniation of the diencephalon structures, such as the thalamus), (3) uncal herniation, and (4) upward or downward herniation of brain tissue of the posterior fossa (Box 8.2).

Cingulate herniation is often asymptomatic, and typically a diagnosis made by CT scanning or MRI. It most frequently is a prelude to central or uncal herniation, when masses shift brain tissue even more. The cingulate gyrus is squeezed under the falx, but unless the anterior cerebral artery occludes (producing infarction and edema with frontal release signs and abulia), no major neurologic manifestation can be expected.

Central or diencephalic herniation occurs when a mass located medially forces the thalamus-midbrain through the tentorial opening. During this downward shift, the brain stem caves in and becomes distorted, and the shearing off of penetrating branches from the basilar artery fixed to the circle of Willis results in irreversible brain stem damage.

Signs of central herniation have been recognized by the evolution of midposition or small bilateral pupils with sluggish light responses. At the

Table 8.6. Diagnostic Considerations in Patients with Single Intracranial Mass

Immunosuppression	No Immunosuppression
Toxoplasma	Astrocytoma
Lymphoma	Oligodendroglioma
Progressive multifocal leukoencephalopathy	Glioblastoma multiforme
	Metastasis
Aspergillus	Bacterial abscess
Mucormycosis	Aneurysm (giant)
Nocardia	Histoplasmosis
Mycobacteria	Coccidioidomycosis
	Blastomycosis
	Multiple sclerosis
	Cysticercosis
	Meningioma
	Echinococcus

Box 8.2. Mechanisms of Herniation

Acute unilateral hemispheric masses may produce herniation syndromes from their volume or from surrounding edema. Whether displacement horizontally or vertically correlates with changes in consciousness and evolution of clinical signs remains a matter of some controversy. An alternative provocative but meritorious view is that horizontal shift measured by CT or MRI correlates better with early changes in consciousness in acute unilateral masses.[18,19] The diencephalic structures are compressed and dislocated toward the opposite side of the mass lesion. Bilateral masses "pinch" the upper brain stem rather than push it down. In addition, direct destructive damage of the thalamus with compression of the opposite dorsal thalamus may produce in the process bilateral involvement of the ARAS and may cause coma despite an impressive shift in all directions (e.g., large, destructive putamen hematomas).[19] The significance of vertical displacement thus may be vastly overrated, and early thalamus damage may be key. However, advances in neuroimaging studies have allowed us to identify the development of mesencephalon ischemia from progressive vertical shift or disappearance of the fourth ventricle from brain stem impaction, suggesting that rostrocaudal deterioration is key in the development of progressive stages of herniation.[20] However, it is not certain whether these changes on MRI are the defining moment of irreversibility.

same time, respiration becomes rapid, often with intermittent Cheyne-Stokes breathing. Patients barely localize pain stimuli and may fidget with bed linen or show a withdrawal response. Further progression results in extensor posturing and development of midposition pupils (diameter 5–6 mm) unresponsive to light, disappearance of oculocephalic reflexes, and irregular gasping. Central herniation may progress to a midbrain stage in a matter of hours but then halts or very slowly progresses further (Fig. 8.13). Central herniation may progress rapidly, but it is possible that the earlier signs of drowsiness, increased respiratory drive, and development of worsening motor responses are not appreciated by the physician or wrongly attributed to a new insult to the opposite hemisphere (e.g., in patients with a recent ischemic stroke).

Uncal herniation denotes displacement of the uncal gyrus, which is part of the temporal lobe, into the incisura tentorii. Uncal herniation has a more apparent presentation, with sudden appearance of a wide pupil with loss of light response. Ptosis, adduction paralysis, and diminished elevation of the affected eye are seen. Level of consciousness is reduced further when the uncus forces itself through the tentorium, flattening the midbrain and shifting it to the opposite direction. Contralateral hemiparesis occurs when the brain stem truly is squeezed against the opposite tentorial edge, damaging the pyramidal long tracts (classically named after Kernohan, Kernohan's notch). The midbrain displaces horizontally and may rotate if the compression is off center. The process can progress only more vertically, or the brain stem buckles and is squashed (Fig. 8.14). Compression of the brain stem causes smaller pupils (often misinterpreted as "improvement of the blown pupil" after administration of mannitol). Damage to the pons may lead to a transient locked-in syndrome.[21] Many of these features can be recognized on neuroimaging.

Acute cerebellar masses (e.g., hematoma) are manifested by vertigo, acute inability to walk, and excruciating headache. Vomiting is common, and many patients can only crawl to the bathroom. Approximately 60% of patients have a noticeable ataxia and nystagmus on examination before level of consciousness deteriorates from upward or tonsillar herniation.

Upward herniation occurs when the brain stem is lifted upward or when cerebellar tissue, particularly the vermis, is squeezed through the tentorial notch into the supracerebellar cisterns. The effects of brain stem compression and upward herniation are almost impossible to distinguish clinically. Patients deteriorate with progressive paralysis of upward gaze and further lapse into a deeper coma. Pupils become asymmetric and finally contract to pinpoint size when pontine compression advances. MRI can document these anatomic changes with accuracy (Fig. 8.15).[22]

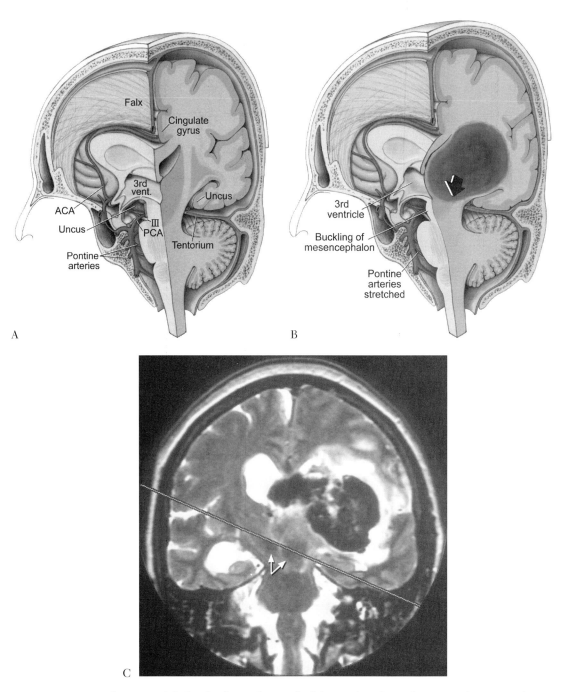

Figure 8.13 Normal anatomy (*A*), sketch of central or diencephalic herniation (*B*), and corresponding magnetic resonance image (*C*). Note downward movement of the brain stem. The red nuclei (only visible using spin echo sequences), usually horizontally aligned, have tilted (*arrows*). Ischemic brain stem lesions are the result of tearing of the penetrating arteries. ACA, anterior cerebral artery; PCA, posterior cerebral artery; vent., ventricle; III, third cranial nerve.

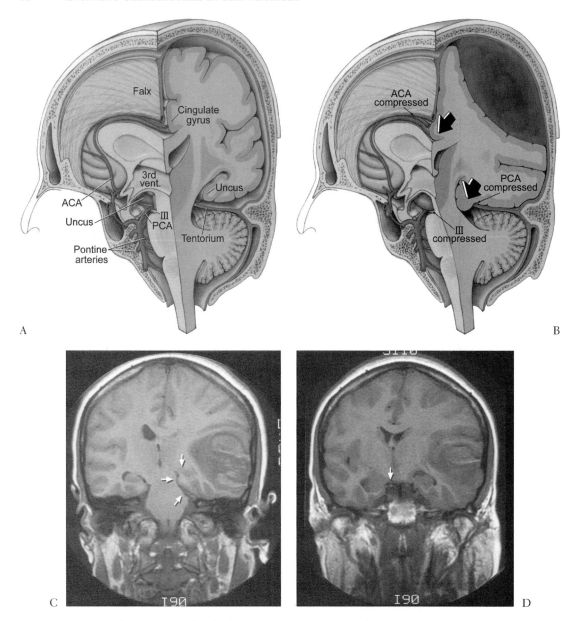

Figure 8.14 Normal anatomy (*A*), sketch of uncal herniation (*B*), and corresponding magnetic resonance image (*C,D*). Note uncal herniation (*C*) (*arrows*) and disappearance of the oculomotor nerve due to compression (*D*) (*arrow* points to opposite oculomotor nerve). ACA, anterior cerebral artery; PCA, posterior cerebral artery; vent., ventricle; III, third cranial nerve.

Assessment of Patients with Poisoning or Drug Abuse Causing Coma

Intentional poisoning and drug abuse are common causes of coma in patients admitted to emergency departments (Box 8.3). The distribution of causes may reflect the geographic location of the hospital. The most common substances used for self-inflicted death by poisoning are tricyclic antidepressants, salicylates (particularly children), and street drugs. In the elderly, suicide attempts and unintentional intoxication through misjudgment of dose remain leading circumstances.

This section reviews the most commonly encountered poisonings causing coma. It is hardly possible to discuss all drugs that may cause coma;

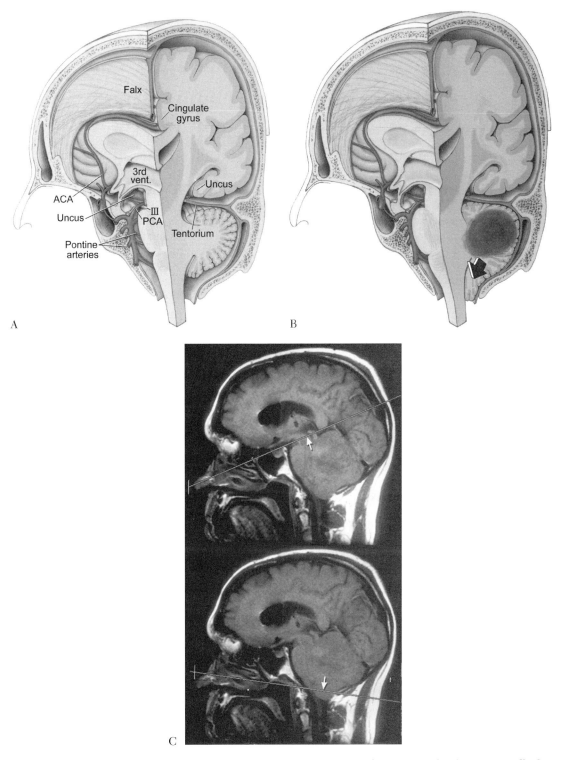

A

B

C

Figure 8.15 Normal anatomy (*A*), sketch of tonsillar herniation (*B*), and magnetic resonance images (*C*) (*arrows* point to orientation lines). The iter of the aqueduct, usually located on the horizontal line drawn from the anterior tuberculum sellae to the confluence of the straight sinus and great vein of Galen, is upwardly displaced. The cerebellar tonsils are herniated below the line of the foramen magnum. ACA, anterior cerebral artery; PCA, posterior cerebral artery; vent., ventricle; III, third cranial nerve.

Box 8.3. Mechanisms of Toxin-Induced Coma

Coma induced by poisoning may result from at least five mechanisms. First, a chief factor may be hypoglycemia. Because many toxins cause profound hypoglycemia, early intravenous administration of glucose in any comatose patient has been advocated. Common examples are salicylates, β-adrenergic blockers, and ethanol.

Second, in other toxins, hypoxia is the main mechanism underlying coma and is produced by interference of oxygen transport, tissue utilization of oxygen, or simply displacement of oxygen by another gas, such as an industrial gas. Hypoxia can also be produced by acute pulmonary edema (e.g., cocaine) or aspiration pneumonitis (e.g., after seizures).

Third, a major mechanism of coma is depression of neuronal function involving the γ-aminobutyric acid (GABA)–benzodiazepine chloride iodophor receptor complex. The mechanism of ac-

tion through GABA, one of the major CNS neurotransmitters, is increased output of GABA, which also leads to reduction of the turnover of acetylcholine, dopamine, and serotonin, culminating in a marked hypnotic-depressant effect. Opioids, however, exert their depressant effects on the CNS through a different set of receptors.

Fourth, toxins may cause seizures, usually as a terminal manifestation, which may be followed by a postictal decreased level of consciousness or nonconvulsive status epilepticus.

Fifth, structural CNS lesions may be caused by the toxin itself or traumatic head injury. Coma in poisoning or drug abuse may be due to spontaneous intracranial hematoma (e.g., amphetamine or cocaine overdose) or hemorrhagic brain contusions associated with a fall.

in fact, many do when ingested in enormous quantities. Polydrug abuse or intentional intoxication often results in widely different clinical presentations. Many of the drug overdose cases are so complicated and difficult to diagnose that physicians are left with a dizzying array of possibilities. There is a potential flaw in presenting these intoxications in a simplistic fashion, but some clinical patterns are truly characteristic and should be recognized at first appearance.[23]

Central Nervous System Depressants

CNS depressants first impair vestibular and cerebellar function. Therefore, nystagmus, ataxia, and dysarthria accompany or even precede the first signs of impaired consciousness.

Diagnosing an overdose of CNS depressant agents remains difficult, and one should appreciate the dangerous potential of some agents (e.g., tricyclic antidepressants).

Ethanol
Alcohol intoxication is a frequent cause of reduced arousal. Alcohol ingestion can be fatal, but for death to occur, extreme quantities of ethanol should have been consumed, and more often an alcoholic binge is combined with consumption

of other depressant drugs, leading to respiratory arrest or respiratory airway obstruction from vomiting.[24,25]

The development of acute alcohol intoxication depends not only on the blood alcohol concentration but also on the rapidity of the increase in blood and on tolerance, which is significantly increased in heavy drinkers (typically, they are able to "drink someone under the table"). The clinical features of alcohol intoxication in relation to blood alcohol level are thus unreliable and apply only to naive drinkers. The clinical presentation of alcohol intoxication is well known and involves ataxia, dysarthria, loss of rapid reaction to sudden danger, and a feeling of high self-esteem that can lead to a series of misjudgments, including driving despite warnings from passengers. Aggression to well-intended restraint may lead to fist fights in susceptible persons and significant head injury or epidural hematoma due to acute skull fracture (see Chapter 20) overlying the middle meningeal artery.

Seizures are uncommon as a direct result of alcohol consumption but may be associated with severe hyponatremia (e.g., after consumption of large quantities at "beer fests"). Alcohol intoxication may mimic or coincide with many neurologic disorders, including hepatic encephalopathy, hypoglycemia, subdural hematoma, fulminant bacterial meningitis, and central pontine myelinolysis. Progressive confusion and combativeness in a previously alcoholic person, particularly if associated with tremors, marked (often initially unexplained) hypertension, and tachycardia, may indicate alcohol withdrawal and delirium. Recognition of profound alcohol withdrawal may become difficult, particularly if patients have passed well into a stage of agitation and decreased alertness.

The diagnosis of acute drunkenness seems straightforward, but laboratory confirmation and exclusion of confounding metabolic derangements are needed. Crucial laboratory tests should include measurement of serum alcohol level, arterial blood gases (to exclude hypoventilation), electrolytes, blood glucose (alcohol reduces gluconeogenesis and causes hypoglycemia in a predisposed patient), calcium and magnesium, and serum osmolality. A large osmolar gap is compatible with alcohol intoxication. Routine drug screens should be performed at all times to rule out other ingested drugs of abuse. When truly measured, the legal limit in many states is 80 mg alcohol/100 mL blood, but toxic levels are usually more than 200 mg alcohol/100 mL blood.

Management of patients in stupor or coma from alcohol intoxication consists of endotracheal intubation to protect the airway, thiamine intravenously, rewarming, liberal intravenous fluids, treatment of recurrent seizures, if any, and frequent assessment and management of potential hypoglycemia.

Barbiturates

Barbiturates are hypnotic-sedative agents that should be considered a cause of coma in drug addicts rushed into emergency departments. It is not surprising to find that barbiturates have been taken with other street drugs, and they may considerably deepen the level of coma.

Barbiturates significantly differ in duration of action (Table 8.7). They are very powerful stimulants of the inhibitory neurotransmitter GABA, resulting in early depression of respiratory drive. In the event of overdose, these differences often determine the time on the mechanical ventilator.

Depending on the degree of CNS depression, barbiturate overdose produces flaccid coma with initially small reactive pupils advancing to light-fixed, dilated pupils in near-fatal doses, often with associated profound hypotension from direct myocardial depression, clammy skin, and hypothermia. Bullous skin lesions ("coma blisters," Fig. 8.2) can be seen at pressure points and are very uncommon at other sites, suggesting skin necrosis from ischemia rather than a specific cutaneous toxicity.

The depth of coma can be estimated by measurement of barbiturate levels and by an electroencephalogram, which in severe cases may show isoelectric tracing mimicking brain death, but more commonly displays a burst suppression pattern.

Management of barbiturate coma is supportive, with full mechanical ventilation until cough reflexes return. Vasopressors, such as dopamine, are needed to support blood pressure. Forced alkaline diuresis and hemodialysis with high blood flow rate should be considered.[26]

With the improvement in intensive care support and hemodialysis, outcome is difficult to predict on the basis of depth of coma. A landmark study by Reed et al.[27] found that mortality was high in patients with respiratory failure, hypotension, and coma for more than 36 hours; but these data may not apply in modern times.

Table 8.7. Classification of Barbiturates

Ultra-short-acting (DA, 0.3 hour)
Thiopental
Thiamylal
Methohexital
Short-acting (DA, 3 hours)
Hexobarbital
Pentobarbital°
Secobarbital†
Intermediate-acting (DA, 3–6 hours)
Amobarbital‡
Aprobarbital
Butabarbital
Long-acting (DA, 6–12 hours)
Barbital
Mephobarbital
Phenobarbital§
Primidone

DA, duration of action.
°Also known as "yellow jackets."
†Also known as "red devils."
‡Also known as "blue heavens."
§Also known as "purple hearts," "goofballs," and "downs."

Tricyclic Antidepressants

The prescription of antidepressant drugs for patients with severe depression may lead to use by the patient for a suicide attempt. This is possibly also related to the observation that it takes 2–3 weeks to achieve the antidepressant effect, and thus, patients with suicidal tendencies may take all of the medication at once. Tricyclic overdose is one of the principal causes of death in intensive care unit series of drug overdosing.[28] By virtue of the profound cardiac toxicity of the drugs, death can be imminent in some patients on arrival in the emergency department.

Coma from tricyclic antidepressant toxicity may progress to a loss of all brain stem reflexes and apnea, mimicking brain death. However, coma with no response to painful stimuli occurred in only 13% of 225 patients with tricyclic overdose.[29] Tricyclic overdose may be manifested by delirium from cholinergic blockade, and some patients have other manifestations, such as dry skin, hyperthermia, and dilated pupils.[30] Seizures are common within hours of ingestion, often emerge at peak serum concentration, but seldom evolve into status epilepticus.[31]

A widened QRS interval on the electrocardiogram is a common manifestation, and at least initially cardiac arrhythmias may be absent. In a significant overdose, the management of cardiac arrhythmia determines care and can involve a temporary pacemaker. Sodium bicarbonate (50 mEq of $NaHCO_3$, 1 mEq/mL) should be administered to produce alkalosis, which inhibits sodium channel blockade by tricyclic antidepressants, a mechanism thought to be responsible for cardiac arrhythmia. Seizures can be managed with intravenous administration of phenytoin or fosphenytoin, but because of its own risk of producing cardiac arrhythmias, this agent probably is indicated only if seizures recur.

Lithium

Toxic manifestations of lithium are most often a result of incorrect dosage. Anticholinergic manifestations are common, including flushing of the face, dilated pupils, fever, and dry skin.[32]

With increasing blood levels, a rather slowly progressive clinical picture seems to emerge, characterized by myoclonus, hand tremor, and slurring of speech. This may further progress to delirium, acute mania, dystonic movements, ocu-logyric crises, facial grimacing, and, finally, stupor. Serum lithium levels are reasonably correlated with the severity of toxicity, which is serious when these levels reach or exceed 2.5 mEq/L.[32]

Restoration of sodium and water balance, which is disturbed by lithium-induced nephrogenic diabetes insipidus, is key in its management. Hemodialysis or peritoneal dialysis should be instituted immediately in most cases.

Benzodiazepines

Patients with a benzodiazepine overdose (slang: downs, nerve pills, tranks) seldom are in need of a long hospital stay unless coingestions have occurred. Massive exposure to benzodiazepines results in coma, but with appropriate support, neurologic morbidity is rare. Coma can be profound, but most patients awaken within 2 days; recovery times are longer with increasing age.[33]

The clinical presentation of benzodiazepine poisoning is nonspecific, and coma with extreme flaccidity is common.[34] Respiratory depression may not be evident, and hypoxic respiratory drive often becomes clear only when a pulse oximeter is connected to the patient on arrival in the emergency department. Not uncommonly, oxygen administration with high flow may then produce hypercarbia and hyperoxemia. Many patients may need to be intubated, but adjustment of the O_2 source and rate-controlled, noninvasive ventilation may be effective in some instances.

The use of flumazenil is controversial because seizures from acute withdrawal have been reported. A more recent study in 110 patients contradicted these risks and demonstrated that flumazenil is safe.[35]

Abuse of Illicit Drugs

It is not possible to gather all illicit drugs under one umbrella and discuss them in a few paragraphs. This section discusses some of the most commonly encountered examples of drug overdose. For complex problems, readers should refer to major toxicology textbooks,[36] available in most emergency departments, or a neurology text.[37] Not infrequently, these unfortunate, poorly nourished, shelterless patients are found hypothermic or next to an empty syringe, bottle of liquor, or unlabeled pill vial.

Phencyclidine

Phencyclidine (slang, "angel dust") is rising in popularity among illicit drug users and users in college students, and thus the prevalence of phencyclidine overdose is increasing in emergency departments. Phencyclidine is usually packed in tablets and sold as powder or mixed with marijuana (slang, "wacky weed").[36]

Phencyclidine is a potent anesthetic agent, acting on both GABA and dopamine systems. Its clinical manifestations are highly unusual, with deep anesthesia and coma but a facial appearance of being fully awake.[35] Typically, a strong pain stimulus is not registered by the patient, and this sign should immediately point to phencyclidine as a toxin. Commonly, phencyclidine produces hypertension, tachycardia, salivation, sweating, and bidirectional nystagmus. Many patients act violently, demonstrate bizarre behavior, and speak endlessly.[38] Distortion of body image and vivid visual hallucinations may occur, and some patients are catatonic, which additionally may lead to rhabdomyolysis. When the patient's condition progresses to coma, cholinergic signs are obvious, with significant frothing, flushing, sweating (often with typical strings of large sweat droplets on the forehead), and miosis.[38,39]

Many patients recover fully with adequate ventilator support, but some may continue to manifest a schizophrenia-like picture of withdrawal, negativism, and delusions, which suggests chronic use of phencyclidine.

Cocaine

Cocaine (slang: blow, snow, toot, coke, rock) blocks the presynaptic uptake of norepinephrine and dopamine and causes excitation.[40] Its recreational use is widespread, either by intranasal snorting or by smoking after dissolution in water and the addition of a strong base (so-called crack).

The clinical presentation after inhalation, smoking, or intravenous injection is characteristic. Patients have hypertension, widely dilated pupils, and tachypnea. Seizures often occur after the initial "rush."[41] In severely intoxicated patients, progression to generalized tonic-clonic epilepticus is not unusual.[42,43]

Coma from cocaine overdose may have other origins. These are cardiac arrest, producing a profound anoxic-ischemic encephalopathy; intracerebral or subarachnoid hemorrhage from brief malignant hypertension. Outcome is worse in aneurysmal subarachnoid hemorrhage associated with cocaine.[44] Up to 50% of patients harbor a vascular malformation or aneurysm. Bilateral cerebral infarcts can be a result of diffuse vasoconstriction[45,46] or long-standing occlusive disease of major cerebral arteries.[47]

General measures for cocaine overdose often include management of hyperthermia with cooling blankets or fans, α-adrenergic blockade or lidocaine to treat ventricular tachycardia, and careful monitoring for the possible development of acute myocardial infarction and recognition of status epilepticus.

Opiates

Acute opiate overdose may be produced by heroin (diacetylmorphine [slang: "H," speedball]) or deliberate use of massive doses of narcotic drugs used for pain control. Fentanyl dermal patches, particularly, have become popular for pain control, and the absorption of this very potent opioid is so erratic that rapidly progressive stupor may occur.[48]

The clinical manifestations of opiate overdose include miosis, hypoventilation, and flaccidity. Brain stem reflexes may become lost, and the preserved light reflex in patients with extremely small pupils may be impossible to discern. Severe hypoxia from hypoventilation or florid pulmonary edema may be a major contributory factor to coma. Seizures appear more commonly with meperidine and propoxyphene.

Management of opioid poisoning has been facilitated by the use of naloxone. This opiate antagonist is without major adverse effects, and dramatic reversal of coma is seen.

Arterial blood gas values are supportive in opioid overdose, demonstrating marked hypoxia and hypercapnia from hypoventilation. A point that cannot be emphasized strongly enough is that because serum drug screens do not identify opioids, urine samples are needed for detection. For other examples, see Appendix 8.1.

Naloxone is administered in doses of 0.4–2.0 mg repeated at 1- to 2-minute intervals. The effect is brief. An intravenous drip of naloxone is justified only in patients with a profound overdose resulting in hypotension and ventricular tachyarrhythmias.

Environmental and Industrial Toxins

Exposure to these toxins, whether intentional or accidental, frequently alters consciousness and produces prolonged coma long after the toxin has been eliminated, washed out, or neutralized. Important clues to environmental poisoning are dead pets and distinctive odors (from often-added sulfur-containing compounds) detected by neighbors.

The effect of these toxins on the CNS can be catastrophic, with a high probability of poor neurologic outcomes.

Carbon Monoxide Poisoning

Carbon monoxide remains one of the leading causes of death by poisoning. Exposure to this odorless gas is possible at the time of a fire, from poorly vented fireplaces, from furnaces, and in any closed space where internal combustion engines have been used without ventilation. In most instances, suicide can be implicated, but one-third of admitted patients are victims of accidental circumstances.

Carbon monoxide readily binds to hemoglobin, with a 200 times greater attraction than oxygen. The cerebral injury due to carbon monoxide poisoning, however, is an accumulation of factors. Early animal studies by Ginsberg[49] clearly showed that the pathognomonic lesions can be produced only by carbon monoxide and hypotension and not by inhalation of carbon monoxide alone.

Carbon monoxide poisoning causes a shift of the hemoglobin dissociation curve to the left, which reduces oxygen unloading (Haldane effect). Through binding with myoglobin, carbon monoxide may trigger cardiac arrhythmias, hypotension, and hypoxemia from pulmonary edema, adding to the injury.[50]

The neuropathologic changes (selected from the most severe cases at autopsy) are predominant in the white matter, with demyelination and edema, and in the hippocampus, cerebellum, and globus pallidus. These lesions may be detected on CT scans;[51] they predict a severely disabled state as the best possible outcome.[52,53] MRI may more clearly delineate these abnormalities, which emerge even within hours of exposure, but only in patients with levels high enough to lead to coma (virtually always more than 50% carboxyhemoglobin levels).[54]

The symptoms preceding coma from carbon monoxide poisoning are nonspecific and vague, including headache, dizziness, and shortness of breath, all suggesting a developing viral illness. A cherry red appearance of the skin is very uncommon; it signals a near-fatal exposure.[49] Other clinical findings are retinal hemorrhages, dark color of retinal arteries and veins, and pulmonary edema. Rhabdomyolysis may be related to pressure necrosis in patients immobilized for an unknown length of time.

The most important laboratory test is the determination of a carbon monoxide hemoglobin level, which may be "falsely low" if oxygen has been administered in the emergency room or if the time between exposure and blood testing is more than 6 hours, which is approximately the half-life of carboxyhemoglobin (a 5% level of hemoglobin carbon monoxide can be attributed to smoking). Other laboratory test results that are more or less supportive are metabolic acidosis, increased creatine kinase, and myocardial ischemia on electrocardiography.

Management of carbon monoxide poisoning is treatment with 100% oxygen with a sealed face mask. Hyperbaric oxygen increases the amount of dissolved oxygen 10 times and may significantly shorten the duration of coma.[55] Hyperbaric oxygen is not routinely available, but there are hard data that prove a better outcome with this therapy. A recent clinical trial held three sessions within a 24-hour period consisting of 100% oxygen at 3 atmospheres followed by 2 atmospheres.[56] Cognitive damage was almost halved, although number of treatments and time window are not exactly known. Benefit may still be possible 6–12 hours after exposure.[56] Additional factors, such as hypotension, are equally important in carbon monoxide's damaging effect. Hyperbaric oxygen therapy is the preferred approach in nonintubated comatose patients and patients with significant myocardial ischemia despite initial breathing of 100% oxygen.

Cyanide

Cyanide poisoning should be entertained in any coma of undetermined cause, particularly in laboratory or industrial workers.[57] A well-recognized intentional cause is the ingestion of nail polish removers.[58] Prevalence of cyanide poisoning is low, but its effects can be reversed with antidotes.

Cyanide has an unusual mechanism of action.

By interacting with cytochrome oxidase (an essential enzyme in the mitochondrial electron transport chain), it greatly reduces production of adenosine triphosphate. Consequently, significant lactic acidosis results from a shift in anaerobic metabolism. Additionally, cyanide, like carbon monoxide, shifts the hemoglobin dissociation curve to the left and directly binds with the iron of hemoglobin, reducing the delivery of oxygen to the brain and other vital organs.[59]

Coma from cyanide poisoning is often accompanied by hypoventilation from central inhibition of the respiratory centers, severe lactic acidosis, bradycardia, hypotension, and rapidly developing pulmonary edema. A bitter almond or musty smell has been linked to cyanide poisoning, but recognition of its odor is impossible for many physicians.[59]

The supportive laboratory finding is metabolic acidosis, which may be combined with respiratory alkalosis from hyperventilation to overcome hypoxia or respiratory acidosis from hypoventilation. Plasma cyanide can be measured, but correlation with the degree of coma is poor, thus making testing impractical.

Cyanide poisoning has a good outcome when treated with the Lilly cyanide antidote kit. This contains amyl nitrite (by crushing of pellets and inhalation by patients), sodium nitrite, and sodium thiosulfate (intravenous, 50 mL of a 25% solution). The effect is based on conversion of hemoglobin into methemoglobin, which combines with cyanide but easily breaks down into free cyanide, which then combines with sodium thiosulfate and is eventually eliminated in the urine.

Reliable neurologic data on outcome are not available. Parkinsonism and dystonia have been reported, with associated lesions in the basal ganglia detected by CT scanning but with improvement in some instances.[60,61]

Toxic Alcohols

Methanol, ethylene glycol, and isopropyl alcohol are used in many commercial products, including antifreeze (ethylene glycol) and solvents (methanol). Isopropyl alcohol is best known as rubbing alcohol. The alcohols produce virtually similar laboratory effects, the most noticeable of which is a high anion gap metabolic acidosis.[62]

Methanol infrequently causes coma, but a fatal outcome is likely if it occurs. Methanol more commonly produces delirium and blurred vision.

Careful examination reveals hyperemia of the optic disk, and blindness may follow as a result of the toxic effect of formaldehyde on retinal ganglion cells. Bilateral necrosis of the putamen is highly characteristic, frequently becoming apparent on neuroimaging studies in comatose patients only after several weeks.[63] However, the brains of patients dying of methanol poisoning may be normal or variably show congestion, edema, petechiae, and necrosis of the cerebellar white matter.

Several features of methanol poisoning are of interest. First, a latent period (up to 12 hours) is typical, making it very difficult for bystanders to understand the sudden occurrence of a lapse into coma. Second, prominent restlessness with vomiting and doubling over from abdominal cramps may be followed by seizures before a lapse into unresponsiveness. Treatment is focused on correction of the acidosis with bicarbonate, but in comatose patients extracorporeal hemodialysis is imperative. Although the outcome can be very satisfactory, permanent neurologic disability may occur.[64]

Ethylene glycol is most commonly known as a major component of antifreeze and many detergents.[65] Suicide is the most common reason for ingestion, and then mortality is high. The metabolites produce toxicity, and the clinical features preceding coma are dramatic. Marked gait ataxia, nystagmus, paralysis of the extraocular muscles, and ocular bobbing are followed by generalized tonic-clonic seizures or profound myoclonus and, because of severe hypocalcemia, tetanic contractions. Lactic acidosis and an osmolar gap are characteristic laboratory features, but diagnosis is confirmed with the demonstration of calcium oxalate crystals in the urine.[65] Ethylene glycol poisoning is often treated with hemodialysis and high doses of ethanol up to intoxication of the patient (plasma ethanol target is 1000 μg/mL). In a recent study, an inhibitor of alcohol dehydrogenase (fomepizole) was successful in preventing renal damage by inhibiting toxic metabolites such as oxalate. Fomepizole is an expensive alternative to ethanol but is without toxic effects. Intravenous loading of 15 mg/kg is followed by 10 mg/kg every 12 hours for 2 days, with a further increase to 15 mg/kg every 12 hours until the plasma ethylene glycol concentration is less than 20 mg/dL.[66]

Finally, isopropyl alcohol is rather potent, producing rapidly developing coma, always with severe hypotension from cardiomyopathy. The typical acetone breath should point to this toxin. The characteristic oxalate crystals in ethylene glycol are not found in isopropyl poisoning. Management involves gastric lavage; because the onset of coma is rapid, recovery of the substance from the stomach can still be substantial.

Miscellaneous Intoxications

In this section, poisonings that are of great clinical importance and proportionally frequent or that produce striking clinical features are discussed.

Salicylates

As a result of safety packaging, the incidence of salicylate poisoning has substantially decreased, but it is still prevalent in children.

Salicylates may take some time to dissolve in the acidic stomach milieu but then are rapidly absorbed, and blood levels are maximal within 1 hour. After exposure to a massive dose, the pharmacokinetics are different, and through a complex mechanism the half-life of salicylates increases to 15–20 hours from a baseline level of 2–4 hours in therapeutic doses.[67]

Salicylates equilibrate rapidly with CSF, and the levels of salicylates in CSF appear to correlate better with outcome than do serum levels.[68] Determination of salicylate levels in CSF, however, is cumbersome. Salicylates significantly interfere with platelet function and prolong prothrombin time and may preclude lumbar puncture.

The mechanism of action of salicylates is not entirely clear. It may involve (1) uncoupling of the oxidative phosphorylation and blocking of glycolysis, producing a metabolic acidosis; (2) direct stimulation of the brain stem respiratory centers, leading to respiratory alkalosis, independent of an already compensatory response to the induced acidosis; and (3) increased metabolic demand from increased glycolysis to compensate for the uncoupling in (1), which may result in profound hypoglycemia.[67]

Salicylate poisoning should always be considered in restless, hyperventilating patients. Hyperthermia and purpura due to platelet dysfunction in the eyelids and neck may occur, simulating fulminant acute meningococcal meningitis. Pulmonary edema may occur and may become rapidly life-threatening. Severe acidemia caused by increased lipid solubility of salicylates in an acidic environment facilitates the entry of salicylates into the brain.

The laboratory features of increased anion gap, metabolic acidosis, and respiratory alkalosis are well appreciated and should lead to measurement of serum salicylate levels or, more practically, ferric chloride testing of the urine. Purple discoloration of the urine is diagnostic, and the test has good predictive value. A plasma salicylate level of 6 mg/dL usually is correlated with seizures and coma.

Management of salicylate poisoning involves gastric lavage, activated charcoal, and forced alkaline diuresis. Alkalization is performed with sodium bicarbonate or, in less severe cases, acetazolamide.

Acetaminophen

Acetaminophen is a substance in many nonprescription drugs, and as a result, poisoning is common. Usually, however, extremely large doses (plasma level >800 $\mu g/mL$) are required to directly depress consciousness; more likely, the development of acute hepatic necrosis or hepatorenal syndrome causes coma.[68]

Overdose of acetaminophen proceeds in phases, but liver damage can occur within 24 hours after ingestion. The biochemical basis for acute liver necrosis has been elucidated and is the rationale for therapy with N-acetylcysteine. In normal situations, acetaminophen is metabolized in the liver through either sulfation or glucuronidation and only a small fraction through the P-450 oxidase system, which produces an active metabolite that has the potential for liver necrosis. Overloading of the glucuronidation system by large ingestion of acetaminophen increases the formation of toxic metabolites. Decreased glutathione stores, as in patients with long-term antiepileptic drug use or chronic alcoholism, may increase the probability of liver necrosis after acetaminophen intoxication.[69,70]

Clinical features of acetaminophen overdose are nausea, vomiting, diaphoresis, and abdominal pain in the right upper quadrant but no depression in consciousness unless hepatic failure develops. Hepatic encephalopathy, with its characteristic asterixis and myoclonus, develops approximately 4 days after ingestion. Brain edema may become a feature in fulminant hepatic failure when patients lapse into stupor.

Together with N-acetylcysteine loading, management is largely supportive. N-Acetylcysteine is metabolized to cysteine, which functions as a precursor for glutathione and restores the glutathione scavenging. Acetaminophen half-lives may vary from 4–120 hours depending on the severity of liver necrosis.[71]

Liver transplantation may be needed, and its consideration leads to an ethical quagmire in patients who used acetaminophen for a suicide attempt.

Antiepileptic Drugs

Overdose with antiepileptic drugs is most often intentional, but every now and then a prescription blunder or drug interaction that reduces metabolism can be implicated. Coma from antiepileptic drug overdose is not common, and most often nonspecific signs, such as dizziness, tremor, nystagmus, and profound ataxia, occur. Paradoxically, antiepileptic drug overdose may produce seizures, and the risk, at least in carbamazepine overdose, is increased in patients with a seizure disorder.[72]

Acute overdose of phenytoin (estimated serum levels >50 μg/mL) is characterized by rapid ataxia, dysarthria with combative behavior, and hallucinations, very seldom followed by generalized tonic-clonic seizures and progression to flaccid coma. Management is supportive, with mechanical ventilation, charcoal to minimize further absorption, and benzodiazepines (e.g., lorazepam) or barbiturates (e.g., phenobarbital) in the rare event that seizures occur.

Carbamazepine is widely used in neurologic disorders. Its side effects are reminiscent of those of tricyclic antidepressants because of structural similarities, and neurologists, who are usually the primary health-care providers, should appreciate this potential threat to life.[73–75] Respiratory depression is common in carbamazepine overdose, and prospective studies have found a median duration of 18 hours. Coma occurs in 20%–50% of the reported series of carbamazepine overdose.[73,74] Fatal outcome may reach 15% of patients, most often affecting those in coma, with seizures, and with resuscitation for cardiac arrest;

ingestion often exceeds 100 tablets.[73,76] Other manifestations of carbamazepine overdose are hypothermia, hypotension, tachycardia, and a diverse range of cardiac arrhythmias from its anticholinergic properties.[73,76] Overdose with controlled-release carbamazepine may lead to peak toxicity 4 days postdigestion, and whole-bowel irrigation may be needed.[77]

Typically, management is focused on cardiac manifestations, and problems similar to those in tricyclic antidepressant overdose should be anticipated. Recovery from carbamazepine overdose can be protracted, with fluctuating levels of consciousness for many days.

Valproate toxicity is notable for its association with acute liver failure, but this devastating side effect has occurred only in young children and with concomitant use of other antiepileptic agents.[78] Hyperammonemia may be a major mechanism for stupor.[79] Massive ingestions (>200 mg/kg) produce coma with pinpoint pupils and hypertonia. As in acetaminophen poisoning, fulminant hepatic failure may produce many of the earlier manifestations of asterixis, myoclonus, and nystagmus. Valproate-associated hyperammonemia is treated with L-carnitine,[80] which could mitigate its effect (50–100 mg/kg daily).[81,82]

Assessment of Acute Metabolic or Endocrine Causes of Coma

Acute metabolic derangements may produce reduced arousal and, when unrecognized, coma. Typical examples are hypoglycemia, hyponatremia, acute uremia, and acute liver failure. Overt hemiparesis, pupil abnormalities, and gaze preference are conspicuously absent on neurologic examination, but asterixis, tremor, and myoclonus predominate when deep coma sets in. Hyperglycemic nonketotic hyperosmolar coma is a notable exception, probably because of previous strokes in these patients with severe cerebrovascular risk factors. The mechanisms of these conditions causing hypometabolism in the brain are poorly understood, but many of these disorders cause diffuse cerebral edema (see Chapter 9); seizures intervene or cardiorespiratory resuscitation results in diffuse anoxic-ischemic damage (see Chapter 10). Endocrine crises, such as rarely encountered Hashimoto's thyroiditis (thyroid coma), Addison's disease, and panhypopitu-itarism, may be responsible for coma; and hor-mones of the hypothalamic pituitary axis should be measured in unexplained coma. The laboratory values compatible with marked impairment of consciousness are shown in Table 8.8. Coma should be attributed to other causes if the bio-chemical derangement is less severe.

Neuroimaging and Laboratory Tests

CT scanning of the brain is particularly useful when the neurologic examination reveals localiz-ing symptoms. Acute lesions in the brain stem and cerebellum may not be visualized on CT. Patients with acute basilar artery occlusion or evolving cerebellar infarction often have normal CT find-ings on admission, and MRI is needed to resolve

Table 8.8. Laboratory Values Compatible with Coma° in Patients with Acute Metabolic and Endocrine Derangements

Derangement	Serum
Hyponatremia	≤110 mmol/L
Hypernatremia	≥160 mmol/L
Hypercalcemia	≥3.4 mmol/L
Hypermagnesemia	≥5 μg/L
Hypercapnia	≥70 mm Hg
Hypoglycemia	≤40 mg/dL
Hyperglycemia	≥800 mmol/L

° Sudden decline in value is obligatory.

the cause of the coma (Fig. 8.16A). It may also demonstrate sparing of the ARAS in locked-in syndrome (Fig. 8.16B).

CT findings in patients with altered conscious-ness, hemiparesis, or gaze preference are often

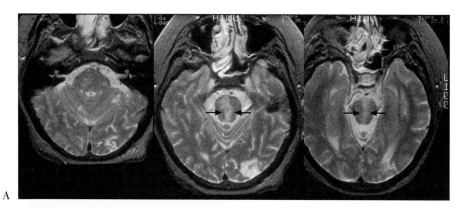

A

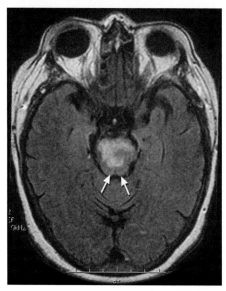

B

Figure 8.16 A: Linear hyperintensity (*arrows*) on magnetic resonance imaging (T$_2$-weighted) in a patient with basilar artery occlusion. B: Locked-in syndrome. Note sparing of tegmentum (*arrows*).

abnormal. One should particularly evaluate whether basal cisterns are present on CT scans because they may be filled in early uncal herniation (Fig. 8.17).[83] Contralateral hydrocephalus may be present, usually caused by compression at the level of the foramen of Monro.[83] The ambient cistern is usually effaced, and an enlargement of the temporal horn is seen.

CT of the brain defines the existence of a mass, its remote effect, and edema and may hint at a cause. However, because of multiplanar views, MRI is more sensitive for recording the extension of the mass and may reveal necrosis, pigments (deoxyhemoglobin, melanin), or fat, which may suggest the underlying pathologic condition. MRI clearly identifies giant aneurysms that may mimic tumors on CT.

In the emergency department, the CT scan appearance of a mass is most often characteristic enough to determine an early plan of action. Solitary lesions in nonimmunosuppressed patients most commonly represent intra-axial brain tumors or abscess. On unenhanced images, low density may represent tumor with edema. The degree of edema may reflect the degree of malignancy; rapidly growing tumors, such as glioblastoma, produce much more surrounding edema. Edema is also comparatively common in metastasis.

Most intracranial masses are hypodense, but hyperdense masses may point to a meningioma, lymphoma, or hemorrhage into a tumor. Speckled calcification inside a mass, an important CT scan finding, is present in more than 50% of patients with an oligodendroglioma but may point to an inflammatory cause, particularly parasite infestation, such as cysticercosis, and less common disorders, such as paragonimiasis and echinococcosis.[84,85] They are often seen in areas other than the cystic mass, indicating calcium deposits in necrotic brain tissue.

Intracranial mass of inflammatory origin has become a much more common presentation in the emergency department from the increase in transplantation surgery and the acquired immunodeficiency syndrome (AIDS) epidemic.

Brain abscesses, usually from toxoplasmosis, are very commonly associated with AIDS infection. Toxoplasmosis seldom appears as a single mass, although one large mass may predominate. Basal ganglia localization is typical, and hemorrhage may occur. Tuberculoma or aspergillosis should be considered as well.[52] MRI can be helpful because a dark (hypointense) T_2 signal inside the mass is often found. The most common CT and MRI findings in comatose patients are summarized in Table 8.9.

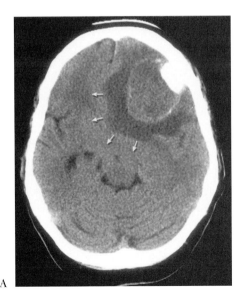
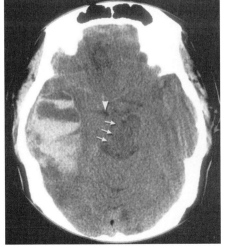

Figure 8.17 Patterns of herniation on computed tomographic scans. *A:* Meningioma with massive edema causing distortion of the diencephalon (*arrows*) and cingulate herniation (*arrows*). *B:* Large intracranial hematoma in the temporal lobe causing shift of the temporal lobe (see tip of temporal horn, *arrowhead*) and brain stem distortion (*arrows*) typical of uncal herniation.

Table 8.9. Frequent Abnormalities on Neuroimaging Studies in Coma

Findings	Suggested Disorders
Computed Tomography	
Mass lesion (brain shift, herniation)	Hematoma, hemorrhagic contusion, MCA territory infarct (see also Table 8.6)
Hemorrhage in basal cisterns	Aneurysmal SAH, cocaine abuse
Intraventricular hemorrhage	Arteriovenous malformation
Multiple hemorrhagic infarcts	Cerebral venous thrombosis
Multiple cerebral infarcts	Endocarditis, coagulopathy, CNS vasculitis
Diffuse cerebral edema	Cardiac arrest, fulminant meningitis, acute hepatic necrosis, encephalitis
Acute hydrocephalus	Aqueduct obstruction, colloid cyst, pineal region tumor
Pontine or cerebellum hemorrhage	Hypertension, arteriovenous malformation, cavernous malformation
Shear lesions in the white matter	Head injury
Magnetic Resonance Imaging	
Bilateral caudate and putaminal lesions	Carbon monoxide poisoning, methanol
Hyperdense signal along sagittal, straight, and transverse sinuses	Cerebral venous thrombosis
Lesions in corpus callosum, white matter	Severe head injury
Diffuse confluent hyperintense lesions in white matter, basal ganglia	Acute disseminated encephalomyelitis, immunosuppressive agent or chemotherapeutic agent toxicity, metabolic leukodystrophies
Pontine trident-shaped lesion	Central pontine myelinolysis
Thalamus, occipital, pontine lesions	Acute basilar artery occlusion
Temporal, frontal lobe hyperintensities	Herpes simplex encephalitis

CNS, central nervous system; MCA, middle cerebral artery; SAH, subarachnoid hemorrhage.

Normal findings on neuroimaging, with no clinical evidence of an acute cerebellar infarction or acute basilar artery occlusion, should prompt immediate examination of the CSF to search for possible CNS infection. Failure to exclude a potentially treatable CNS infection may have devastating consequences. The evaluation of CSF findings in meningitis and encephalitis is further discussed in Chapters 7, 16, and 17.

Neuroimaging is an obligatory study in patients who may be brain dead. The results of neuroimaging studies or CSF examination should be generally compatible with the diagnosis of brain death. Thus, one should expect a large mass lesion producing brain tissue shift with herniation or an intracranial hemorrhage with enlarged ventricles. Other validating CT scan findings are multiple, large, acute cerebral infarcts, massive cerebral edema, multiple hemorrhagic contusions, and cerebellar-pontine lesions compressing or destroying the brain stem.

Normal brain images in brain death can be seen immediately after cardiac arrest, carbon monoxide poisoning, asphyxia, acute encephalitis, and cyanide or other fatal poisoning.

Abdominal radiographs can be helpful in establishing whether the patient has ingested any tablets or foreign objects. Examples of radiopaque pills are chloral hydrate, trifluoperazine, amitriptyline, and enteric-coated tablets; however, many tablets may have dissolved before the patient is admitted to the emergency department.

Electrocardiography can be useful, and results are nearly always abnormal if intoxication is due to phenothiazines, quinidine, procainamide, or tricyclic antidepressants. Tricyclic antidepressant overdose characteristically produces widening of the QRS complex and QT prolongation. Widening of the QRS complex considerably increases the risk of seizures associated with tricyclic antidepressant overdose.[31] Electrocardiographic findings are also important in confirming hypothermia as a cause of coma (typically, the QRS complex widens and ST elevation occurs, also known as a "camel's hump").

When poisoning is strongly considered as a cause of coma, laboratory tests are essential before time-consuming toxicologic screening is performed. However, most poisons and illicit drugs do not cause significant laboratory derangements. In fact, if abnormalities are found in a comatose patient, they may be more representative of poor nutrition, dehydration, or a rapidly developing febrile illness.

Acid-base abnormalities, however, may point to certain toxins.[23] A high anion gap acidosis is most common. The most prevalent toxins are shown in Table 8.10. Often, a high anion gap acidosis indicates ethylene glycol or methanol ingestion. Increased lactate, particularly when venous lactate can entirely account for a decrease in serum bicarbonate, may point to previous, often undetected, seizures, shock, and early sepsis.

The anion gap is calculated from the serum electrolytes. Normally, more cations (sodium and potassium) than anions (chloride and bicarbonate) are present, causing an anion gap of 11–13 mEq/L. Generally, potassium is deleted from the equation because its extracellular contribution in the anion gap is minimal; therefore, the equation becomes as follows: anion gap = $(Na^+ - [Cl^- + HCO_3^-])$. Increases in the anion gap result from the additional presence of an anion. Most of the time, it is lactate that increases in serum and creates an anion gap, often originating from poor tissue perfusion.

Salicylates usually produce a combined acid-base abnormality, and respiratory acidosis is often present.[67] The partial pressure of CO_2 ($PaCO_2$) decrease in metabolic acidosis can be calculated ($PaCO_2 = [1.5 \times (HCO_3)] + 8 \pm 2$), and a lower $PaCO_2$ should point to additional respiratory alkalosis.

Osmol gap is a useful test to determine accumulation of osmotically active solutes. The normal osmol gap is calculated with the equation $2 \times Na + (glucose/18) + (blood\ urea\ nitrogen/2.8)$. This calculated osmolality is less than the measured osmolarity (the so-called osmol gap) and should be less than 10 mOsm/L. Alcohols of any kind increase the osmol gap, and blood levels can be estimated by multiplying the osmol gap with the molecular weight of the alcohol (46 for ethanol) and dividing the result by a factor of 10.

Urine testing for salicylates is important and can be done with a 10% ferric chloride solution, which turns urine purple if salicylates are present. Urine should be tested for ketones. Ketones in combination with a marked anion gap immediately suggest salicylate poisoning, but this combination can also be observed in alcohol- or diabetes-induced ketoacidosis. The absence of ketones in a patient with anion gap metabolic acidosis suggests ingestion of methanol or ethylene glycol. Urinalysis is also important, specifically in looking for calcium oxalate crystals associated with ethylene glycol (antifreeze) ingestion. The use of Wood's lamp (if available) may be important because fluorescein is added to many antifreeze products.

Many hospitals have laboratories that can provide drug screens.[86,87] Their value often lies in the demonstration of the toxin rather than quantification. The blood levels of many sedatives and alcohol correlate poorly with depth of coma, duration of mechanical ventilation, and time in the intensive care unit. This lack of correlation applies particularly to patients who attempt suicide with a medication they have taken long enough to cause tolerance.

Many smaller hospitals use thin-layer chromatography, which is less reliable, operator-dependent, and unable to quantitate the toxin.[86] Most academic centers can measure with gas

Table 8.10. Blood Gas Abnormalities Due to Toxins

Metabolic Acidosis (Anion Gap)	Respiratory Acidosis
Methanol	Barbiturates
Ethanol	Benzodiazepines
Paraldehyde	Botulism toxin
Isoniazid	Opioids
Salicylates (other combined)	Strychnine
	Tetrodotoxin

Metabolic Alkalosis	Respiratory Alkalosis
Diuretics	Salicylates
Hyperglycemic nonketotic coma	Amphetamines
Lithium	Anticholinergics
	Cocaine
	Cyanide
	Paraldehyde
	Theophylline
	Carbon monoxide

chromatography and mass spectrometry. This laboratory investigative tool is powerful and quantitates the toxin. The spectrum of drugs measured in serum is depicted in Appendix 8.1. Physicians assessing patients with poisoning and drug abuse should be well informed about the hospital laboratory practices available. Laboratory confirmation of the clinical diagnosis is often very desirable and may also serve a medicolegal purpose. Delay in the performance of these tests remains a major limitation, and often the information becomes available too late to be useful in guiding treatment in daily practice.

Blood tests that should be performed include a full hematologic screen and differential cell count, blood glucose, serum osmolality, liver function panel, electrolytes, and renal function tests (Table 8.11). Arterial blood gas measurements further assist in categorizing the major classes of acid-base imbalance, if present.

Initial Management of Vital Signs in Coma

One of the fundamental responsibilities of the physician faced with the care of a comatose patient is to maintain or correct the vital signs, such as oxygenation, gas exchange, blood pressure, pulse rate, cardiac rhythm, and temperature.

Table 8.11. Laboratory Tests in the Evaluation of Coma

Hematocrit, white blood cell count
Electrolytes (Na, K, Cl, CO_2, Ca, PO_4)
Glucose
Urea, creatinine
Aspartate transaminase (AST) and γ-glutamyltransferase (GGT)
Osmolality
Arterial blood gases (pH, PCO_2, PO_2, HCO_3, HbCO) (optional)
Platelets, smear, fibrinogen degeneration products, activated partial thromboplastin time, prothrombin time (optional)
Plasma thyrotropin (optional)
Blood and cerebrospinal fluid cultures (optional)
Toxic screen in blood and urine (optional)
Cerebrospinal fluid (protein, cells, glucose, India ink stain, and cryptococcal antigen, viral titers) (optional)

PO_2/PCO_2, partial pressure of O_2/CO_2; HbCO, carbon monoxide hemoglobin.

Airway Assessment and Gas Exchange

The basic principles of airway management apply and have been discussed in Chapter 1. The need for intubation remains difficult to judge in comatose patients, but tachypnea, desaturation on pulse oximetry (<95%), or emerging pulmonary abnormalities on examination or chest X-ray are clear indications. Seizures do not warrant intubation, but status epilepticus does if second-line drugs are contemplated. Vomiting could be a reason for intubation to protect the airway, certainly if the patient has poor reflexive cough. In patients with minor intoxications that seem to be resolving, noninvasive ventilation with rate control may be useful to bridge the period of elimination of the drug. Early intubation in severe traumatic head injury is probably justified and allows better control of the airway and oxygenation. Early tracheostomy may be needed when the face and neck are severely injured, increasing the risk of loss of airway (in facial fractures of LeFort type, posterior displacement may seriously obstruct the airway).[88]

Assessment of Circulation and Blood Pressure

Dehydration resulting in reduced intravascular volume is often a cause of hypotension. Hypotension should be corrected by placing the patient in the Trendelenburg position and infusing isotonic saline or blood when indicated in traumatized patients. If blood pressure is not reversed with these measures, hypotension may indicate that the patient has (1) toxic effects from ingestion of a drug that produces vasodilation or myocardial depression, (2) major abdominal trauma, or (3) a life-threatening illness, such as myocardial infarction, pulmonary embolus, or sepsis. It is a misconception to attribute hypotension to catastrophic damage to the brain, which occurs only in patients who are brain dead or who have severe spinal cord injury. Vasoparalysis in brain death results in marked hypotension and may be noted acutely in a rapidly progressing catastrophe. Hypertension, however, is very common in a patient with an acute structural lesion in the CNS. Usually, hypertension is caused by a sympathoadrenal discharge or is part of the Cushing response, particularly when the brain stem is distorted. Acute severe hypertension (MAP >140 mm Hg) may also have its origin in poisoning caused by such agents as amphetamines, cocaine, phencyclidine, and cyclic antidepressants. Often, hypertension in these types of intoxication is associated with significant tachycardia.

The management of acute hypertension in comatose patients is complex. At least theoretically, untreated hypertension may exacerbate cerebral edema in injured areas from increased cerebral blood flow. Too rapid correction of blood pressure may introduce ischemic areas surrounding acute mass lesions from reduction of cerebral perfusion pressure. In patients with longstanding hypertension, the autoregulation curve has shifted to the right, and this further increases the risk of decreased cerebral blood flow, with a decrease in blood pressure at this juncture. One should probably avoid extremes, and persistent surges of blood pressure (MAP >120 mm Hg) can be treated with a short-acting α- or β-adrenergic blocking drug, such as labetalol (40 mg at 10-minute intervals).

Miscellaneous Care

Patients with hypothermia (defined as core temperature <34°C) should be gradually warmed. Physicians should be aware that noxious stimuli applied to patients with moderate hypothermia to assess responsiveness can potentially trigger ventricular fibrillation. Virtually all brain stem reflexes are lost when the core temperature reaches 27°C, and they can entirely return after rewarming.

Patients with a core temperature of 32°C–35°C need to be warmed with blankets, those with a core temperature of 30°C–32°C are warmed with IV infusions, and those with a core temperature <30°C may need peritoneal lavage with heated dialysate.

In patients comatose after cardiac resuscitation, induced hypothermia could be beneficial and subnormal temperatures should be tolerated.[89] The effect of superficial cooling in patients with devastating anoxic-ischemic injury to the brain appears promising, but much larger clinical trials are needed to prove its effect.[89] It remains unclear

what its effect could be in traumatic brain injury. Some more recent studies continue to suggest 35°–35.5°C reduces intracranial pressure while maintaining cerebral perfusion pressure[90] despite lack of effect in the National Brain Injury Hypothermic Study (see Chapter 19).

All patients in coma for whom the diagnosis is very unclear should receive concentrated dextrose (50% dextrose, 50 mL, 25 g IV). The well-known adrenergic symptoms from the counterregulating hormone epinephrine, such as sweating, tremor, and tachycardia, may not be present when hypoglycemia has developed more or less gradually. However, its use in patients in whom the proximate cause of coma is known is ill-advised.

Wernicke's encephalopathy is a rare cause of coma.[91] However, if chronic alcohol abuse or malnourishment is suspected during the physical examination, a "routine" glucose infusion may precipitate acute Wernicke's encephalopathy. To prevent this, 100 mg of thiamine should be administered IV (slowly over 5 minutes) or intramuscularly. Indiscriminate use of thiamine in comatose patients is potentially dangerous because of acute anaphylactic reactions and acute pulmonary edema.

Cardiac arrhythmias often define the severity of the intoxication in patients with an overdose of a cyclic antidepressant drug. Sodium bicarbonate, 1–2 mEq/kg IV, is advised when the QRS interval narrows. In patients with sympathomimetic agent intoxication resulting in tachycardia, esmolol can be used: 500 μg/kg over 1 minute, followed by an infusion of 50 μg/kg per minute for 4 minutes; maximum maintenance dose is 200 μg/kg per minute. If tachycardia is caused by an anticholinergic overdose, physostigmine, 0.01–0.03 mg/kg IV, is used.[92] Patients with ventricular fibrillation or ventricular tachycardia associated with amphetamines or overdose should be treated with lidocaine, 1–3 mg/kg IV up to 300 mg in a 1-hour period.

Management in Specific Causes of Coma

Supratentorial Mass Lesions

Patients with a mass lesion that causes shift of brain structures need immediate management of increased intracranial pressure. If available, an intracranial pressure monitoring device should be inserted to measure increases in intracranial pressure and possible development of plateau waves that indicate imminent decompensation of brain compliance. Transfer to a neurologic or neurosurgical intensive care unit is imperative.

The most successful method of decreasing intracranial pressure is the brief use of hyperventilation (aiming at a partial pressure of arterial CO_2 [$PaCO_2$] of 30 mm Hg) and equally effective use of osmotic diuretics, such as mannitol (aiming at an increase in plasma osmolality of 310 mOsm/L). Hyperventilation results in profound vasoconstriction from hypocapnia and reduces cerebral blood flow, thus contributing to reduction of the intracranial volume. One may expect cerebral blood flow to decrease 40% in 30 minutes if the $PaCO_2$ is reduced by 15–20 mm Hg.[93] However, the physiologic effects of hyperventilation are less significant after several hours because efficient buffering systems rapidly correct changes in CSF pH. Its effect is short, probably hours.[94]

Hyperventilation can be easily instituted by changing the respiratory rate on the mechanical ventilator. The respiratory rate should be increased to approximately 20 breaths/minute while a normal tidal volume is maintained. Increasing minute ventilation by changing both components is ill-advised because it may lead to high airway pressures and increases the risk of barotrauma.

In addition, hyperosmolar agents, preferably mannitol, should be administered, starting with a 20% solution at a dose of 1 g/kg.[95] The effect on intracranial pressure is rapid and may last for at least 4 hours. Mannitol essentially decreases brain volume by extracting water from brain tissue.[96] This influx to the intravascular compartment is generated by an osmotic gradient. Mannitol, therefore, expands the blood volume just before its diuretic action, hence the name "osmotic diuretic." First, a bolus of 1 g/kg of body weight is given. If no effect is seen after 15 minutes, a double dose is administered. The effect of mannitol is at least twofold. First, infusion of mannitol produces an osmotic gradient between the intravascular component and the brain. Second, a more complex mechanism of mannitol is a possible rheologic effect.[97] Mannitol reduces hematocrit and blood viscosity, thereby increasing cerebral blood flow. Vasoconstriction becomes a compensatory reflex and reduces cerebral blood volume. This

mechanism rather than diuresis, which usually is seen at a later stage, may be the prime means by which mannitol causes a rapid response. Mannitol may cause significant changes in electrolytes, particularly increase in serum potassium and acute renal failure from altered glomerular hemodynamics. Mannitol, when extravasated, could produce a compartmental syndrome.[98]

Failure of the patient to improve with hyperventilation and mannitol indicates that surgical evacuation of the mass should be considered. When swelling of one hemisphere is prominent, decompressive craniotomy with duraplasty can be considered. Preliminary studies in patients with encephalitis and a large hemispheric infarction have shown promise.

Corticosteroids should be considered in patients who have edema surrounding a cerebral metastatic lesion or primary brain tumor. There is no proof that corticosteroids improve outcome in patients with other mass lesions, such as intracranial hematoma, closed head injury, infarction, and cerebral abscess.[99,100] Corticosteroid therapy is usually initiated with a single 100-mg dose of dexamethasone given IV, and this is followed by a 16-mg daily dose.

The management of acute supratentorial mass lesions is summarized in Table 8.12.

Subtentorial Lesions

Acute posterior fossa lesions that evolve into coma from a compressive brain stem lesion need immediate neurosurgical evacuation. Only occasionally does decreased level of consciousness result from an evolving hydrocephalus, and then ventriculostomy improves the degree of responsiveness. A cerebellar hematoma or cerebellar infarct is a neurosurgical emergency, and craniotomy is necessary to remove the hematoma or necrotic tissue.

An intrinsic lesion of the brain stem is usually best initially treated medically with endotracheal intubation and mechanical ventilation. Patients with acute basilar artery occlusion should be placed in a flat body position to augment blood pressure, and intra-arterial thrombolysis, if available, should be considered. We have been able to reverse a virtually locked-in syndrome in acute basilar occlusion by using intra-arterial thrombolysis with urokinase but not when pontomesen-

Table 8.12. Management of Acute
Supratentorial Mass with Brain Shift

Stabilizing measures
  Protect airway: intubate
  Correct hypoxemia with O_2 nasal catheter, 3–4 L/min,
    or face mask
  Elevate head to 30 degrees
  Treat extreme agitation with lorazepam, 2 mg
    intravenously, or propofol, 0.3 mg/kg/hr
  Correct coagulopathy with fresh-frozen plasma, vitamin K
    (if applicable)
Specific medical measures
  Hyperventilation: increase respiratory rate to 20
    breaths/minute, aim at $PaCO_2$ of 25–30 mm Hg
  Mannitol 20%, 1 g/kg; if no effect, 2 g/kg; aim at plasma
    osmolality of 310 mOsm/L
  Dexamethasone, 100 mg intravenously (in tumors only)
Specific surgical measures
  Evacuation of hematoma
  Placement of drain in abscess
  Decompressive craniotomy in brain swelling of one
    hemisphere

PCO_2, partial pressure of CO_2.

cephalic reflexes have been lost. Criteria for intra-arterial thrombolysis in the posterior circulation are further discussed in Chapter 15. Specific management in subtentorial lesions is summarized in Table 8.13.

Infectious Disorders

Comatose patients with infectious disease have fever and meningeal irritation at presentation. If focal neurologic signs are present, the three steps

Table 8.13. Management of Acute
Subtentorial Mass or Brain Stem Lesion

Stabilizing measures
  Intubation and mechanical ventilation
  Correct hypoxemia with 3 L of O_2/min
  Flat body position (in acute basilar artery occlusion)
Specific medical measures
  Intra-arterial urokinase (in basilar artery occlusion)
  Mannitol 20%, 1 g/kg (in acute cerebellar mass)
  Hyperventilation to PCO_2 of 25–50 mm Hg (in acute
    cerebellar mass)
Specific surgical measures
  Ventriculostomy
  Suboccipital craniotomy

PCO_2, partial pressure of CO_2.

to take are (1) an immediate IV infusion with antibiotics and dexamethasone (bacterial meningitis), (2) a CT scan to exclude an abscess, and (3) a lumbar puncture for final culture of the offending organism.

Patients with acute viral encephalitis may be in a coma at presentation without any other localizing neurologic signs. The history obtained from family members may reveal fluctuating aphasia, seizures, or significant confusion before the lapse into unresponsiveness. It is important to immediately start an infusion of acyclovir. In herpes simplex encephalitis, outcome is largely determined by early treatment; however, the prospects for full recovery remain small in patients in stupor or coma.

With the emergence of immunosuppression (particularly in the human immunodeficiency virus population), toxoplasma encephalitis should be considered. Initial treatment remains empiric and includes pyrimethamine and sulfadiazine, particularly in patients with multiple abscesses. In endemic areas, patients in coma may have cysticercosis associated with *Taenia solium* infestation, and immediate treatment with praziquantel is required. It is important to start these treatments early, after consulting an infectious disease specialist. The initial management in these acute inflammatory conditions of the CNS is summarized in Table 8.14.

Acute Metabolic Derangements and Poisoning

No harm is done if patients with a high likelihood of hypoglycemia are given 50 mL of a 50% glucose solution. Immediate awakening during infusion is highly indicative of severe hypoglycemia.

Table 8.14. Empirical Antibiotic and Antiviral Therapy in Patients in Coma Associated with Inflammatory Conditions

Antibacterial	Cefotaxime 2 g every 6 hours
	Vancomycin 2 g every 12 hours
Antiviral	Acyclovir 10 mg/kg every 8 hours
Antiparasitic	Pyrimethamine 75 mg p.o.
	Sulfadiazine 2–8 g p.o. divided
	every 6 hours
	Praziquantel 75 mg/kg daily

See also Chapters 16 and 17.

Failure to awaken after hypoglycemia, however, may indicate that hypoglycemia has been lengthy and has caused significant brain damage leading to prolonged or no recovery.

Management of severe hyponatremia involves hypertonic saline and furosemide (3% hypertonic saline, 0.5 mL/kg hourly) with frequent serum sodium surveillance. Overcorrection ($\geq$140 μg/L) and rapid correction (within 12 hours) have been linked to the development of central pontine myelinolysis.

Hypercalcemia is adequately corrected by saline rehydration infusion (3–4 L) followed by the parenteral bisphosphonate pamidronate (infused at 60 mg over 24 hours).

The use of a "coma cocktail" in assessing and managing coma of undetermined cause must be questioned.[101] Usually, this cocktail consists of a combination of hypertonic dextrose, thiamine hydrochloride, naloxone hydrochloride, and, recently, flumazenil.[102] Its use must be discouraged simply because of the possible side effects of naloxone and flumazenil. Naloxone has great efficacy but also potentially serious side effects, such as aspiration from rapid arousal and development of a florid withdrawal syndrome[103] characterized by agitation, diaphoresis, hypertension, dysrhythmias, and pulmonary edema.[103,104] In addition, after 30 minutes, the patient may again lapse into coma, which if unwitnessed may cause significant respiratory depression and respiratory arrest. A more prudent approach is to prophylactically intubate the patient and to gradually reverse the overdose of opiates by use of naloxone, 0.4–2 mg every 3 minutes by incremental doubling.[105] At the first sign of relapse, 0.4–4 mg of naloxone can be given IV[106] or an infusion of 0.8 mg/kg hourly started. Failure to reverse coma from alleged opiate overdose has many causes, and they are summarized in Table 8.15.

Flumazenil reverses the effect of any benzodiazepine but has the same major disadvantages as naloxone: rapid arousal and risk of life-threatening aspiration pneumonitis. In addition, when high doses of flumazenil are administered, seizures may occur.[106,107] Therefore, flumazenil is contraindicated in patients with a seizure disorder and in patients in whom concomitant tricyclic antidepressant intoxication is suspected.[13,106] When flumazenil is administered, cardiac arrhythmias may occur, and status epilepticus has been re-

Table 8.15. Differential Diagnosis in Failure to Reverse Coma from Alleged Opiate Overdose

Head injury, traumatic intracerebral hematoma
Hypoglycemia
Anoxic-ischemic encephalopathy
Mixed overdose with drug in another category (e.g., cocaine, ethanol)
Central nervous system infection, systemic infection, sepsis
Seizures, nonconvulsive status epilepticus (rare)

Source: Goldfrank et al.[36]

ported in patients who had an overdose of tricyclic antidepressants and received treatment with flumazenil.[106] The recommended dose of flumazenil, by slow IV administration, is 0.2 mg/minute up to a total dose of 1 mg.[35] We seldom use flumazenil to reverse coma. Benzodiazepine overdose, in general, is not life-threatening and can be managed by supportive care only.

Inducing emesis in a patient who is stuporous from poisoning may be a mistake because of the significant danger of aspiration. Gastric lavage, which is possible if a comatose patient is protected by endotracheal intubation, should be done if the suspicion of a massive overdose is great. Also, activated charcoal (60–100 g) can be delivered through the gastric tube. Placement of the tube in the stomach before administration of charcoal should be confirmed by radiography because charcoal deposition in the lung is often fatal. The technique of gastric lavage includes placement of the patient in the left lateral decubitus position after intubation of the trachea with a cuffed endotracheal tube. This position greatly facilitates drainage. The largest possible gastric tube should be inserted through the nose or mouth into the stomach and checked often with air insufflation while the physician listens over the stomach. The stomach aspirate should be investigated for possible toxins, and activated charcoal should be administered before lavage is started. Charcoal absorbs material that cannot be removed by active suctioning and that may enter the intestine. Lukewarm tap water or saline in 200 mL aliquots up to a total of 2 L is infused and aspirated until no pills or toxic material is observed.

Elimination of the toxin can also be enhanced by hemodialysis and hemoperfusion, and many drugs and toxins can be cleared (the most common are acetaminophen, amitriptyline, lithium, and salicylates).

Coma of Unknown Origin

In some patients it may seem very difficult to pinpoint the exact grounds of coma. The management of coma of undetermined cause is full intensive care support and observation over time while a more detailed history and laboratory test results are awaited. When no cause of decreased arousal or coma is found and results of laboratory tests including CT scan or MRI and CSF examination are negative, unidentified toxin exposure, plant or berry ingestion or other type (such as tetrodotoxin from puffer fish),[108] should be considered. However, toxin exposure may have resulted in significant hypoxemic-ischemic damage, which may cause persistent coma.[109] Electroencephalography may be helpful to exclude nonconvulsive status epilepticus or prolonged postictal state despite no documentation of a seizure.

Basilar artery migraine may produce drowsiness, confusion, and prolonged amnesia and may progress to coma.[110] Typically, a strong family history of common migraine exists. Of the patients originally reported by Bickerstaff,[110] about 80% had a positive family history. Basilar artery migraine is more prevalent in children but may persist through adulthood, often converting later into common migraine. The clinical presentation is impressive. Visual hallucinations, bilateral zig-zag forms or photopsia, and even sudden blindness or grayouts may occur as a result of hypoperfusion of the occipital lobes. Most of the time, patients present with vertigo, ataxia, diplopia, dysarthria, and tinnitus from ischemia to the brain stem. Bilateral throbbing headache may last for hours, commonly with vomiting, after resolution of the neurologic deficits. Coma remains uncommon in basilar migraine. More commonly, patients with migraine become drowsy or stuporous from overmedication, particularly with narcotics. A retrospective review in a large series of patients noted stupor or coma in 24% of 49 patients and more often "somnolence."[110] Bickerstaff's original descriptions[110] highlight gradual onset of a dream-like state. Seizures may occur and can be documented on electroencephalograms at the time of a full-blown attack. The precise nature of the disorder is unresolved. Unfortunately, brain stem infarcts may occur, with a fatal outcome.[111]

A recently reported disorder characterized by spells of sudden coma has been linked to increased endogenous production of benzodiazepines (endozepine stupor, idiopathic recurrent stupor). Patients may awaken immediately after administration of flumazenil. The prevalence of this disorder is unknown.[112]

Psychogenic unresponsiveness should always be considered after all laboratory test results are negative. Unfortunately, many of these patients have already received a battery of laboratory tests even though the discrepancies with detailed clinical examination are very obvious. Most often, psychogenic unresponsiveness lasts for only 1 or 2 days, with characteristic sudden unexpected "awakening" and often complete amnesia for the episode and for events during many months preceding hospital admission.

Malignant neuroleptic syndrome and catatonia may produce decreased responsiveness and are fatal if untreated. Profound rigidity and continuous autonomic storm with impressive tachycardia, hypertension, and profuse sweating may result in cardiac arrest (from subendocardial and myocardial hemorrhages) or renal failure (due to severe acidosis from massive rhabdomyolysis). Therapy is discussed in Chapter 5.

Hereditary metabolic disorders may be manifested by impaired consciousness during adolescence. These disorders are exceptionally uncommon but should be excluded when the cause of coma is unknown. These disorders are acute porphyria (psychosis rather than coma and seizures in some), mitochondrial encephalopathies, and necrotizing encephalopathy of Leigh. Acute porphyria often has resulted in earlier visits to the emergency department because of "abdominal colic" or a chronic pain syndrome. It can be diagnosed by demonstrating increased δ-aminolevulinic acid and porphobilinogen in the urine.

It is highly unusual when a patient presents comatose with markedly elevated venous ammonia, respiratory alkalosis, and normal anion gap. In the vast majority of cases, these patients can be eventually diagnosed with a heterozygotic form of ornithine transcarbamylase deficiency. (This X-linked disorder in homozygotes is commonly fatal.) Twenty percent of female carriers may become symptomatic. Known triggers are delivery, gastrointestinal bleed, infection, surgical procedure, and antiepileptic medication (e.g., valproate). In these instances, the liver is overwhelmed by ex-

Box 8.4. Hyperammonemic Coma

Deficiencies of urea cycle enzymes increase serum ammonia. The most common, albeit rare in adults, is X-linked ornithine transcarbamylase (OTC) deficiency, the second enzyme in the urea cycle located in the liver mitochondria matrix (Fig. 8.18). Multiple pathologic mutations of the *OTC* gene are known. Prior early symptoms could have been present (seizures, migraine, vomiting episodes). Ironically, antiepileptic agents for seizures are known triggers (e.g., valproate). Presentation may be typi-

cal in the teenage years, but patients 50–60 years old have been reported.

The diagnosis is confirmed by increased urine levels of orotic acid, particularly after loading with allopurinol treatment in hemodialysis, IV sodium benzoate, and occasionally liver transplantation. An inefficient carnitine reserve may be present in valproate-associated hepatotoxicity, and L-carnitine should be supplied.

cess nitrogen load. Hyperammonemia may lead to cytotoxic brain edema and death if untreated (Box 8.4).[79,113–115]

The mitochondrial encephalopathies include MELAS syndrome (mitochondrial encephalopathy, lactic acidosis, and stroke-like episodes), Kearns-Sayre syndrome, and Leigh's disease. Lactic acidosis with increased lactate and pyruvate as well as typical MRI abnormalities (MELAS, cortical T_2-weighted hyperintensities in both cerebral hemispheres, with a predilection for the posterior regions and the cerebellum; Leigh, bilateral putaminal lesions) should suggest

the diagnosis. Evaluation is very complex and outside the scope of this book. Most recently, confusion and coma have been described as an unusual presentation of cerebral autosomal dominant arteriopathy with subcortical infarct and leukoencephalopathy (CADASIL). Prior migraine and family history of stroke or dementia in combination with profound confluent white matter lesions could suggest the diagnosis. Most reported cases have resolved slowly.[116,117] All of these causes for coma are exceptional and rarely observed. In many elderly patients, transient stupor or coma remains unexplained.

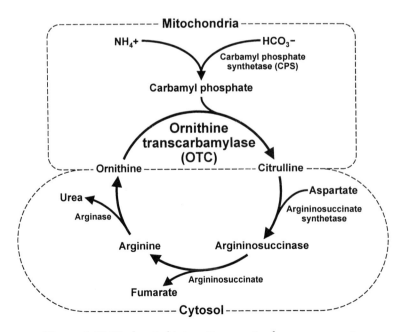

Figure 8.18 Biochemical interactions causing hyperammonemia.

REFERENCES

1. Oberndorfer S, Grisold W, Hinterholzer G, et al.: Coma with focal neurological signs caused by *Datura stramonium* intoxication in a young man. *J Neurol Neurosurg Psychiatry* 73:458, 2002.

2. Dunn C, Held JL, Spitz J, et al.: Coma blisters: report and review. *Cutis* 45:423, 1990.

3. Maguiness S, Guenther L, Shum D: Coma blisters, peripheral neuropathy, and amitriptyline overdose: a brief report. *J Cutan Med Surg* 6:438, 2002.

4. Tsokos M, Sperhake JP: Coma blisters in a case of fatal theophylline intoxication. *Am J Forensic Med Pathol* 23:292, 2002.

5. Bauby J-D: *The Diving Bell and the Butterfly*, Translated from French by J Leggatt (trans). New York: Alfred A Knopf, 1997.

6. Teasdale G, Jennett B: Assessment of coma and impaired consciousness. A practical scale. *Lancet* 2:81, 1974.

7. Teasdale G, Knill-Jones R, van der Sande J: Observer variability in assessing impaired consciousness and coma. *J Neurol Neurosurg Psychiatry* 41:603, 1978.

8. Jennett B: The history of the Glasgow Coma Scale: an interview with professor Bryan Jennett. Interview by Carole Rush. *Int J Trauma Nurs* 3:114, 1997.

9. Wijdicks EFM: Temporomandibular joint compression in coma. *Neurology* 46:1774, 1996.

10. Wijdicks EFM, Kokmen E, O'Brien PC: Measurement of impaired consciousness in the neurological intensive care unit: a new test. *J Neurol Neurosurg Psychiatry* 64:117, 1998.

11. Thomas KE, Hasbun R, Jekel J, Quagliarello VJ. The diagnostic accuracy of Kernig's sign, Brudzinski's sign, and nuchal rigidity in adults with suspected meningitis. *Clin Infect Dis* 35:46, 2002.

12. Wijdicks EFM: Determining brain death in adults. *Neurology* 45:1003, 1995.

13. Chern TL, Hu SC, Lee CH, et al.: Diagnostic and therapeutic utility of flumazenil in comatose patients with drug overdose. *Am J Emerg Med* 11:122, 1993.

14. Wijdicks EFM: The diagnosis of brain death. *N Engl J Med* 344:1215, 2001.

15. Plum F, Posner JB: *The Diagnosis of Stupor or Coma*, 3rd ed. Philadelphia: FA Davis, 1982.

16. Wijdicks EFM: Intracranial hemorrhage. In GB Young, AH Ropper, CF Bolton (eds), *Coma and Impaired Consciousness: A Clinical Perspective*. New York: McGraw-Hill, 1998, p. 131.

17. Kwon SU, Lee SH, Kim JS: Sudden coma from acute bilateral internal carotid artery territory infarction. *Neurology* 58:1846, 2002.

18. Ropper AH: A preliminary MRI study of the geometry of brain displacement and level of consciousness with acute intracranial masses. *Neurology* 39:622, 1989.

19. Ropper AH, Gress D: Computerized tomography and clinical features of large cerebral hemorrhages. *Cerebrovasc Dis* 1:38, 1991.

20. Wijdicks EFM, Miller GM: MR imaging of progressive downward herniation of the diencephalon. *Neurology* 48:1456, 1997.

21. Wijdicks EFM, Miller GM: Transient locked-in syndrome after uncal herniation. *Neurology* 52:1296, 1999.

22. Wijdicks EFM, Maus TP, Piepgras DG: Cerebellar swelling and massive brain stem distortion: spontaneous resolution documented by MRI. *J Neurol Neurosurg Psychiatry* 65:400, 1998.

23. Nice A, Leikin JB, Maturen A, et al.: Toxidrome recognition to improve efficiency of emergency urine drug screens. *Ann Emerg Med* 17:676, 1988.

24. Charness ME, Simon RP, Greenberg DA: Ethanol and the nervous system. *N Engl J Med* 321:442, 1989.

25. Klatsky AL, Friedman GD, Siegelaub AB: Alcohol and mortality. A ten-year Kaiser-Permanente experience. *Ann Intern Med* 95:139, 1981.

26. Palmer BF: Effectiveness of hemodialysis in the extracorporeal therapy of phenobarbital overdose. *Am J Kidney Dis* 36:640, 2000.

27. Reed CE, Driggs MF, Foote CC: Acute barbiturate intoxication: a study of 300 cases based on a physiologic system of classification of the severity of the intoxication. *Ann Intern Med* 37:290, 1952.

28. Henderson A, Wright M, Pond SM: Experience with 732 acute overdose patients admitted to an intensive care unit over six years. *Med J Aust* 158:28, 1993.

29. White A: Overdose of tricyclic antidepressants associated with absent brain-stem reflexes. *CMAJ* 139:133, 1988.

30. Hultén BA, Heath A: Clinical aspects of tricyclic antidepressant poisoning. *Acta Med Scand* 213:275, 1983.

31. Boehnert MT, Lovejoy FH Jr: Value of the QRS duration versus the serum drug level in predicting seizures and ventricular arrhythmias after an acute overdose of tricyclic antidepressants. *N Engl J Med* 313:474, 1985.

32. Sansone ME, Ziegler DK: Lithium toxicity: a review of neurologic complications. *Clin Neuropharmacol* 8:242, 1985.

33. Greenblatt DJ, Allen MD, Noel BJ, et al. Acute overdosage with benzodiazepine derivatives. *Clin Pharmacol Ther* 21:497, 1977.

34. Greenblatt DJ, Shader RI, Abernethy DR: Drug therapy. Current status of benzodiazepines. *N Engl J Med* 309:354, 1983.

35. Weinbroum A, Rudick V, Sorkine P, et al.: Use of flumazenil in the treatment of drug overdose: a double-blind and open clinical study in 110 patients. *Crit Care Med* 24:199, 1996.

36. Goldfrank LR, Flomenbaum NE, Lewin NA, et al.: *Goldfrank's Toxicologic Emergencies*, 7th ed. New York: McGraw-Hill Professional, 2002.

37. Brust JCM: *Neurological Aspects of Substance Abuse*. Boston: Butterworth-Heinemann, 1993.

38. McCarron MM: Phencyclidine intoxication. *NIDA Res Monogr* 64:209, 1986.

39. Aniline O, Pitts FN Jr: Phencyclidine (PCP): a review and perspectives. *Crit Rev Toxicol* 10:145, 1982.

40. Gawin FH, Ellinwood EH Jr: Cocaine and other stimu-

lants. Actions, abuse, and treatment. *N Engl J Med* 318:1173, 1988.

41. Dhuna A, Pascual-Leone A, Langendorf F, et al. Epileptogenic properties of cocaine in humans. *Neurotoxicology* 12:621, 1991.

42. Choy-Kwong M, Lipton RB: Seizures in hospitalized cocaine users. *Neurology* 39:425, 1989.

43. Lowenstein DH, Massa SM, Rowbotham MC, et al.: Acute neurologic and psychiatric complications associated with cocaine abuse. *Am J Med* 83:841, 1987.

44. Howington JU, Kutz SC, Wilding GE, Awasthi D. Cocaine use as a predictor of outcome in aneurysmal subarachnoid hemorrhage. *J Neurosurg* 99:271, 2003.

45. Levine SR, Brust JC, Futrell N, et al.: Cerebrovascular complications of the use of the "crack" form of alkaloidal cocaine. *N Engl J Med* 323:699, 1990.

46. Wojak JC, Flamm ES: Intracranial hemorrhage and cocaine use. *Stroke* 18:712, 1987.

47. Storen EC, Wijdicks EFM, Crum B, et al.: Moyamoya-like vasculopathy from cocaine dependency. *AJNR Am J Neuroradiol* 21:1008, 2000.

48. Pasternak GW: Pharmacological mechanisms of opioid analgesics. *Clin Neuropharmacol* 16:1, 1993.

49. Ginsberg MD: Carbon monoxide intoxication: clinical features, neuropathology and mechanisms of injury. *J Toxicol Clin Toxicol* 23:281, 1985.

50. Krantz T, Thisted B, Strom J, et al.: Acute carbon monoxide poisoning. *Acta Anaesthesiol Scand* 32:278, 1988.

51. Miura T, Mitomo M, Kawai R, et al.: CT of the brain in acute carbon monoxide intoxication: characteristic features and prognosis. *AJNR Am J Neuroradiol* 6:739, 1985.

52. Carrazana EJ, Rossitch E Jr, Morris J: Isolated central nervous system aspergillosis in the acquired immunodeficiency syndrome. *Clin Neurol Neurosurg* 93:227, 1991.

53. Sawada Y, Takahashi M, Ohashi N, et al.: Computerized tomography as an indication of long-term outcome after acute carbon monoxide poisoning. *Lancet* 1:783, 1980.

54. Horowitz AL, Kaplan R, Sarpel G: Carbon monoxide toxicity: MR imaging in the brain. *Radiology* 162:787, 1987.

55. Ziser A, Shupak A, Halpern P, et al.: Delayed hyperbaric oxygen treatment for acute carbon monoxide poisoning. *BMJ* 289:960, 1984.

56. Weaver LK, Hopkins RO, Chan KJ, et al.: Hyperbaric oxygen for acute carbon monoxide poisoning. *N Engl J Med* 347:1057, 2002.

57. Mutlu GM, Leikin JB, Oh K, et al.: An unresponsive biochemistry professor in the bathtub. *Chest* 122:1073-1076, 2002.

58. Losek JD, Rock AL, Boldt RR: Cyanide poisoning from a cosmetic nail remover. *Pediatrics* 88:337, 1991.

59. Vogel SN, Sultan TR, Ten Eyck RP: Cyanide poisoning. *Clin Toxicol* 18:367, 1981.

60. Carella F, Grassi MP, Savoiardo M, et al.: Dystonic-parkinsonian syndrome after cyanide poisoning: clinical and MRI findings. *J Neurol Neurosurg Psychiatry* 51:1345, 1988.

61. Rosenberg NL, Myers JA, Martin WR: Cyanide-induced parkinsonism: clinical, MRI, and 6-fluorodopa PET studies. *Neurology* 39:142, 1989.

62. Peterson CD, Collins AJ, Himes JM, et al.: Ethylene glycol poisoning: pharmacokinetics during therapy with ethanol and hemodialysis. *N Engl J Med* 304:21, 1981.

63. Rubinstein D, Escott E, Kelly JP: Methanol intoxication with putaminal and white matter necrosis: MR and CT findings. *AJNR Am J Neuroradiol* 16:1492, 1995.

64. Guggenheim MA, Couch JR, Weinberg W: Motor dysfunction as a permanent complication of methanol ingestion. Presentation of a case with a beneficial response to levodopa treatment. *Arch Neurol* 24:550, 1971.

65. Jacobsen D, Hewlett TP, Webb R, et al.: Ethylene glycol intoxication: evaluation of kinetics and crystalluria. *Am J Med* 84:145, 1988.

66. Brent J, McMartin K, Phillips S, et al.: Fomepizole for the treatment of ethylene glycol poisoning. *N Engl J Med* 340:832, 1999.

67. Hill JB: Salicylate intoxication. *N Engl J Med* 288:1110, 1973.

68. Flanagan RJ, Mant TG: Coma and metabolic acidosis early in severe acute paracetamol poisoning. *Hum Toxicol* 5:179, 1986.

69. Bray GP, Harrison PM, O'Grady JG, et al.: Long-term anticonvulsant therapy worsens outcome in paracetamol-induced fulminant hepatic failure. *Hum Exp Toxicol* 11:265, 1992.

70. Lauterburg BH, Velez ME: Glutathione deficiency in alcoholics: risk factor for paracetamol hepatotoxicity. *Gut* 29:1153, 1988.

71. Schiodt FV, Ott P, Christensen E, et al.: The value of plasma acetaminophen half-life in antidote-treated acetaminophen overdose. *Clin Pharmacol Ther* 71:221-225, 2002.

72. Stilman N, Masdeu JC: Incidence of seizures with phenytoin toxicity. *Neurology* 35:1769, 1985.

73. Schmidt S, Schmitz-Buhl M: Signs and symptoms of carbamazepine overdose. *J Neurol* 242:169, 1995.

74. Sullivan JB Jr, Rumack BH, Peterson RG: Acute carbamazepine toxicity resulting from overdose. *Neurology* 31:621, 1981.

75. Weaver DF, Camfield P, Fraser A: Massive carbamazepine overdose: clinical and pharmacologic observations in five episodes. *Neurology* 38:755, 1988.

76. Spiller HA, Krenzelok EP, Cookson E: Carbamazepine overdose: a prospective study of serum levels and toxicity. *J Toxicol Clin Toxicol* 28:445, 1990.

77. Graudins A, Peden G, Dowsett RP: Massive overdose with controlled-release carbamazepine resulting in delayed peak serum concentrations and life-threatening toxicity. *Emerg Med* 14:89, 2002.

78. Dreifuss FE, Langer DH, Moline KA, et al.: Valproic acid hepatic fatalities. II. US experience since 1984. *Neurology* 39.201, 1989.

79. Schwarz S, Georgiadis D, Schwab S: Fulminant progression of hyperammonaemic encephalopathy after treatment with valproate in a patient with ureterosigmoidostomy. *J Neurol Neurosurg Psychiatry* 73:90, 2002.

80. Barrueto F Jr, Hack JB. Hyperammonemia and coma without hepatic dysfunction induced by valproate therapy. *Acad Emerg Med* 8:999, 2001.

81. Bohan TP, Helton E, McDonald I: Effect of L-carnitine treatment of valproate-induced hepatotoxicity. *Neurology* 56:1405, 2001.

82. DeVivo DC: Effect of L-carnitine treatment for valproate-induced hepatotoxicity. *Neurology* 58:507, 2002.

83. Osborn AG: Diagnosis of descending transtentorial herniation by cranial computed tomography. *Radiology* 123:93, 1977.

84. Rodriguez JC, Gutierrez RA, Valdes OD, et al.: The role of computed axial tomography in the diagnosis and treatment of brain inflammatory and parasitic lesions: our experience in Mexico. *Neuroradiology* 16:458, 1978.

85. Sotelo J, Guerrero V, Rubio F: Neurocysticercosis: a new classification based on active and inactive forms. A study of 753 cases. *Arch Intern Med* 145:442, 1985.

86. Helliwell M, Hampel G, Sinclair E, et al.: Value of emergency toxicological investigations in differential diagnosis of coma. *BMJ* 2:819, 1979.

87. Hepler BR, Sutheimer CA, Sunshine I: The role of the toxicology laboratory in emergency medicine. II. Study of an integrated approach. *J Toxicol Clin Toxicol* 22:503, 1984.

88. Ng M, Saadat D, Sinha UK. Managing the emergency airway in Le Fort fractures. *J Craniomaxillofac Trauma* 4:38, 1998.

89. Bernard SA, Gray TW, Buist MD, et al.: Treatment of comatose survivors of out-of-hospital cardiac arrest with induced hypothermia. *N Engl J Med* 21:557, 2002.

90. Tokutomi T, Morimoto K, Miyagi T, et al.: Optimal temperature for the management of severe traumatic brain injury: effect of hypothermia on intracranial pressure, systemic and intracranial hemodynamics, and metabolism. *Neurosurgery* 52:102, 2003.

91. Kearsley JH, Musso AF: Hypothermia and coma in the Wernicke-Korsakoff syndrome. *Med J Aust* 2:504, 1980.

92. Nattel S, Bayne L, Ruedy J: Physostigmine in coma due to drug overdose. *Clin Pharmacol Ther* 25:96, 1979.

93. Raichle ME, Posner JB, Plum F: Cerebral blood flow during and after hyperventilation. *Arch Neurol* 23:394, 1970.

94. Muizelaar JP, van der Poel HG, Li ZC, et al.: Pial arteriolar vessel diameter and CO_2 reactivity during prolonged hyperventilation in the rabbit. *J Neurosurg* 69:923, 1988.

95. Marshall LF, Smith RW, Rauscher LA, et al.: Mannitol dose requirements in brain-injured patients. *J Neurosurg* 48:169, 1978.

96. Nath F, Galbraith S: The effect of mannitol on cerebral white matter water content. *J Neurosurg* 65:41, 1986.

97. Muizelaar JP, Wei EP, Kontos HA, et al.: Mannitol causes compensatory cerebral vasoconstriction and vasodilation in response to blood viscosity changes. *J Neurosurg* 59:822, 1983.

98. Edwards JJ, Samuels D, Fu ES: Forearm compartment syndrome from intravenous mannitol extravasation during general anesthesia. *Anesth Analg* 96:245, 2003.

99. Braakman R, Schouten HJ, Blaauw-van Dishoeck M, et al.: Megadose steroids in severe head injury. Results of a prospective double-blind clinical trial. *J Neurosurg* 58:326, 1983.

100. Dearden NM, Gibson JS, McDowall DG, et al.: Effect of high-dose dexamethasone on outcome from severe head injury. *J Neurosurg* 64:81, 1986.

101. Hoffman RS, Goldfrank LR: The poisoned patient with altered consciousness. Controversies in the use of a "coma cocktail." *JAMA* 274:562, 1995.

102. Votey SR, Bosse GM, Bayer MJ, et al.: Flumazenil: a new benzodiazepine antagonist. *Ann Emerg Med* 20:181, 1991.

103. Hoffman JR, Schriger DL, Luo JS: The empiric use of naloxone in patients with altered mental status: a reappraisal. *Ann Emerg Med* 20:246, 1991.

104. Prough DS, Roy R, Bumgarner J, et al.: Acute pulmonary edema in healthy teenagers following conservative doses of intravenous naloxone. *Anesthesiology* 60:485, 1984.

105. Goldfrank L, Weisman RS, Errick JK, et al.: A dosing nomogram for continuous infusion intravenous naloxone. *Ann Emerg Med* 15:566, 1986.

106. Gueye PN, Hoffman JR, Taboulet P, et al.: Empiric use of flumazenil in comatose patients: limited applicability of criteria to define low risk. *Ann Emerg Med* 27:730, 1996.

107. Spivey WH: Flumazenil and seizures: analysis of 43 cases. *Clin Ther* 14:292, 1992.

108. Auerbach PS: *Wilderness Medicine,* 4th ed. St. Louis: Mosby Year Book, 2001.

109. Blans MJ, Vos PE, Faber HJ, et al.: Coma in a young anorexic woman. *Lancet* 357:1944, 2001.

110. Bickerstaff ER: Basilar artery migraine. *Handbook Clin Neurol* 48:135, 1986.

111. Caplan LR: Migraine and vertebrobasilar ischemia. *Neurology* 41:55, 1991.

112. Lugaresi E, Montagna P, Tinuper P, et al.: Endozepine stupor: recurring stupor linked to endozepine-4 accumulation. *Brain* 121:127, 1998.

113. Arn PH, Hauser ER, Thomas GH, et al.: Hyperammonemia in women with mutation at the ornithine carbamoyltransferase locus. A cause of postpartum coma. *N Engl J Med* 322:1652, 1990.

114. Leao M: Valproate as a cause of hyperammonemia in heterozygotes with ornithine-transcarbamylase deficiency. *Neurology* 45:593, 1995.

115. Legras A, Labarthe F, Maillot F, et al.: Late diagnosis of ornithine transcarbamylase defect in three related female patients: polymorphic presentations. *Crit Care Med* 30:241, 2002.

116. Chabriat H, Tournier-Lasserve E, Vahedi K, et al.: Autosomal dominant migraine with MRI white-matter abnormalities mapping to the CADASIL locus. *Neurology* 45:1086, 1995.

117. Schon F, Martin RJ, Prevett M, et al.: "CADASIL coma": an underdiagnosed acute encephalopathy. *J Neurol Neurosurg Psychiatry* 74:249, 2003.

Appendix 8.1.

Drug Screening Tests (Chromatographic Techniques)

Analgesics

Acetaminophen°
Acetylsalicylate
Chlorzoxazone
Codeine
Dicyclomine
Fenoprofen
Flurbiprofen
Hydrocodone
Ibuprofen
Indomethacin
Ketoprofen
Meperidine
Methaqualone
Morphine
Naproxen°
Pentazocine
Propoxyphene°
Salicylate°
Tramadol

Antidepressants

Amitriptyline°
Bupropion
Clomipramine°
Desipramine°
Doxepin°

Fluoxetine°
Imipramine°
Maprotiline
Nortriptyline°
Sertraline°
Trazodone°
Trimipramine
Venlafaxine°

Stimulants

Amphetamine
Benzoylecgonine
Benztropine
Caffeine
Cocaine
Cyclobenzaprine
Ethyl-benzoylecgonine
Methamphetamine
Phencyclidine
Phentermine
Strychnine

Sympathomimetics

Brompheniramine
Chlorpheniramine
Diphenhydramine°

Doxylamine
Ephedrine
Hydroxyzine
Phenylephrine
Phenylpropanolamine
Phenyltoloxamine
Pseudoephedrine

Antiepileptics

Carbamazepine°
N-Desmethylmethsux-
    imide
Ethosuximide°
Felbamate°
Lamotrigine
Mephobarbital°
Methsuximide°
Phenobarbital°
Phenytoin°
Primidone°
Valproic acid°

Cardioactive Agents

Diltiazem
Lidocaine°

Quinidine°
Verapamil

Tranquilizers

Chlordiazepoxide°
Chlorpromazine
Clozapine
Desalkyl flurazepam
Diazepam°
Flunitrazepam
Flurazepam
Hydroxyethyl
    flurazepam
Lorazepam
Midazolam
Nordiazepam
Oxazepam
Prochlorperazine
Promethazine
Temazepam
Thioridazine°
Trifluoperazine

Hypoglycemics

Acetohexamide
Chlorpropamide

Tolazamide
Tolbutamide

**Sedatives and
Hypnotics**

Allobarbital
Amobarbital°
Aprobarbital

Barbital
Butabarbital°
Butalbital°
Carisoprodol
Ethchlorvynol
Glutethimide
Meprobamate°
Metharbital
Methyprylon
Pentobarbital°

Secobarbital°
Thiopental
Zolpidem

Other

Dextromethorphan
Gemfibrozil
Methadone

Metoclopramide
Metronidazole
Pentoxifylline
Phenylbutazone
Sulfadiazine
Sulfamethoxazole
Sulfapyridine
Sulfisoxazole
Theophylline°
Ticlopidine

If serum is submitted for analysis, quantitative reports often are issued for the drugs marked by an asterisk, with a therapeutic, toxic, or potentially lethal range referenced on the report. Drugs in italics can be detected only in urine. If serum is submitted for analysis, these drugs will not be detected, even at toxic levels.

Source: Porter WH, Moyer TP: Clinical toxicology. In CA Burtis, ER Ashwood (eds), *Tietz Textbook of Clinical Chemistry*, 3rd ed. Philadelphia: WB Saunders, 1999, p. 906.

Chapter 9
Brain Edema

Brain edema at its core, particularly when profound and widespread, displaces brain tissue and results in compression of the diencephalic structures and in impairment of consciousness.

Edema may also occur in one hemisphere and be proportionally more severe than the primary lesion (e.g., brain metastasis). In contrast, brain edema may be rather inconsequential, as in anoxic-ischemic-related brain swelling, and an inevitable result of widespread brain damage. The complexity of diagnosis and management of acute cerebral edema warrant a separate discussion. Outcome in many instances is somber because of the rapid emergence of irreversible damage to the brain stem.

Classification and Presentation of Brain Edema

The structure and workings of the blood–brain barrier have been partly elucidated. A brief discussion is found in Box 9.1.

Brain edema has been conveniently classified, but the types are clinically indistinguishable. For comparative purposes, the different types are summarized in Table 9.1.[1] Brain edema has been classified by Klatzo[2] into (1) vasogenic edema, which is a consequence of damage to the blood–brain barrier leading to increased capillary permeability, and (2) cytotoxic edema, which is a consequence of a direct cellular insult leading to swelling without abnormalities in capillary permeability. An additional category has been pro-

posed by Fishman,[1] who includes interstitial or hydrocephalic edema caused by obstruction of the cerebrospinal fluid (CSF) pathways (Fig. 9.1).

Milhorat[3] suggested an alternative classification, categorizing specific compartmental increases that cause enlargement of brain bulk. Enlargement of brain bulk is an increase in brain volume that may take place in one of three major compartments: the vascular compartment (by arterial dilatation or venous obstruction), the astrocytes (by ischemia or intoxication), or the interstitium, including the CSF compartment (by tumors, infections, trauma, or obstructive hydrocephalus).[3]

Any classification of brain edema suffers from the fact that many acute insults to the brain involve multiple compartments. In addition, the clinical manifestations are a consequence of brain tissue shift, and neither the initial presentation nor the evolution of clinical signs is much different among the different categories. The pathophysiology of brain edema is discussed in Box 9.2.

Diffuse cerebral edema commonly is rapid in onset and results in coma; focal cerebral edema can go largely unnoticed.

Clinical manifestations of brain edema in fulminant hepatic failure are dramatic.[16] Often, patients rather suddenly lapse into coma and may exhibit significant extensor responses, sometimes with progression to brain death. When intracranial pressure is monitored, extreme increases with reduction in cerebral perfusion pressure are typical.

Cerebral edema in diabetic ketoacidosis usually is a devastating complication with high mortality,

Box 9.1. The Blood–Brain Barrier

The exchange of fluids and solute between blood and brain in both directions is governed by multiple mechanisms. Exchange is determined by an anatomical restriction (in the true sense, a barrier), transport systems to rapidly provide the main energy source (e.g., facilitated glucose transport system), and osmolality. Breakdown of the blood–brain barrier, therefore, may not be an anatomical defect but may involve any of these control systems.

The blood–brain barrier is located at the capillary level, and its morphology is unique. A characteristic feature is the crowding of the capillary with astrocyte processes. These astrocyte feet initially appeared to define the barrier, but electron microscopic studies clearly demonstrated an open intercellular space. The physiologic function of these astrocyte foot processes is not entirely known, and their influence on the barrier may be only to moderate permeability rather than to define it anatomically. The capillary consists of a single layer of endothelial cells with a well-organized basement membrane. The endothelial cells are continuous, connected with tight junctions, and without true gaps. Structures that appear to be gaps are in fact very thin layers suggesting an opening, but the membranes are intact, securing impermeability.

more often, unfortunately, in children and adolescents with juvenile diabetes. The clinical presentation is often without warning: rapidly developing stupor is soon followed by extensor posturing and fixed, dilated pupils. Many patients fulfill the clinical criteria for brain death in a matter of hours.[17–19]

Focal cerebral hemisphere edema is manifested by one of the herniation syndromes (see Chapter 8) or, in less severe cases, only with more obvious drowsiness. Notably, edema surrounding neoplasms can be clinically silent. In general, degree of impaired consciousness and degree of focal edema may be very poorly related.

Cerebellar softening and swelling may quickly compress the upper brain stem, leading to sudden pontomedullary dysfunction and respiratory arrest. However, the critical threshold of tolerable swelling is not known, and we have observed dramatic swelling with spontaneous resolution.[20]

Different types of edema can be visualized by computed tomography (CT) scanning or magnetic resonance imaging (MRI). CT is not very sensitive to global cerebral edema in early stages, but the severity of edema can be graded by a simple system that characterizes different areas of involvement (Table 9.2). Most difficult in the evaluation of edema is the absence of sulci. This often becomes an issue in young persons who have a catastrophic illness that may produce edema but that may be difficult to appreciate because of an age-related lack of sulci (Fig. 9.2).

Vasogenic edema produces increased signal intensity on T_2-weighted images, particularly in the

Table 9.1. Types of Brain Edema

	Vasogenic	Cytotoxic	Interstitial
Pathophysiologic mechanism	Proteinaceous plasma filtrate in extracellular space	Cellular swelling from influx of water and sodium	Cerebrospinal fluid migration from increased ventricular pressure
Location	Preferentially white matter (often sparing gray matter)	Preferentially gray matter (often adjacent white matter)	Preferentially periventricular white matter
Disorders	• Primary or metastatic brain tumor • Inflammation • Head injury	• Cerebrovascular disorders • Global anoxic-ischemic insult • Fulminant hepatic failure • Water intoxication, dysequilibrium syndrome	Obstructive hydrocephalus
Capillary permeability	Increased	Normal	Normal

Source: Modified from Fishman.[1] By permission of WB Saunders Company.

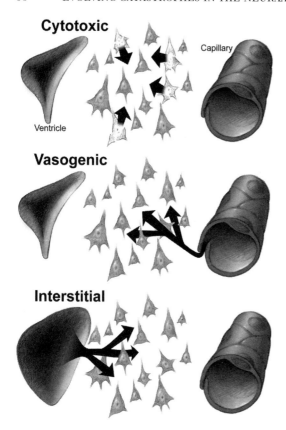

Figure 9.1 Changes in brain tissue with cytotoxic edema, vasogenic edema, and interstitial edema.

white matter. Cytotoxic edema in stroke increases the T_2 signal as well but often is found in the boundary zone of the infarct between the central area of infarction and the surrounding normal brain tissue. Diffusion-weighted MRI specifically measures free water diffusion. The apparent diffusion coefficient (ADC value) can be calculated. Elevated ADC values indicate vasogenic edema (Fig. 9.3). Restricted diffusion with reduced ADC values indicates cytotoxic edema due to neuronal injury, be it trauma or ischemia. Normal ADC values may indicate intravoxel averaging of ADC values when both mechanisms are present.[21,22]

Specific Clinical Circumstances of Brain Edema

Brain Edema in Postanoxic-Ischemic Encephalopathy

Brain edema usually affects both hemispheres and invariably is present in comatose patients. Brain edema in anoxic-ischemic injury is a global astroglial swelling involving the entire hemisphere. Tissue necrosis results in the development of brain edema several days later, and its appearance is not associated with a significant increase in intracranial pressure. Therefore, brain edema in postanoxic-ischemic encephalopathy, whether from cardiac arrest or asphyxia, is a measure of the severity of the insult and implies a poor prognosis.[23]

Brain edema in survivors of cardiopulmonary resuscitation is noted only when CT scanning is performed several days after the event. Brain edema on CT scans is more common in patients with absent motor responses or extensor posturing responses, abnormal cranial nerve reflexes, and generalized myoclonus. These patients are often in cardiogenic shock and need progressively higher doses of vasopressors.

Brain edema in postanoxic-ischemic encephalopathy rarely results in further clinical deterioration in these already ravaged patients. In some patients, however, further progression to brain death may occur and is accompanied by further worsening of brain edema revealed by CT scans. CT scanning often shows loss of definition of cortical sulci, lack of gray and white matter differentiation, and, in the most severe cases, obliteration of the basal cisterns (Fig. 9.4).[24] In some patients, the initial CT scans may show hypodensity of the basal ganglia (caudate and putamen), which are fields of terminal vascular supply, or of the thalamus. MRI may be useful in delineating the extent of abnormalities, but experience is limited.[22]

Brain Edema from Acute Metabolic Derangements and Organ Failure

The water content of the brain may increase significantly as a result of changes in plasma osmolality. Brain edema may also occur as a result of an increased osmotic effect of a toxic intermediate, as in acute liver failure.[25,26] Fulminant hepatic failure has been associated with the development of brain edema, and its emergence has been linked to early mortality.[27]

Experiments in hepatectomized rats found that an increase in cortical glutamine may act as an osmotically active molecule (osmolyte), increasing brain water and resulting in astrocyte swelling. The increase in astrocyte content of glutamine in hepatic failure correlates with an increase in arterial

Box 9.2. Brain Edema: Physiology and Pathology

In vasogenic edema, the breakdown of the barrier results in fluid accumulation into the white matter. Myelin sheets are swollen and filled with vacuoles, which may further result in myelin breakdown, and cysts appear in the white matter. The astrocytes are swollen at a later stage. The breakdown of the blood–brain barrier is most illustrative in vasogenic edema. Whatever disorder triggers the insult, the result is transudation of plasma into the extracellular white matter space. With this flooding of the white matter, however, cerebral blood flow remains unaffected, and cellular mechanisms remain intact.[4]

In cytotoxic or cellular edema, a preferential astrocyte swelling (gemistocyte) is observed, often maximal in the astrocyte foot processes. Because cytotoxic edema represents intracellular swelling, gray matter is more involved than white matter.

The mechanisms of cytotoxic edema are more complex than opening of the blood–brain barrier. Experimental studies have indicated that compounds blocking the release of excitatory amino acids reduce the water content of the brain, an in-

direct suggestion that glutamate has a potential role. Free radicals, prostaglandins, arachidonic acid, and possibly leukotrienes may potentiate cerebral swelling.[5-7] Other evidence indicates that initial cellular acidity could activate ion antiport channels, such as Na^+/H^- and Cl^-/HCO_3^-, to extrude H^+ but at the expense of an increase in osmolarity.

Clearing of brain edema occurs predominantly through the CSF. Clearance of extravasated proteins by the glial cells is also closely linked to resolution of edema fluid; this suggests a major role for colloid osmotic pressure generated by the proteins.[8,9] Edema spreads through bulk flow and a downhill pressure gradient between the white matter and the CSF compartment, a mechanism that may be further facilitated when CSF pressure is reduced.[10] A centrally located atrial natriuretic factor has been found to moderate the brain water content, and it might decrease edema formation.[11-14] Another mechanism may be due to water channel proteins (aquaporins), widely expressed in the brain. Up-regulation of aquaporin-4 has been found in contusional brain lesions.[15]

ammonia. An increase in glutamine may therefore reflect an attempt by astrocytes to detoxify themselves from ammonia by producing glutamine, creating an osmolyte. The development of brain

Table 9.2. Calculation of Brain Edema Severity Score on the Basis of CT Findings in Patients with Fulminant Hepatic Failure

Feature	Score
Visibility of cortical sulci	
3 CT scan slices of upper cerebral area (L/R)	6
Visibility of white matter	
Internal capsule (L/R)	2
Centrum semiovale (L/R)	2
Vertex (L/R)	2
Visibility of basal cisterns	
Sylvian fissure (horizontal–vertical, L/R)	4
Frontal interhemispheric fissure	1
Quadrigeminal cistern	1
Paired suprasellar cisterns (L/R)	2
Ambient cistern (L/R)	2
Maximal total°	22

CT, computed tomographic; L/R, left and right cerebral hemispheres.

°In CT scan with normal findings.

Source: Wijdicks et al.[16] By permission of Mayo Foundation for Medical Education and Research.

edema may be further amplified by changes in cerebral blood flow. Increased arterial ammonia may induce vasodilatation, and a relative increase in cerebral blood flow despite the decreased metabolic demand from encephalopathy (so-called luxury perfusion) may increase the development of vasogenic edema.[28,29] Other potential mechanisms are inhibition of Na^+,K^+–adenosine triphosphatase, which may result in astrocyte swelling. This explanation is supported by one study in which serum from patients with fulminant hepatic failure inhibited this pump.[30]

CT scans may demonstrate disappearance of the sylvian fissures, and later, complete compression of the basal cisterns and loss of white–gray matter differentiation may be seen (Fig. 9.5). These abnormalities may reverse entirely with control of intracranial pressure and after liver transplantation.[24]

Brain edema is rarely present in patients with fluctuating drowsiness; it is usually not visualized on CT until patients become stuporous. A linear relationship between the severity of cerebral edema and the degree of hepatic encephalopathy has been found[16] and implies that brain edema is the final common pathway by which coma occurs.

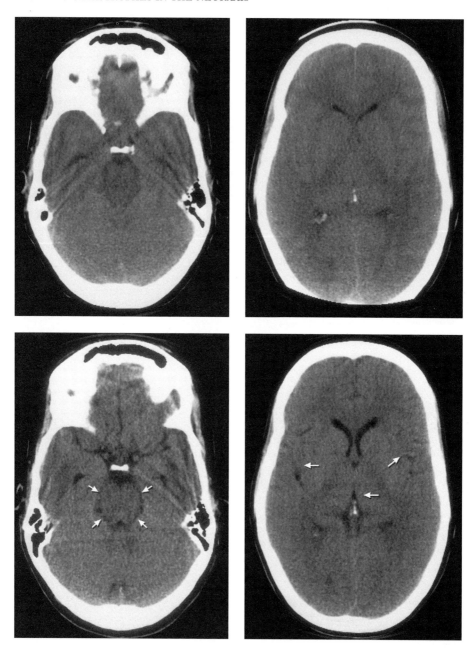

Figure 9.2 Resolving brain edema in encephalitis. Virtual lack of sulci and sylvian fissures, poor white–gray matter differentiation, and effacement of basal cistern and third ventricle with improvement (*arrows*).

Cerebral edema may develop in acute, often dramatic, sodium and glucose derangements. Hyperosmolality can be brought on by severe dehydration or from infusion of hypertonic solutions. This may lead to shrinkage of the endothelial cells, causing gaps and possible rupture of the interendothelial connection that result in increased permeability. Its effect is brief and reversed in a matter of hours.[31]

Acutely induced hypo-osmolality or hyponatremia of a sufficient degree (usually 110 mmol/L or less) may induce significant cerebral edema. Cerebral edema in this hypo-osmolar state has been noted in young healthy women after general

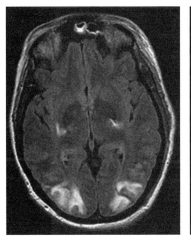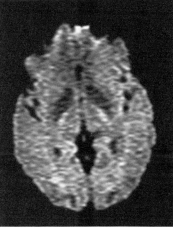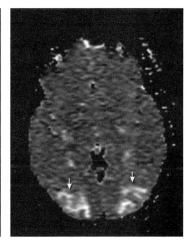

Figure 9.3 Series of magnetic resonance sequences (fluid attenuation inversion recovery [FLAIR], diffusion-weighted imaging [DWI], perfusion-weighted imaging [PWI]) showing increased apparent diffusion coefficient values in hypertensive encephalopathy indicative of edema (*arrows*).

anesthesia and in patients with polydipsia, predominantly in schizophrenia. Excessive administration of free water results in acute onset of massive brain edema,[32] rapid displacement of the diencephalon, and respiratory arrest.

Nonetheless, brain edema is uncommon after acute severe hyponatremia and may be explained by a corrective mechanism due to rapid loss of organic osmolytes. Loss of osmolytes permits transport of potassium outside the cell and leads to reduction in the content of intracellular solute, minimizing the risk of cell swelling induced by this rapid osmotic change. A linear correlation between the degree of hyponatremia and the loss of important osmolytes, such as taurine, glutamate, and aspartame, by the brain has been documented.[33] Reduction in the number of osmolytes was already detectable 3 hours after the onset of

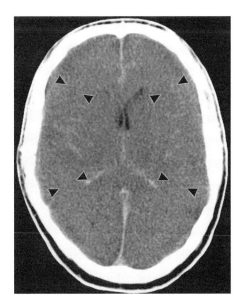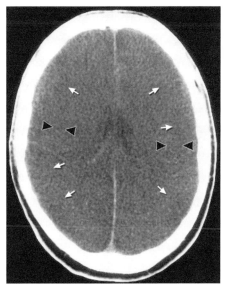

Figure 9.4 Anoxic-ischemic encephalopathy with generalized brain edema. *Arrowheads* indicate loss of gray–white matter definition. *Arrows* point to absence of sulci.

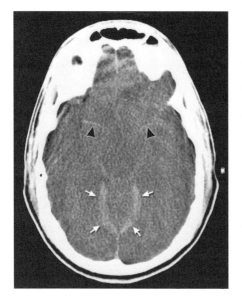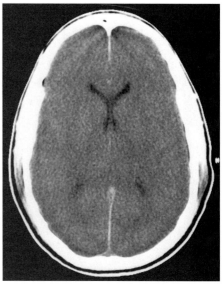

Figure 9.5 Cerebral edema in fulminant hepatic failure. *Left:* Note pseudo-subarachnoid hemorrhage, which occurs when the brain tissue becomes very low in attenuation and the dura and blood vessels appear comparatively hyperdense (*arrowheads* point to the basal cisterns and *arrows* to the tentorium region). *Right:* Loss of sylvian fissures and loss of cortical sulci.

hyponatremia, decreasing to a minimal concentration in 24 hours.

The mechanism of brain edema in diabetic ketoacidosis may be related to rapid fluid management to correct the ketoacidosis and dehydration, but this is not clear. At least theoretically, rapid administration of fluid may lead to intracellular shift of water because of osmotically active molecules that are intrinsically present to protect the brain from excessive shrinkage. Rapid administration of fluid may override the washout of osmolytes when plasma osmolality rapidly corrects itself. Alternatively, insulin administration may activate the Na^+/H^+ pump, enhancing sodium and water influx.[34] Cerebral edema may be more prevalent than appreciated, and serial CT scan studies have shown the development of clinically unrecognizable cerebral edema.[35,36] In one study, increased serum urea nitrogen concentrations, more severe hypocapnia, and treatment with bicarbonate emerged as important factors, even more important than rate of fluid, sodium, and insulin infusion. The vasoconstrictive effect of hypocapnia and extreme dehydration could cause anoxic-ischemic injury, leading to cerebral edema.[37] In clinical practice, brain edema may also be related to anoxic-ischemic damage from acidosis-related cardiopulmonary arrest.

Treatment with osmotic diuretic agents is often unsuccessful, evidence that massive cerebral edema has resulted in irreversible herniation.

Brain Edema and Acute Bacterial Meningitis

Brain edema in acute bacterial meningitis may complicate the clinical course and almost certainly increases mortality.

The true prevalence of brain edema in bacterial meningitis is not known, and reported series have been biased toward autopsy material. Brain edema occurs early in the course of bacterial meningitis but is not invariably the cause of early death. In a series of 29 patients with bacterial meningitis, 15 had pathologic evidence of cerebral edema by the appearance of tonsillar herniation at autopsy.[38]

There may be several mechanisms of brain edema in inflammatory disorders. It has been proposed that granulocyte ("granulocytic brain edema") products may induce edema.[39] Cytokines originating from leukocytes may cause endothelial alterations that can lead to vasogenic edema.[39,40] In addition, it has been documented that high doses of these chemotactically active agents administered intrathecally increased brain water content, but it is not clear whether this experiment, which used very high doses, reflected the changes in vivo.[41,42] The cytokine–endothelium–leukocyte interaction is currently an active field of research, and recent studies have shown that both dexamethasone and monoclonal antibodies against leukocyte adhesion receptors attenuate meningeal inflammation and brain edema in rats inoculated with *Haemophilus influenzae*.[43]

CT scanning of brain edema in acute bacterial meningitis typically shows generalized edema, with edematous white matter and cortical effacement. The ventricles may become extremely small. In contrast-enhanced CT scans, enhancement of the basal cisterns due to hypervascularity or gyral configurations in cortical zones may represent extensive meningitis. MRI may document pus (see Chapter 16).

Brain Edema Associated with Hemispheric Mass

Brain edema often only surrounds a hemispheric mass irrespective of whether it is an intraparenchymal hematoma, a large territorial infarct, or a tumor.

Intracranial hematomas, when located in the basal ganglia, often have a perihematoma rim of edema that invariably represents vasogenic edema. Its significance is unknown, and an increase in the volume of edema is common within the first 24 hours after the ictus.[44] Secondary clinical deterioration from progressive perihematoma swelling commonly occurs in lobar hematomas. The products of degraded erythrocytes are responsible for edema. Hemoglobin breakdown products take time to form, which explains delayed edema in most cases. Hemin, bilirubin, and $FeCl_2$ produce brain edema and leave the way open to explore the use of iron-chelating agents in patients with intracerebral hematomas.[45–47]

Brain edema from a cerebral arteriovenous malformation (AVM) most commonly is associated with recent hemorrhage. Brain edema may also be correlated with increased pressure on the draining veins and marked dilatation or varices of the draining veins. Acute venous occlusion may be another mechanism of venous outflow.[48] However, brain edema can be explained by seizures in patients with documented AVM and is most often seen on MRI. The focal hyperintensity on T_2-weighted images in the white matter may disappear after control of seizures.

Large hemispheric infarcts may swell, usually after 3–5 days.[49] In many patients, brain swelling is heralded by increasing headache and a fluctuating level of consciousness. Outcome in patients with brain stem involvement from herniation is invariably poor (Fig. 9.6). Tumor-associated edema most likely involves multiple mechanisms (Box 9.3, Fig. 9.7). A preliminary study suggested that reduced brain tissue oxygenation improves with decompression in peritumoral brain edema.[56]

Brain Edema Associated with Head Injury

Diffuse brain swelling is more common in children than in adults. Brain swelling is present commonly in comatose patients with closed head injury and rarely in patients who remain alert. Subsequent deterioration from diffuse brain swelling in a previously alert patient is uncommon (<5%). It has been reported after repeated brain injury—the second impact syndrome—but its mechanism and risk factors are not known.[57] Brain swelling occurs more often in patients who suffered a systemic insult, such as hypotension or pre-hospital hypoxemia. Brain swelling often is evident on CT scans and may involve absence of the third ventricle and basal cisterns in most cases. Intracranial pressure is almost always significantly increased.[58] Brain swelling in adults with closed head injury is often associated with multiple parenchymal contusions, shearing lesions, and traumatic subarachnoid hemorrhage.[58–62]

Management of Brain Edema

Acute brain edema is associated with high morbidity and mortality, and results of aggressive intervention have not been encouraging. In the course of several hours, brain shift may be extensive, resulting in permanent damage even after the water content of the brain has been ameliorated.

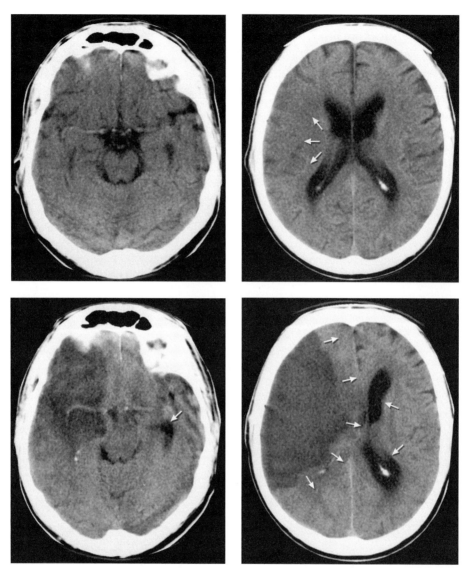

Figure 9.6 Cerebral swelling associated with middle cerebral artery territory infarct. *Top row:* Initial scan with hypodensity and loss of sulci in the middle cere-bral artery territory (*arrows*). *Bottom row:* Massive edema and shift with contralateral hydrocephalus and enlargement of temporal horn (*arrows*).

Osmotic diuretics, such as mannitol or hypertonic saline, may be useful initially, while the true value of intracranial pressure is determined by placement of a monitor. Continuous infusion with 3% hypertonic saline should be considered if a bolus of mannitol (1 g/kg) is unsuccessful in head trauma, intracranial hematoma, or cerebral infarct. The dose is increased until serum sodium concentrations are 145–155 mmol/L.[63] A pilot study suggested an effect from intravenous bolus administration of 23.4% saline in refractory increased intracranial pressure. Cerebral perfusion pressure was augmented as well, and intravascular volume was not depleted.[64]

Treatment in diabetic ketoacidosis would be normal saline 10 mL/kg in the first hour, followed by 3.5–5 mL/kg hourly infusion. Insulin could be added at 0.1 unit/kg hourly. However, with cerebral edema, decreased partial pressure of arterial CO_2 ($PaCO_2$) should be corrected to normal val-

Box 9.3. Edema in Brain Tumors

Four processes have been suggested that may be related to edema associated with primary brain tumors or metastasis:[50] (1) tumor angiogenesis of vessels with defective blood–brain barrier, characterized by large interendothelial gaps;[51] (2) increased microvascular permeability from production of mediators, such as prostaglandin E_2 and thromboxane B_2, in this process;[52] (3) an immunologic mechanism such as interleukin-2, which when injected has resulted in brain edema in experimental studies;[53] and

(4) less likely, an inflammatory mechanism through substances, such as platelet-activating factor, released from polynuclear leukocytes surrounding the tumor-associated edema. Other factors that may potentiate tumor-associated edema are seizures, chemotherapeutic agents, and therapeutic radiation.[54] Plasma osmolality may play an important role, and one experimental study found a direct relation between plasma osmolality and formation of brain edema.[55]

---

ues, intravenous fluid and insulin infusion should be markedly reduced, and mannitol 1–2 g/kg should be added.[65] Corticosteroids are useful only in metastasis or glioma with mass effect from perilesional edema. Corticosteroids (10 mg of dexamethasone intravenously) should be considered in brain edema from fulminant bacterial meningitis (see Chapter 16). The major beneficial effect is improvement of CSF dynamics, predominantly the CSF outflow tract over the convexity. Corticosteroids have no documented value in brain edema from endocrine or hepatic disturbances.

Focal hemispheric edema is more difficult to manage, and craniectomy with duraplasty greatly increases the possibility for swelling outside the skull, relieving pressure. Removal of additional swollen brain tissue (anterior temporal lobectomy or frontal lobectomy) is optional but considered only if the primary lesion is in this location (e.g., temporal lobe swelling from herpes simplex encephalitis,[66] metastasis with malignant edema).

Surgical decompression in patients with head injury but retained brain stem reflexes has been advocated but only in young patients (<40 years), with reimplantation of bone flaps as early as 6 weeks after surgery. In one experience, results were "surprisingly good."[67] The craniotomy is extensive (frontotemporoparietal), leaving a bone rim on top of the superior sagittal sinus.

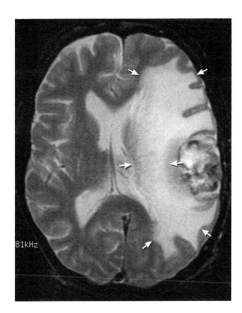

Figure 9.7 Peritumoral edema (*arrows*) in mass lesion (glioma).

REFERENCES

1. Fishman RA: *Cerebrospinal Fluid in Diseases of the Nervous System*, 2nd ed. Philadelphia: WB Saunders, 1992.
2. Klatzo I: Presidential address. Neuropathological aspects of brain edema. *J Neuropathol Exp Neurol* 26:1, 1967.
3. Milhorat TH. *Cerebrospinal Fluid and the Brain Edemas*. New York: Neuroscience Society of New York, 1987.
4. Sutton LN, Barranco D, Greenberg J, et al.: Cerebral blood flow and glucose metabolism in experimental brain edema. *J Neurosurg* 71:868, 1989.
5. Ikeda Y, Long DM: The molecular basis of brain injury and brain edema: the role of oxygen free radicals. *Neurosurgery* 27:1, 1990.
6. Ito U, Baethmann A, Hossmann KA, et al.: Brain edema IX. *Acta Neurochir* 60:1, 1993.
7. Kimelberg HK: Current concepts of brain edema. Review of laboratory investigations. *J Neurosurg* 83:1051, 1995.

8. Marmarou A, Hochwald G, Nakamura T, et al.: Brain edema resolution by CSF pathways and brain vasculature in cats. *Am J Physiol* 267:H514, 1994.

9. Marmarou A, Nakamura T, Tanaka K: The kinetics of fluid movement through brain tissue. *Semin Neurol* 4:439, 1984.

10. Reulen HJ, Graham R, Spatz M, et al.: Role of pressure gradients and bulk flow in dynamics of vasogenic brain edema. *J Neurosurg* 46:24, 1977.

11. Doczi T, Joó F, Szerdahelyi P, et al.: Regulation of brain water and electrolyte contents: the possible involvement of central atrial natriuretic factor. *Neurosurgery* 21:454, 1987.

12. Nakao N, Itakura T, Yokote H, et al.: Effect of atrial natriuretic peptide on ischemic brain edema: changes in brain water and electrolytes. *Neurosurgery* 27:39, 1990.

13. Rosenberg GA, Estrada EY: Atrial natriuretic peptide blocks hemorrhagic brain edema after 4-hour delay in rats. *Stroke* 26:874, 1995.

14. Vajda Z, Pedersen M, Doczi T, et al.: Effects of centrally administered arginine vasopressin and atrial natriuretic peptide on the development of brain edema in hyponatremic rats. *Neurosurgery* 49:697, 2001.

15. Sun MC, Honey CR, Berk C, et al.: Regulation of aquaporin-4 in a traumatic brain injury model in rats. *J Neurosurg* 98:565, 2003.

16. Wijdicks EFM, Plevak DJ, Rakela J, et al.: Clinical and radiologic features of cerebral edema in fulminant hepatic failure. *Mayo Clin Proc* 70:119, 1995.

17. Clements RS Jr, Prockop LD, Winegrad AI: Acute cerebral edema during treatment of hyperglycaemia. An experimental model. *Lancet* 2:384, 1968.

18. Fitzgerald MG, O'Sullivan DJ, Malins JM: Fatal diabetic ketosis. *BMJ* 2:247, 1961.

19. Young E, Bradley RF: Cerebral edema with irreversible coma in severe diabetic ketoacidosis. *N Engl J Med* 276:665, 1967.

20. Wijdicks EFM, Maus TP, Piepgras DG: Cerebellar swelling and massive brain stem distortion: spontaneous resolution documented by MRI. *J Neurol Neurosurg Psychiatry* 65:400, 1998.

21. Albers GW: Diffusion-weighted MRI for evaluation of acute stroke. *Neurology* 51:S47, 1998.

22. Wijdicks EFM, Campeau NG, Miller GM: MR imaging in comatose survivors of cardiac resuscitation. *AJNR Am J Neuroradiol* 22:1561, 2001.

23. Lupton BA, Hill A, Roland EH, et al.: Brain swelling in the asphyxiated term newborn: pathogenesis and outcome. *Pediatrics* 82:139, 1988.

24. Wijdicks EFM, Parisi JE, Sharbrough FW: Prognostic value of myoclonus status in comatose survivors of cardiac arrest. *Ann Neurol* 35:239, 1994.

25. Hilgier W, Olson JE: Brain ion and amino acid contents during edema development in hepatic encephalopathy. *J Neurochem* 62:197, 1994.

26. Olafsson S, Gottstein J, Blei AT: Brain edema and intracranial hypertension in rats after total hepatectomy. *Gastroenterology* 108:1097, 1995.

27. Blei AT, Olafsson S, Therrien G, et al.: Ammonia-induced brain edema and intracranial hypertension in rats after portacaval anastomosis. *Hepatology* 19:1437, 1994.

28. Butterworth RF: Hepatic encephalopathy and brain edema in acute hepatic failure: does glutamate play a role? *Hepatology* 25:1032, 1997.

29. Durham S, Yonas H, Aggarwal S, et al.: Regional cerebral blood flow and CO_2 reactivity in fulminant hepatic failure. *J Cereb Blood Flow Metab* 15:329, 1995.

30. Seda HW, Hughes RD, Gove CD, et al.: Inhibition of rat brain Na^+,K^+-ATPase activity by serum from patients with fulminant hepatic failure. *Hepatology* 4:74, 1984.

31. Cserr HF, DePasquale M, Patlak CS: Volume regulatory influx of electrolytes from plasma to brain during acute hyperosmolality. *Am J Physiol* 253:F530, 1987.

32. Arieff AI: Hyponatremia, convulsions, respiratory arrest, and permanent brain damage after elective surgery in healthy women. *N Engl J Med* 314:1529, 1986.

33. Sterns RH, Baer J, Ebersold S, et al.: Organic osmolytes in acute hyponatremia. *Am J Physiol* 264:F833, 1993.

34. Van der Meulen JA, Klip A, Grinstein S: Possible mechanism for cerebral oedema in diabetic ketoacidosis. *Lancet* 2:306, 1987.

35. Hoffman WH, Steinhart CM, el Gammal T, et al.: Cranial CT in children and adolescents with diabetic ketoacidosis. *AJNR Am J Neuroradiol* 9:733, 1988.

36. Krane EJ, Rockoff MA, Wallman JK, et al.: Subclinical brain swelling in children during treatment of diabetic ketoacidosis. *N Engl J Med* 312:1147, 1985.

37. Glaser N, Barnett P, McCaslin I, et al.: Risk factors for cerebral edema in children with diabetic ketoacidosis. The Pediatric Emergency Medicine Collaborative Research Committee of the American Academy of Pediatrics. *N Engl J Med* 344:264, 2001.

38. Dodge PR, Swartz MN: Bacterial meningitis—a review of selected aspects. II. Special neurologic problems, postmeningitic complications and clinicopathological correlations. *N Engl J Med* 272:954, 1965.

39. Fishman RA, Sligar K, Hake RB: Effects of leukocytes on brain metabolism in granulocytic brain edema. *Ann Neurol* 2:89, 1977.

40. Montesano R, Orci L, Vassalli P: Human endothelial cell cultures: phenotypic modulation by leukocyte interleukins. *J Cell Physiol* 122:424, 1985.

41. Niemöller UM, Täuber MG: Brain edema and increased intracranial pressure in the pathophysiology of bacterial meningitis. *Eur J Clin Microbiol Infect Dis* 8:109, 1989.

42. Täuber MG, Borschberg U, Sande MA: Influence of granulocytes on brain edema, intracranial pressure, and cerebrospinal fluid concentrations of lactate and protein in experimental meningitis. *J Infect Dis* 157:456, 1988.

43. Sáez-Llorens X, Jafari HS, Severien C, et al.: Enhanced attenuation of meningeal inflammation and brain edema by concomitant administration of anti-CD18 monoclonal antibodies and dexamethasone in experimental *Haemophilus* meningitis. *J Clin Invest* 88:2003, 1991.

44. Gebel JM Jr, Jauch EC, Brott TG, et al.: Natural history of perihematomal edema in patients with hyperacute

spontaneous intracerebral hemorrhage. *Stroke* 33: 2631, 2002.

45. Huang FP, Xi G, Keep RF, et al.: Brain edema after experimental intracerebral hemorrhage: role of hemoglobin degradation products. *J Neurosurg* 96:287, 2002.

46. Xi G, Hua Y, Bhasin R, et al.: Mechanisms of edema formation after intracerebral hemorrhage: effects of extravasated red blood cells on blood flow and blood–brain barrier integrity. *Stroke* 32:2932, 2001.

47. Xi G, Reiser G, Keep RF: The role of thrombin and thrombin receptors in ischemic, hemorrhagic and traumatic brain injury: deleterious or protective? *J Neurochem* 84:3, 2003.

48. Miyasaka Y, Kurata A, Tanaka R, et al.: Mass effect caused by clinically unruptured cerebral arteriovenous malformations. *Neurosurgery* 41:1060, 1997.

49. Wijdicks EFM, Diringer MN: Middle cerebral artery territory infarction and early brain swelling: progression and effect of age on outcome. *Mayo Clin Proc* 73:829, 1998.

50. Del Maestro RF, Megyesi JF, Farrell CL: Mechanisms of tumor-associated edema: a review. *Can J Neurol Sci* 17:177, 1990.

51. Coomber BL, Stewart PA, Hayakawa K, et al.: Quantitative morphology of human glioblastoma multiforme microvessels: structural basis of blood-brain barrier defect. *J Neurooncol* 5:299, 1987.

52. Cooper C, Jones HG, Weller RO: Production of prostaglandins and thromboxane by isolated cells from intracranial tumours. *J Neurol Neurosurg Psychiatry* 47:579, 1984.

53. Saris SC, Patronas NJ, Rosenberg SA, et al.: The effect of intravenous interleukin-2 on brain water content. *J Neurosurg* 71:169, 1989.

54. Posner JB: *Neurologic Complications of Cancer.* Philadelphia: FA Davis, 1995.

55. Hansen TD, Warner DS, Traynelis VC, et al.: Plasma osmolality and brain water content in a rat glioma model. *Neurosurgery* 34:505, 1994.

56. Pennings FA, Bouma GJ, Kedaria M, et al.: Intraoperative monitoring of brain tissue oxygen and carbon dioxide pressures reveals low oxygenation in peritumoral brain edema. *J Neurosurg Anesthesiol* 15:1, 2003.

57. McCrory PR, Berkovic SF: Second impact syndrome. *Neurology* 50:677, 1998.

58. Eisenberg HM, Gary HE Jr, Aldrich EF, et al.: Initial CT findings in 753 patients with severe head injury. A report from the NIH Traumatic Coma Data Bank. *J Neurosurg* 73:688, 1990.

59. Lang DA, Teasdale GM, Macpherson P, et al.: Diffuse brain swelling after head injury: more often malignant in adults than children? *J Neurosurg* 80: 675, 1994.

60. Pearl GS: Traumatic neuropathology. *Clin Lab Med* 18:39, 1998.

61. Feldman Z, Zachari S, Reichenthal E, et al.: Brain edema and neurological status with rapid infusion of lactated Ringer's or 5% dextrose solution following head trauma. *J Neurosurg* 83:1060, 1995.

62. Shapira Y, Artru AA, Cotev S, et al.: Brain edema and neurologic status following head trauma in the rat. No effect from large volumes of isotonic or hypertonic intravenous fluids, with or without glucose. *Anesthesiology* 77:79, 1992.

63. Qureshi AI, Suarez JI, Bhardwaj A, et al.: Use of hypertonic (3%) saline/acetate infusion in the treatment of cerebral edema: effect on intracranial pressure and lateral displacement of the brain. *Crit Care Med* 26:440, 1998.

64. Suarez JI, Qureshi AI, Bhardwaj A, et al.: Treatment of refractory intracranial hypertension with 23.4% saline. *Crit Care Med* 26:1118, 1998.

65. Bohn D, Daneman D: Diabetic ketoacidosis and cerebral edema. *Curr Opin Pediatr* 14:287, 2002.

66. Ebel H, Kuchta J, Balogh A: Operative treatment of tentorial herniation in herpes encephalitis. *Childs Nerv Syst* 15:84, 1999.

67. Guerra W, Gaab MR, Dietz H: Surgical decompression for traumatic brain swelling: indications and results. *J Neurosurg* 90:187, 1999.

Chapter 10
Status Epilepticus and Recurrent Seizures

Status epilepticus is a multifaceted neurologic emergency. It may present suddenly in the setting of other clinical neurologic conditions (e.g., acute bacterial meningitis and herpes simplex encephalitis) for which therapeutic interventions are urgently indicated. The tasks at hand need to be well executed because long-standing morbidity in many patients has been linked to lapses in aggressive control of seizure activity. Thus, rapid termination of seizures and simultaneous treatment of the underlying illness are of utmost priority in tonic-clonic status epilepticus, and this undisputed urgency must be appreciated by any physician faced with this illness. Status epilepticus lasting 1 hour or more increases morbidity 10-fold. Furthermore, neurogenic pulmonary edema or life-threatening cardiac arrhythmia[1] may occur, but more likely prolonged apnea and anoxia may result in an additional ischemic-anoxic injury and persistent coma, emphasizing the need for early intubation and airway control.

Concurrent destructive brain lesions are common in adult status epilepticus and, thus, in most cases are responsible for morbidity and mortality. Regrettably, outcome studies in status epilepticus include comatose patients with myoclonus status epilepticus, a phenomenon indicative of profound injury to the cortex and associated with cardiac arrest. These causes may account for 30%–40% of the cases, thus skewing the results toward an unfavorable outcome.[1–3] Conversely, albeit uncommonly, unprovoked status epilepticus may have an excellent neurologic outcome.

Status epilepticus in adults can be distinguished in several forms, each of which is discussed in detail. Potentially important differences in effect may exist with different antiepileptic agents. Why they differ in their ability to abort status epilepticus is not initially clear. In this chapter, an approach is presented that is based on the integration of position papers[4–6] and systematic reviews.[7,8]

Classification and Presentation of Status Epilepticus

Convulsive status epilepticus can be divided into four major categories, and nonconvulsive status epilepticus can be further divided into complex partial and absence types (Fig. 10.1). The distinction has relevance because the initial choice of antiepileptic agents may be different, management may not involve antiepileptic agents (as in myoclonus status epilepticus and psychogenic seizures), and outcome may differ from category to category.

Persistence of seizure activity is an important discriminating factor because it is directly linked to cumulative development of neurological and medical complications. The risk of neuronal dropout resulting in morbidity is related not only to the duration of status epilepticus but also to age and systemic complications, such as severe hypoxemia from aspiration. Autonomic storm resulting in tachyarrhythmias and hyperthermia probably does not directly contribute to brain damage.

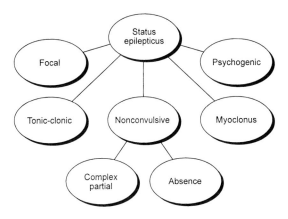

Figure 10.1 Classification of status epilepticus.

Tonic-Clonic Status Epilepticus

Tonic-clonic status epilepticus has typically been defined as repetitive generalized tonic-clonic seizures lasting 30 minutes or longer or seizures without full return of consciousness between episodes. However, the evolution of seizures into status epilepticus often becomes clear within 10–15 minutes, and the time criterion should not be applied rigorously.

The tonic phase involves flexion of the axial muscles, upward gaze, and marked widening of the pupil diameter with sluggish light responses. Flexion occurs in the arms and legs and is soon followed by extension, clenching of teeth, and forced expiration for several seconds. Sweating may be profuse, with an increase in blood pressure and pulse. The clonic phase begins with a tremor or shivering but gives way to uninterrupted jerking, which dies out gradually and may result in urinary and fecal incontinence after the sphincter muscles relax from a forceful contraction during the clonic phase. Usually, a generalized tonic-clonic seizure lasts 1–2 minutes and is followed for up to 5 minutes by a dazed state or agitation resulting in labored breathing and deep sleep. Most patients gradually awaken but never to a point that conversation is understood or simple commands are followed. Then, tonic spasm may occur again with a similar pattern of jerking and resolution.

Electrographic recordings, if available, typically show rhythmic spike- or sharp-wave complexes or sharp- and slow-wave discharges with a generalized distribution. Clinically, the distinction between a postictal confusional state emerging from a generalized tonic-clonic seizure and convulsive status epilepticus is difficult in the emergency department. Subtle eyelid or limb twitching in a stuporous patient may indicate continuous epileptic activity, but the distinction may require electroencephalographic recording.

Typical clinical findings are tongue bite (large purple hematoma or erosion at the lateral border of the tongue, which should be carefully inspected while the tongue is pushed out or sideways with a tongue depressor) (Fig. 10.2) and, occasionally, petechial hemorrhages in the conjunctiva, chest, and neck. Other complications are tachycardia, hyperglycemia, bone fractures, posterior shoulder dislocation, pulmonary aspiration, and, rarely if ever, neurogenic pulmonary edema. Prolonged

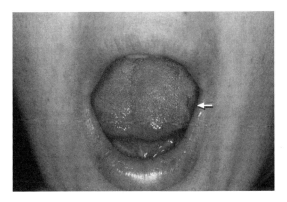
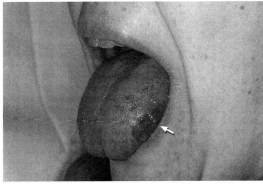

Figure 10.2 Tongue bite much more evident when tongue pushed out.

Table 10.1. Causes of Status Epilepticus

Change in antiepileptic drugs
Withdrawal of benzodiazepines (NCSE)
Drugs or alcohol
Bacterial meningitis or intracranial abscess
Encephalitis
Intracranial tumor or metastasis
Stroke
Arteriovenous or cavernous malformation
Hyperglycemia
Hypoglycemia
Hyponatremia
Preeclampsia
Intravenous contrast agent (NCSE)
Electroconvulsive therapy (NCSE)

NCSE, nonconvulsive status epilepticus.

status epilepticus may produce fever (up to 42°C), even on the day after presentation. The most common causes of status epilepticus are shown in Table 10.1. Withdrawal of antiepileptic agents in patients with established seizure disorder is most common.[9–11] In de novo status epilepticus, no overriding cause may be apparent, but an acute brain lesion is common. In one urban hospital study, the most common causes for status epilepticus were alcohol-related.[10,12]

Nonconvulsive Status Epilepticus

Delayed diagnosis is common because behavioral abnormalities are mistaken for a postictal state or psychiatric disorder.[13] Nonconvulsive status epilepticus is further divided into complex partial status and absence status.[14–16] Complex partial status epilepticus is most prevalent in adults 20–40 years of age.[17] It may occur after a single seizure and after replacement of antiepileptic drugs[18] and is more likely in patients with prior brain injury.[19]

Clinical presentation is diverse, but clinical signs are not always suggestive and may be diagnostically confusing. Consciousness is always impaired. Nonconvulsive status epilepticus results in blank staring, sometimes with tremulousness and subtle periorbital, facial, or limb myoclonus or eye-movement abnormalities such as nystagmus or eye deviation.[19] Patients have decreased or rambling speech output or are mute; thus, the distinction from aphasia with a structural lesion can be difficult. Aggressive behavior is uncommon,[14] and more often patients are mildly agitated and easy to restrain. A waxing and waning state alternating between agitation and obtundation is characteristic. Inappropriate laughing, crying, or even singing may occur. Some patients express a feeling of imminent death. Absence status epilepticus is additionally characterized by reduction in vigilance rather than drowsiness. Attention is absent, and automatisms may occur. Complex status epilepticus can be characterized by hallucinations and a complete amnesia for the attacks.[17]

Focal Status Epilepticus

Focal status epilepticus can be simple (normal level of consciousness) or complex (impaired consciousness but no overt jerking). Focal status epilepticus is probably similar to epilepsia partialis continua. It involves continuous clonic movements of one or two extremities. Jerking of one arm or leg can be directly observed by the patient, who should be unable to influence its jerking frequency. Hemiparesis (which may last for days) may result if the condition is treated late. The disorder often is related to an acute hemispheric lesion (e.g., hemorrhage in cavernous hemangioma or metastasis, spontaneous lobar hematoma).

Psychogenic Status Epilepticus

Pseudoseizures can be very difficult to differentiate from true seizures and may occur comparatively frequently in patients with proven seizure disorder. The incidence was 40% in one referral hospital,[20] but this appears inflated. The assessment of psychogenic seizures can be complicated because previous indiscriminate administration of a benzodiazepine may cloud the neurologic assessment, and electroencephalography often is not immediately available to verify the psychiatric origin of the convulsions.

Several clinical characteristics should increase the likelihood of psychogenic status epilepticus.[21,22] Jerking movements are characteristically out of phase and asynchronous, with a highly typical forward thrusting of the pelvis. Screaming is common. Tongue biting is absent, pupils may be dilated but have retained light responses, and the gag reflex is present.[21–24] Jerking of the extremities may rapidly alternate in tonic-clonic-like movements, and often the arms can be positioned above the patient's face while continuously jerking without falling on the face. The head turns from side to side, and more characteristically, both eyes are consistently deviated from the examiner, occasionally switching with the examiner's position. In between the jerking movements, the patient may speak brief sentences indicating major distress.

All of these manifestations, although very characteristic, may rarely be imitated by nonconvulsive status epilepticus due to a frontal epileptic focus.

Myoclonus Status Epilepticus

Myoclonus status epilepticus is common in emergency departments admitting comatose patients after asphyxia or cardiac arrest. The clinical manifestations of myoclonus status epilepticus are vastly different, but it is still misinterpreted as tonic-clonic seizures.

Myoclonus status epilepticus often consists of synchronous brief jerking in the limbs and face and may involve the diaphragm. Touch, intubation, and placement of catheters may provoke the movements, but continuous jerking is more commonly the rule. An episodic upward gaze of both eyes during a series of myoclonic jerks is typical. Myoclonus status epilepticus can be seen moments after cardiac resuscitation when the pulse has returned and the patient has failed to awaken. Pathologic withdrawal or extensor motor responses are common. Its presence denotes massive laminar cortical necrosis, often in association with ischemic damage to the thalamus and spinal cord.

Other conditions that cause myoclonus status epilepticus, such as environmental injuries (e.g., electrical injury, decompression sickness), are related to severe global anoxia produced by the insult. However, profound myoclonus status epilepticus in comatose patients may be caused by drug intoxication (predominantly lithium but also haloperidol, antiepileptic agents, tricyclic antidepressants, and penicillin), toxic exposure to industrial agents (pesticides) and heavy metals, renal or hepatic failure, or a degenerative condition such as Creutzfeldt-Jakob disease in the final stage.

Neuroimaging in Status Epilepticus

Because withdrawal of antiepileptic drugs remains a commonly recognized cause in adults with a prior seizure disorder, computed tomography (CT) scan or magnetic resonance imaging (MRI) findings are frequently normal in status epilepticus. In refractory epilepsy, the rate of detection of histopathologically proven abnormalities (glioma, hippocampal sclerosis, developmental lesions) is 95% with conventional MRI and much lower with CT scan, with a sensitivity of 32%. CT scan sensitivity for temporal lobe abnormalities is very low.[25] However, CT or MRI may show acute destructive lesions, such as stroke or traumatic injury, metastatic disease, and glioma. CT scanning in myoclonus status epilepticus may show diffuse cerebral edema and, less often, thalamic or cerebral infarcts in watershed territories. An imaging study of cryptic seizures at the Mayo Clinic found mesial temporal sclerosis in 55%, brain tumor in 20%, nonspecific findings in 15%, and neuronal migration disorder, vascular malformation (Fig. 10.3), or head injury–associated sclerosis in 10%.[26] Focal hyperintensities on T_2-weighted images and decrease in apparent diffusion coefficients in complex partial status epilepticus—all reversible—may be seen as a consequence of edema associated with breakdown of the blood–brain barrier.[27] As alluded to earlier, hippocampus or neocortical dropout abnormalities may emerge later and may be a direct correlate of seizures and not of hypoxemia (Box 10.1, Fig. 10.4).[28,29]

Miscellaneous Tests

Physiologic changes are observed in the aftermath of status epilepticus. A single generalized tonic-clonic seizure may produce similar laboratory changes if values are obtained within 1 hour of presentation. Most laboratory changes directly resulting from seizures or status epilepticus are self-limiting and rarely need intervention. However, abnormal laboratory values may suggest a competing systemic illness.

White cell counts may increase up to $30 \times 10^9/L$.[33] Neutrophils usually remain dominant, but equally common is a lymphocyte increase in the differential count. Immature neutrophils can be present. Acute-phase hepatic proteins, glycoproteins, and globulins may transiently increase the erythrocyte sedimentation rate. Plasma glucose concentration may increase but remains in an indeterminate range of <150 mg/dL. Plasma osmolality should be normal or mildly increased

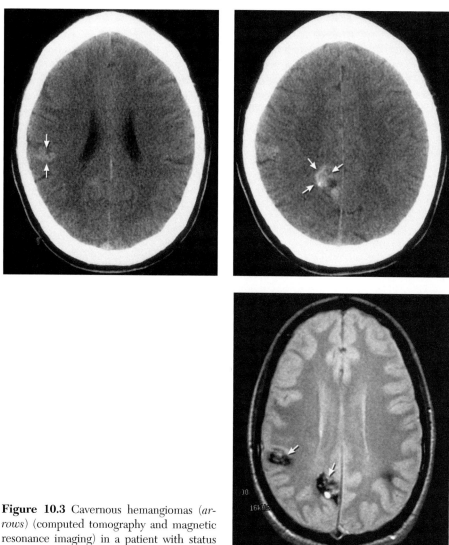

Figure 10.3 Cavernous hemangiomas (*arrows*) (computed tomography and magnetic resonance imaging) in a patient with status epilepticus at presentation.

in patients with dehydration but more significantly increased if recent alcohol abuse contributes to status epilepticus. Plasma osmolalities of 400–600 mOsm could be due to nonketotic hyperosmolar hyperglycemia. Hyponatremia may cause status epilepticus only when values are <120 mmol/L or have decreased at least 20–30 mmol/L within several hours.

Spontaneous hypoglycemia possibly indicates a poison (see Chapter 8) or, less commonly, insulinoma. Acute renal failure should point to possible rhabdomyolysis and prompt measurement of serum creatine kinase, which may reach values in the thousands.

Arterial blood gas should be measured. Respiratory acidosis is as common as metabolic lactic acidosis, but the pH is rarely below 7.0 (Table 10.2).[34] The abnormality is self-limiting and resolves within hours.[35] Cardiac arrhythmias, such as sinus tachycardia, bradycardia, and supraventricular tachycardia, are rarely related to changes in the blood gases. Abnormal QRS complexes are not a manifestation of status epilepticus.

Laboratory results may be helpful in distinguishing between status epilepticus and pseudoseizures. An entirely normal blood gas value while the patient is having convulsions supports pseudoseizures. The serum concentration of prolactin is

Convulsive status epilepticus may greatly increase the excitatory amino acid glutamate, which in turn opens cation channels to calcium through N-methyl-D-aspartate receptors ("excitotoxic theory"). Whether this damage, with a proclivity for the hippocampus, thalamus, cerebellum, and neocortex, is also caused by additional hyperglycemia, anoxia, hyperpyrexia, or severe acidosis in humans remains unresolved. Neuronal dropout in the neocortex is predominantly apparent in inappropriately treated or unrecognized long-standing status epilepticus. It can take the form of dramatic MR changes (arrows in Fig. 10.4). Hippocampal cell damage does not occur after single seizures or nonconvulsive status epilepticus,[30] but hippocampal edema has been demonstrated after febrile seizures.[31] Paradoxically, one study found that hypoxemia protects against edema, possibly because of an early adaptive response involving stress-related transcription factors.[32]

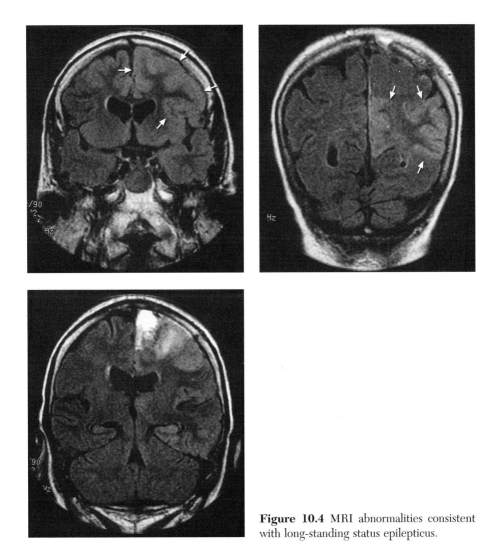

Figure 10.4 MRI abnormalities consistent with long-standing status epilepticus.

Table 10.2. Acid-Base Disorders Associated with Status Epilepticus

Derangement	Number of Patients	pH
Respiratory acidosis	10	7.10–7.25
Respiratory and metabolic acidosis	6	7.11–7.15
Metabolic acidosis	8	7.05–7.13
Respiratory alkalosis	8	7.51–7.55
Normal	6	7.35–7.45

Source: Modified from Wijdicks and Hubmayr.[34] By permission of Mayo Foundation for Medical Education and Research.

increased (peak value 15–20 minutes after onset of seizure) after a single epileptic generalized seizure but seldom after pseudoseizures.[36] However, the discriminatory value in pseudo-status epilepticus has been debated,[37] and prolactin may also be increased after syncope.[38]

In any new-onset status epilepticus, cerebrospinal fluid (CSF) examination should be strongly considered, to exclude acute bacterial meningitis and encephalitis. White blood cell counts in the CSF may increase from seizures but not above 30 mononuclear cells/mL, and CSF protein rarely increases significantly.

Electroencephalography is particularly useful to confirm focal status epilepticus and detect nonconvulsive status epilepticus. Electroencephalography may be helpful when the patient is sedated by antiepileptic drugs and clinical manifestations of electrographic discharges are difficult to detect.[39] The findings should guide further use of antiepileptic agents or an increase in dose until epileptic activity is entirely suppressed. The patterns are shown in Figure 10.5.

Violent seizures may cause bone fractures but also injury to the shoulder. Apart from the typical posterior dislocation (such a characteristic feature that when seen by an orthopedic surgeon should result in referral to a neurologist for possible seizures), tendon injury may cause prolonged shoulder pain. Plain shoulder overviews are normal and in sharp contrast with abnormal MRI findings (Fig. 10.6).

Management of Status Epilepticus

Not only do patients with status epilepticus urgently need antiepileptic agents to reduce morbidity from injurious seizure activity but also the systemic effects are potentially harmful and may evolve into a complex medical emergency. It is important to immediately ventilate with oxygen, secure instruments to intubate quickly, and obtain intravenous access (Box 10.2).

Aspiration is very common in status epilepticus and may be the overriding cause of hypoxemia at presentation. In patients with altered pulmonary defenses, such as those with chronic obstructive pulmonary disease or alcohol abuse, pneumonia develops rapidly. Food particles may obstruct large airways and cause atelectasis and hypoxemia. Adult respiratory failure may follow rapidly and actually evolve in the emergency department. Dyspnea is profound from alveolar flooding, hypoxemia worsens within minutes, and patients with underlying chronic pulmonary disease have hypercapnia as well. These patients need intubation for airway protection and possibly fiberoptic bronchoscopy if early chest X-ray findings so indicate. Aspiration pneumonitis (Mendelson's syndrome) may be due to sterile gastric contents causing chemical injury. Empiric antibiotics are recommended (levofloxacin 500 mg/day, infusion over 1 hour).[43] Neurogenic pulmonary edema from status epilepticus is uncommon but has been linked to sudden death, mostly in children and young adults. Chest X-ray findings are typically widespread "whiteout" infiltrates but resolve after several hours of positive end-expiratory pressure ventilation.

Cardiac arrhythmias may appear only if continuous seizures have resulted in prolonged significant lactic acidosis. Many patients have sinus tachycardia from the sympathetic overdrive state. Only cardiac arrhythmias causing measurable blood pressure reduction need correction with antiarrhythmic agents and bicarbonate infusion. Overzealous use of bicarbonate may cause alkalosis, which may perpetuate status epilepticus by lowering the seizure threshold.

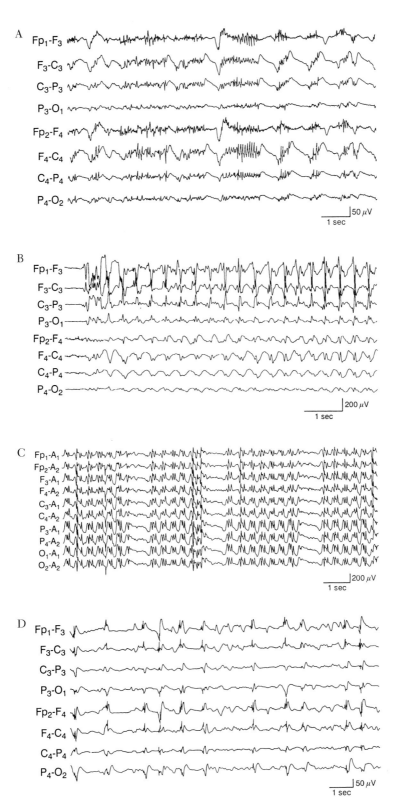

Figure 10.5 Electroencephalographic patterns of different types of status epilepticus. *A:* Generalized tonic-clonic seizures (generalized high-frequency spikes and spike-and-wave discharges). *B:* Focal status epilepticus (rhythmic waves and spikes in one hemisphere). *C:* Non-convulsive status epilepticus (episodes of spike-and-wave discharges coinciding with obtundation). *D:* Myoclonic status epilepticus (continuous epileptiform discharges with a burst-suppression pattern).

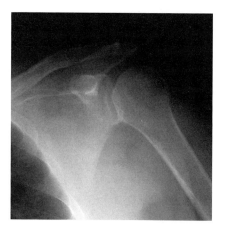
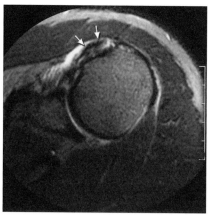
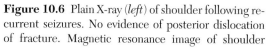

Figure 10.6 Plain X-ray (*left*) of shoulder following recurrent seizures. No evidence of posterior dislocation of fracture. Magnetic resonance image of shoulder

(*right*) shows capsular edema, tear of the posterior labrum, and partial injury to subscapularis and biceps tendon.

Creatine kinase should be measured in each patient because rhabdomyolysis may result in acute renal failure, which can be entirely prevented by liberal intake of fluids.

The sequence of use of antiepileptic agents in status epilepticus continues to evolve.[8] When patients with status epilepticus are referred to large institutions, approximately 30% have a recurrence of seizure after phenytoin loading, and seizures recurred in 40% of patients after a third-line agent. This demonstrates more difficult control with increasing duration. Morbidity will be substantial.[44] An approach with additional precautionary measures is shown in Figure 10.7. Lorazepam 4 mg bolus is more effective than phenytoin for initial therapy.[45] Up to 90% of patients are successfully managed with a combination of benzodiazepines and phenytoin.[46,47] Failure to control seizures probably is related to inappropriate phenytoin loading (the popular "1 g of phenytoin" is almost always inadequate) and to failure to appreciate that a second intravenous bolus of phenytoin may abort status epilepticus. A common sequence is phenytoin (Boxes 10.3, 10.4), midazolam or propofol[49–53] (Boxes 10.5, 10.6), and pentobarbital and phenobarbital (Box 10.7). Newer drugs are ketamine (2 mg/kg bolus, 10–50 mg/kg per minute) or topiramate (300–1600 mg/day) and have aborted status epilepticus when all else fails.[64,65] In addition, inhalation anesthetics can be used. Both isoflurane

and desflurane are effective in controlling electroencephalographic activity, but improvement of the patient is rarely encountered.[66]

A particularly difficult situation is created by epilepsia partialis continua. Treatment is phenytoin loading followed by increasing doses of phenobarbital, starting with 40 mg or, in resistant cases, with intravenous administration of valproate (20 mg/min bolus and 20–50 mg/min infusion).[67] In our experience, focal seizures are commonly treated well with valproate without need for endotracheal intubation due to respiratory depression. If valproate fails, additional doses of phenobarbital can be infused and could achieve control or at least a considerable decrease in manifestations.

Nonconvulsive status epilepticus, when documented by electroencephalography, can be treated under electroencephalographic monitoring with benzodiazepines (lorazepam, 4–8 mg, or diazepam, 10 mg).

The management of seizures in patients with preeclampsia is notably different. Magnesium sulfate remains the standard in prevention and treatment of seizures or status epilepticus.[68,69] Magnesium sulfate is given at a beginning dose of 4–5 g intravenously or 10 g intramuscularly.[70] An intravenous infusion of 1 g/hour is started. Additional antiepileptic agents are not warranted and may cause respiratory depression in the newborn. Magnesium toxicity may, however, also reduce

Box 10.2. No Intravenous Access

Lack of intravenous access can be anticipated in long-term users of intravenous drugs. Intramuscular administration of fosphenytoin (12–20 mg/kg phenytoin equivalent) produces plasma concentrations of phenytoin equal to those with the oral dose within 30 minutes of administration, divided over different ejection sites. If intramuscular fosphenytoin is not available, diazepam should be used rectally (0.5 mg/kg) in repeated doses. Other options are intramuscular use of midazolam (5 mg) and observation for 3 minutes to allow absorption. Alternatively, the intranasal route can be considered for midazolam, with rapid absorption (within minutes, 0.1–0.2 mg/kg).[40–42] Probably the last resort but the most effective way to counter status epilepticus is to use inhalation anesthetic agents. This should be followed by a saphenous vein cutdown at the ankle. The superficial location of the vein and large diameter make it suitable for placement of a large-bore cannula. Phenytoin can then be administered. Administration of isoflurane is started at 0.5% inspired concentration, with a gradual increase while end-tidal concentrations are monitored until a seizure-free electroencephalogram is obtained. Blood pressure most likely requires support with fluid infusions, the Trendelenburg position, and dopamine, phenylephrine, or dobutamine.

mother and child respirations. Reduced tendon reflexes may occur and may indicate imminent toxicity; thus, they are a useful monitoring sign during titration of treatment.

Antiepileptic therapy in myoclonus status epilepticus is usually not effective after cardiac arrest. Clonazepam has been advocated for treatment but has not been consistently effective in our experience. There is no rationale to aggressively treat these myoclonic jerks with a series of antiepileptic drugs. When myoclonus is forceful and causes marked contractions, even hampering

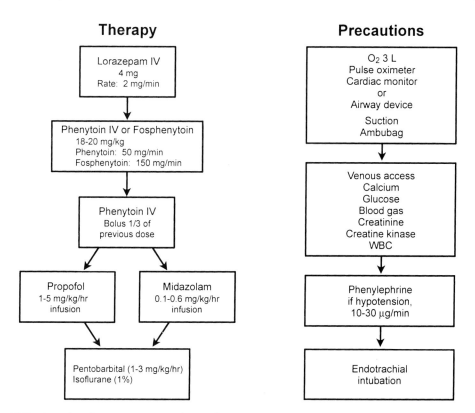

Figure 10.7 Algorithm for management of convulsive status epilepticus. IV, intravenous; WBC, white blood cells.

Box 10.3. Phenytoin

Phenytoin is rapidly distributed to body tissue and the brain. Respiratory depression does not occur in loading doses of 10–20 mg/kg. Sinus bradycardia is the most common cardiac arrhythmia. Transient diastolic pauses may occur and may worsen any heart block. Asystole has been reported. Phenytoin can be mixed only in isotonic saline because it precipitates in glucose. Oral dosage should resume 6–12 hours after infusion.

Box 10.4. Fosphenytoin

Fosphenytoin sodium (Cerebyx) is a prodrug of phenytoin that is rapidly (within minutes) converted by enzymes to phenytoin. Both intravenous and intramuscular administrations of 15–20 mg/kg produce therapeutic total ($\geq$10 μg/mL) and free ($\geq$1 μg/mL) plasma levels. Intramuscular loading (9–12 mg/kg phenytoin equivalent) produces therapeutic levels in 1 hour and can be considered in status epilepticus but only if intravenous access is not available. Fosphenytoin is completely water-soluble. Therefore, phlebitis, hypotension, and cardiac arrhythmias, typically associated with the propylene glycol–based intravenous phenytoin, are infrequent. However, cardiac arrhythmias may still occur when fosphenytoin is infused at rates >150 mg/minute. There is no pharmacokinetic drug interaction with intravenously administered diazepam or lorazepam. Major side effects are nystagmus, headache, ataxia, and drowsiness. Previously unrecognized and highly typical side effects (up to 30%) are transient but very annoying paresthesias and itching in the groin, genitalia, and head and neck.[48]

Box 10.5. Midazolam

It is not clear why midazolam works when benzodiazepines and phenytoin fail to control seizures. The drug is currently also being evaluated for initial management in outpatients.[54] The half-life of midazolam (1–12 hours) is less than that of lorazepam (10–12 hours), and midazolam produces sedation of short duration in status epilepticus. Hourly infusion of 0.1–0.6 mg/kg should be continued for at least 12 hours before the dose is tapered. The cost, comparable with that of lorazepam, is high, approaching $800 for 24 hours of continuous infusion. The absence of propylene glycol solution in midazolam reduces the risk of hypotension, bradycardia, and electrocardiographic changes, which are more common with diazepam and lorazepam.[55] High rates of infusion may produce cardiac depression and hypotension. Often, the mean dose to abolish seizure activity is three times the starting dose. When administration is discontinued, full consciousness is expected in 4–5 hours in most patients.[56–62]

Box 10.6. Propofol

Propofol has been considered controversial because of its association with myoclonic jerking and opisthotonos in humans. However, several studies have confirmed that it inhibits seizure activity. These animal studies included lidocaine-induced seizure activity or pentylenetetrazol-induced epilepsy. Propofol has been used in anesthetic doses to control status epilepticus and has reduced the risk of prolonged seizures in electroconvulsive therapy. A bolus of propofol may cause significant hypotension and is ill-advised. Only case series exist, but clinical experience is very favorable, with good control (1–5 mg/kg/hour). Bradycardia, hypotension, and lactic acidosis are side effects. The caloric intake with propofol is enormous.

Box 10.7. Barbiturates

Failure to control seizures with therapeutic levels of phenytoin (≥25 μg/mL) may justify intravenous administration of phenobarbital. Phenobarbital is much more potent than pentobarbital. Its major drawbacks are direct myocardial depression and vascular dilatation, but these are not treatment-limiting. Phenobarbital also has a very long elimination half-life (24–140 hours) but zero-order elimination at high doses (constant amount of drug elimination per unit of time).

Intravenous pentobarbital (1–3 mg/kg per hour) virtually always controls status epilepticus, but relapse can be substantial, usually preceded by electrographic recurrence of seizure activity.[63] Pentobarbital and phenobarbital are equal in effectiveness. Experience with propofol and midazolam will reduce the use of barbiturates greatly, but barbiturates remain very useful also in partial status epilepticus.

normal ventilator cycling, propofol is needed (starting dose of 0.5 mg/kg per hour with 0.5 mg/kg per hour increments to effect) and is commonly successful. If myoclonus still cannot be controlled, neuromuscular blocking agents should be considered to eliminate the constant generalized jerks until the level of care has been assessed.

Psychogenic epilepticus typically lasts longer but may be aborted almost instantaneously with a supportive suggestion. The diagnosis can be confirmed by an electroencephalogram, but the jerking movements are often so bizarre that it is clear from the outset. A recent study found that psychogenic status epilepticus could be rapidly induced by administering saline intravenously and telling the patients (some of whom had visited many different emergency departments) that the saline solution will provoke seizures.[71] However, the use of these deceptive provocative techniques is ethically questionable.[72]

Management of Recurrent Seizures

A clinical policy for the initial approach to patients with a seizure who do not have status epilepticus has been published by the American College of Emergency Physicians.[73] Four major guidelines are highlighted. First, prolonged altered consciousness should not be attributed to a postictal state. Second, patients with prior epilepsy who are alert and have normal findings on neurologic examination do not require aggressive evaluation other than measurement of antiepileptic drug levels. Third, alcohol-related seizures may indicate serious underlying morbidity. Fourth, the patient should be implicitly told that driving and opera-

tion of machines should be restricted until a reasonable observation period has passed, to prevent future disasters.

Approximately 75% of patients with two or three unprovoked seizures have further seizures within 4 years.[74] In contrast, the risk of a second seizure is approximately 35% in the subsequent 3–5 years.[75] The risk of seizure recurrence is substantially increased (probably doubled) when an identifiable brain lesion is found.

Before a patient is sent out of the emergency department, several diagnostic tests should be done (Table 10.3); but in many instances, admission for intravenous phenytoin loading is advised. The above data suggest treatment in patients with two or more unprovoked seizures.

The recommended drugs for primary generalized tonic-clonic seizures or partial seizures with secondary generalization are phenytoin (300 mg/day in one dose; therapeutic level, 10–20 μg/mL), carbamazepine (300–1200 mg daily; therapeutic level, 4–12 μg/mL), and valproate (600–3000 mg/day; therapeutic level, 50–150 μg/mL). Valproate has notable side effects, particularly platelet dyscrasias and liver failure (1 in 20,000).[76] The first-line agent for absence seizures is valproate

Table 10.3. Diagnostic Tests in Recurrent de Novo Seizures

Computed tomographic scan with contrast
Cervical spine radiograph (if trauma is suspected)
Cerebrospinal fluid (predominantly in immunosuppressed patients, human immunodeficiency virus)
Toxicologic screen, alcohol level
Sodium, calcium, magnesium, blood urea nitrogen, creatinine, complete blood cell count, glucose

(600–3000 mg/day; therapeutic level, 50–150 μg/mL), ethosuximide (20–30 mg/kg per day; therapeutic level, 40–100 μg/mL), or lamotrigine (100–400 mg/day in 2 divided doses). A combination of lamotrigine and valproate is often needed to control recurrent absences.

An alternative medication, mostly if seizures occur with first-line agents at therapeutic levels, could be gabapentin (900 mg/day in three gradually increasing doses) or other second-line antiepileptic drugs (e.g., lamotrigine, topiramate, tiagabine, or levetiracetam).

Specific concerns may arise when seizures are observed during pregnancy without evidence of eclampsia. Antiepileptic drugs for brief treatment of recurrent seizures should be well tolerated when pregnancy is beyond the first trimester and the risk to the infant seems unsubstantiated. Antiepileptic drugs in pregnancy double the risk of congenital malformations, including limb deformities, spina bifida (valproate), and growth retardation. Folic acid, 0.4 mg/day, should be added during pregnancy, but its effect on reducing birth defects probably takes place around conception.[77] Monitoring phenytoin levels in pregnancy is complicated by a decrease in serum albumin levels; thus, the unbound fraction should be measured to manage dosage. In addition, the increased volume of distribution and increased clearance by liver and placenta may force an increase in the total daily dose.

Discontinuation of antiepileptic therapy is considered after a 2-year seizure-free interval, and if this can be achieved, recurrence is very low except in patients with documented brain lesions (e.g., cavernous angioma, cerebral contusion). Sudden withdrawal may increase the risk of recurrence and, in some instances, unfortunately, status epilepticus. Recurrence of seizures cannot be entirely excluded by a normal electroencephalogram before discontinuation is attempted.

REFERENCES

1. Scholtes FB, Renier WO, Meinardi H: Generalized convulsive status epilepticus: causes, therapy, and outcome in 346 patients. *Epilepsia* 35:1104, 1994.
2. Towne AR, Pellock JM, Ko D, et al.: Determinants of mortality in status epilepticus. *Epilepsia* 35:27, 1994.
3. Treiman DM: Generalized convulsive status epilepticus in the adult. *Epilepsia* 34(Suppl 1):S2, 1993.
4. Cascino GD: Generalized convulsive status epilepticus. *Mayo Clin Proc* 71:787, 1996.
5. Gemma M, Cipriani A, Mungo M: Management of status epilepticus. *Intensive Care Med* 20:611, 1994.
6. Runge JW, Allen FH: Emergency treatment of status epilepticus. *Neurology* 46(Suppl 1):S20, 1996.
7. Claasen J, Hirsch LJ, Emerson RG, et al.: Treatment of refractory status epilepticus with pentobarbital, propofol, or midazolam: a systematic review. *Epilepsia* 43:146, 2002.
8. Lawn ND, Wijdicks EFM: Progress in clinical neurosciences. Status epilepticus: a critical review of management options. *Can J Neurol Sci* 29:206, 2002.
9. DeLorenzo RJ, Hauser WA, Towne AR, et al.: A prospective, population-based epidemiologic study of status epilepticus in Richmond, Virginia. *Neurology* 46:1029, 1996.
10. Lowenstein DH, Alldredge BK: Status epilepticus at an urban public hospital in the 1980s. *Neurology* 43:483, 1993.
11. Sung CY, Chu NS: Status epilepticus in the elderly: etiology, seizure type and outcome. *Acta Neurol Scand* 80:51, 1989.
12. Alldredge BK, Lowenstein DH: Status epilepticus related to alcohol abuse. *Epilepsia* 34:1033, 1993.
13. Fagan KJ, Lee SI: Prolonged confusion following convulsions due to generalized nonconvulsive status epilepticus. *Neurology* 40:1689, 1990.
14. Kaplan PW: Nonconvulsive status epilepticus in the emergency room. *Epilepsia* 37:643, 1996.
15. Baykan B, Gokyigit A, Gurses C, et al.: Recurrent absence status epilepticus: clinical and EEG characteristics. *Seizure* 11:310, 2002.
16. Agathonikou A, Panayiotopoulos CP, Giannakodimos S, et al.: Typical absence status in adults: diagnostic and syndromic considerations. *Epilepsia* 39:1265, 1998.
17. Cockerell OC, Walker MC, Sander JW, et al.: Complex partial status epilepticus: a recurrent problem. *J Neurol Neurosurg Psychiatry* 57:835, 1994.
18. Trinka E, Dilitz E, Unterberger I, et al.: Non-convulsive status epilepticus after replacement of valproate with lamotrigine. *J Neurol* 249:1417, 2002.
19. Husain AM, Horn GJ, Jacobson MP: Non-convulsive status epilepticus: usefulness of clinical features in selecting patients for urgent EEG. *J Neurol Neurosurg Psychiatry* 74:189, 2003.
20. Howell SJ, Owen L, Chadwick DW: Pseudostatus epilepticus. *Q J Med* 71:507, 1989.
21. Rosenberg ML: The eyes in hysterical states of unconsciousness. *J Clin Neuroophthalmol* 2:259, 1982.
22. Shen W, Bowman ES, Markand ON: Presenting the diagnosis of pseudoseizure. *Neurology* 40:756, 1990.
23. Jagoda A, Richey-Klein V, Riggio S: Psychogenic status epilepticus. *J Emerg Med* 13:31, 1995.
24. King DW, Gallagher BB, Murvin AJ, et al.: Pseudoseizures: diagnostic evaluation. *Neurology* 32:18, 1982.
25. Bronen RA, Fulbright RK, Spencer DD, et al.: Refractory epilepsy: comparison of MR imaging, CT, and histopathologic findings in 117 patients. *Radiology* 201:97, 1996.

26. Jack CR Jr: Magnetic resonance imaging in epilepsy. *Mayo Clin Proc* 71:695, 1996.

27. Calistri V, Caramia F, Bianco F, et al. Visualization of evolving status epilepticus with diffusion and perfusion MR imaging. *Am J Neuroradiol* 24:671, 2003.

28. Meierkord H, Wieshmann U, Niehaus L, et al.: Structural consequences of status epilepticus demonstrated with serial magnetic resonance imaging. *Acta Neurol Scand* 96:127, 1997.

29. Tien RD, Felsberg GJ: The hippocampus in status epilepticus: demonstration of signal intensity and morphologic changes with sequential fast spin-echo MR imaging. *Radiology* 194:249, 1995.

30. Bertram EH, Lothman EW, Lenn NJ: The hippocampus in experimental chronic epilepsy: a morphometric analysis. *Ann Neurol* 27:43, 1990.

31. Scott RC, Gadian DG, King MD, et al.: Magnetic resonance imaging findings within 5 days of status epilepticus in childhood. *Brain* 125:1951, 2002.

32. Emerson MR, Nelson SR, Samson FE, et al.: Hypoxia preconditioning attenuates brain edema associated with kainic acid-induced status epilepticus in rats. *Brain Res* 825:189, 1999.

33. Barry E, Hauser WA: Pleocytosis after status epilepticus. *Arch Neurol* 51:190, 1994.

34. Wijdicks EFM, Hubmayr RD: Acute acid-base disorders associated with status epilepticus. *Mayo Clin Proc* 69:1044, 1994.

35. Yaffe K, Lowenstein DH: Prognostic factors of pentobarbital therapy for refractory generalized status epilepticus. *Neurology* 43:895, 1993.

36. Laxer KD, Mullooly JP, Howell B: Prolactin changes after seizures classified by EEG monitoring. *Neurology* 35:31, 1985.

37. Tomson T, Lindbom U, Nilsson BY, et al.: Serum prolactin during status epilepticus. *J Neurol Neurosurg Psychiatry* 52:1435, 1989.

38. Oribe E, Amini R, Nissenbaum E, et al.: Serum prolactin concentrations are elevated after syncope. *Neurology* 47:60, 1996.

39. Privitera MD, Strawsburg RH: Electroencephalographic monitoring in the emergency department. *Emerg Med Clin North Am* 12:1089, 1994.

40. Kendall JL, Reynolds M, Goldberg R: Intranasal midazolam in patients with status epilepticus. *Ann Emerg Med* 29:415, 1997.

41. Kofke WA, Young RS, Davis P, et al.: Isoflurane for refractory status epilepticus: a clinical series. *Anesthesiology* 71:653, 1989.

42. Rey E, Delaunay L, Pons G, et al.: Pharmacokinetics of midazolam in children: comparative study of intranasal and intravenous administration. *Eur J Clin Pharmacol* 41:355, 1991.

43. Marik PE. Aspiration pneumonitis and aspiration pneumonia. *N Engl J Med* 344:665, 2001.

44. Mayer SA, Claassen J, Lokin J, et al.: Refractory status epilepticus: frequency, risk factors, and impact on outcome. *Arch Neurol* 59:205, 2002.

45. Treiman DM, Meyers PD, Walton NY, et al.: A comparison of four treatments for generalized convulsive status epilepticus. *N Engl J Med* 339:792, 1998.

46. Mitchell WG: Status epilepticus and acute repetitive seizures in children, adolescents, and young adults: etiology, outcome, and treatment. *Epilepsia* 37(Suppl 1):S74, 1996.

47. Weise KL, Bleck TP: Status epilepticus in children and adults. *Crit Care Clin* 13:629, 1997.

48. Browne TR: Fosphenytoin (Cerebyx). *Clin Neuropharmacol* 20:1, 1997.

49. Borgeat A, Wilder-Smith OH, Jallon P, et al.: Propofol in the management of refractory status epilepticus: a case report. *Intensive Care Med* 20:148, 1994.

50. Kuisma M, Roine RO: Propofol in pre-hospital treatment of convulsive status epilepticus. *Epilepsia* 36:1241, 1995.

51. Mackenzie SJ, Kapadia F, Grant IS: Propofol infusion for control of status epilepticus. *Anaesthesia* 45:1043, 1990.

52. Pitt-Miller PL, Elcock BJ, Maharaj M: The management of status epilepticus with a continuous propofol infusion. *Anesth Analg* 78:1193, 1994.

53. Stecker MM, Kramer TH, Raps EC, et al.: Treatment of refractory status epilepticus with propofol: clinical and pharmacokinetic findings. *Epilepsia* 39:18, 1998.

54. LeDuc TJ, Goellner WE, el-Sanadi N: Out-of-hospital midazolam for status epilepticus. *Ann Emerg Med* 28:377, 1996.

55. Labar DR, Ali A, Root J: High-dose intravenous lorazepam for the treatment of refractory status epilepticus. *Neurology* 44:1400, 1994.

56. Crisp CB, Gannon R, Knauft F: Continuous infusion of midazolam hydrochloride to control status epilepticus. *Clin Pharmacol Ther* 7:322, 1988.

57. Jawad S, Oxley J, Wilson J, et al.: A pharmacodynamic evaluation of midazolam as an antiepileptic compound. *J Neurol Neurosurg Psychiatry* 49:1050, 1986.

58. Kumar A, Bleck TP: Intravenous midazolam for the treatment of refractory status epilepticus. *Crit Care Med* 20:483, 1992.

59. Lal Koul R, Raj Aithala G, Chacko A, et al.: Continuous midazolam infusion as treatment of status epilepticus. *Arch Dis Child* 76:445, 1997.

60. Mayhue FE: IM midazolam for status epilepticus in the emergency department. *Ann Emerg Med* 17:643, 1988.

61. Nordt SP, Clark RF: Midazolam: a review of therapeutic uses and toxicity. *J Emerg Med* 15:357, 1997.

62. Parent JM, Lowenstein DH: Treatment of refractory generalized status epilepticus with continuous infusion of midazolam. *Neurology* 44:1837, 1994.

63. Krishnamurthy KB, Drislane FW: Relapse and survival after barbiturate anesthetic treatment of refractory status epilepticus. *Epilepsia* 37:863, 1996.

64. Sheth RD, Gidal BE: Refractory status epilepticus: response to ketamine. *Neurology* 51:1765, 1998.

65. Towne AR, Garnett LK, Waterhouse EJ, et al.: The use of topiramate in refractory status epilepticus. *Neurology* 60:332, 2003.

66. Sharpe MD, Young GB, Mirsattari S, et al.: Prolonged desflurane administration for refractory status epilepticus. *Anesthesiology* 87:261, 2002.

67. Kaplan PW: Intravenous valproate treatment of generalized nonconvulsive status epilepticus. *Clin Electroencephalogr* 30:1, 1999.

68. Crowther C: Magnesium sulphate versus diazepam in the management of eclampsia: a randomized controlled trial. *Br J Obstet Gynaecol* 97:110, 1990.

69. Belfort MA, Anthony J, Saade GR, et al.: A comparison of magnesium sulfate and nimodipine for the prevention of eclampsia. *N Engl J Med* 348:304, 2003.

70. Lucas MJ, Leveno KJ, Cunningham FG: A comparison of magnesium sulfate with phenytoin for the prevention of eclampsia. *N Engl J Med* 333:201, 1995.

71. Ney GC, Zimmerman C, Schaul N: Psychogenic status epilepticus induced by a provocative technique. *Neurology* 46:546, 1996.

72. Cohen RJ, Suter C: Hysterical seizures: suggestion as a provocative EEG test. *Ann Neurol* 11:391, 1982.

73. American College of Emergency Physicians: Clinical policy for the initial approach to patients presenting with a chief complaint of seizure who are not in status epilepticus. *Ann Emerg Med* 29:706, 1997.

74. First Seizure Trial Group: Randomized clinical trial on the efficacy of antiepileptic drugs in reducing the risk of relapse after a first unprovoked tonic-clonic seizure. *Neurology* 43:478, 1993.

75. Hauser WA, Rich SS, Lee JR, et al.: Risk of recurrent seizures after two unprovoked seizures. *N Engl J Med* 338:429, 1998.

76. Perucca E: Pharmacological and therapeutic properties of valproate: a summary after 35 years of clinical experience. *CNS Drugs* 16:695, 2002.

77. Samren EB, van Duijn CM, Christiaens GC, et al.: Antiepileptic drug regimens and major congenital abnormalities in the offspring. *Ann Neurol* 46:739, 1999.

Chapter 11
Acute Obstructive Hydrocephalus

The cerebrospinal fluid (CSF) is produced in the choroid plexus of the lateral ventricle; circulated throughout a system with critical passages at the foramen of Monro, third ventricle, and aqueduct of Sylvius; and absorbed through arachnoid villi. Any impingement at these sites causes increased hydrostatic pressure in a matter of hours (Box 11.1). Enlargement of the ventricular system may be acutely created by a mass obstructing CSF outflow or by sudden stretching and ballooning out from introduction of a jet of arterial blood. Only ventriculostomy results in adequate diversion of flow and, in fact, may be lifesaving.

There is an urgency when patients present with acute hydrocephalus in the emergency department. This chapter describes clinical presentation, causes, and shunt placement. Definitive management, carefully planned later, could imply resection or debulking of the tumor or permanent placement of a ventriculoperitoneal shunt.

Clinical Presentation

Patients with acute obstructive hydrocephalus have diminished alertness at presentation. Often in retrospect, episodes of headache are said to have been common and frequently intense. Earlier periods of blurred vision and obscuration (sudden grayouts or blackouts lasting seconds) associated with papilledema (due to pressure-induced relative ischemia of the optic nerve) are

reported.[2] Papilledema may occur, implying long-standing increased CSF pressure, but remains an uncommon clinical finding in most intraventricular, pineal, or choroid plexus tumors. Unfortunately, the diagnosis in some patients is made only after symptoms and signs referable to brain stem compression or brain stem shift have occurred.

Decreased consciousness from ventricular enlargement may have several mechanisms. First, hydrocephalus may impair the ascending reticular activating system (ARAS) at the level of the periaqueduct, which pushes against relay nuclei and fibers of the ARAS when it expands. Second, displacement of the upper brain stem by a massively enlarged third ventricle may tilt it backward and kink its structure. Third, when intracranial pressure from increased ventricular pressure rises above the cerebral perfusion pressure, and certainly when the increase in pressure occurs rapidly, global ischemic damage to both hemispheres or herniation of brain tissue bilaterally through the tentorium or foramen magnum produces an advanced stage of coma. Fourth, and by an indirect mechanism, decreased arousal may also be caused by tumor infiltration into paramedian thalamic nuclei or the mesencephalon, which at the same time obstructs normal CSF flow (see Chapter 8). Finally, tumors that obstruct the ventricles may produce clinical signs from compression by the mass effect itself to the brain stem (e.g., pinealoma). These signs may combine to form Parinaud's syndrome, consisting of upward gaze

Box 11.1. Pathophysiology of Acute Hydrocephalus

Acute hydrocephalus occurs when normal physiologic equilibrium is disturbed. CSF (an ultrafiltrate from capillaries) is produced in the choroid plexus and may increase in the plexus papilloma. The circulation of CSF depends on several variables, such as rate of production (400–600 mL/day), choroid plexus pulsations (filling of choroid plexus with each arterial pulse generates a pumping force), resistance (series of conduits, including foramina, aqueduct of Sylvius, and arachnoid villi), and sagittal sinus pressure (CSF pressure is greater, and flow depends on this pressure gradient). Absorption is linearly related to CSF pressure. Some of the CSF is merely recycled.[1] Reduction in CSF volume therefore may be achieved by decreasing CSF production (carbonic anhydrate inhibitors; acetazolamide, which takes hours to achieve the effect), removing obstructing tumor, and improving absorption (e.g., corticosteroids to reduce inflammatory response in arachnoid villi). Enlargement of the ventricles is incremental, with elevation of the corpus callosum after dilation of the lateral ventricles and eventually reduction of the convexity gray matter.

palsy and impaired convergence, with a so-called light-near dissociation of the pupillary light reflex (pupil constriction to accommodation and not to light).[2] The lesion for the classic finding of Parinaud's syndrome is in the dorsal midbrain (pretectum) and interrupts the supranuclear mechanisms for upward gaze. However, the dorsal midbrain can also be distorted by enlargement of the posterior third ventricle and periaqueductal structures.

Pineal gland tumors may directly compress the midbrain, and compression may persist despite CSF diversion methods. Colloid cysts are incidentally found, but they obstruct the foramen of Monro only after reaching a critical size. Intermittent headaches may precede acute deterioration, which can lead to sudden brain death.

Specific Disorders Associated with Acute Hydrocephalus

In a large proportion of patients, the cause of acute hydrocephalus in adults seen in the emergency department is ventricular dilatation associated with subarachnoid hemorrhage, lobar hematoma, primary intraventricular hemorrhage, or, less commonly, malfunctioning ventriculolumbar or peritoneal shunts for previous hydrocephalus. The causes of acute hydrocephalus associated with masses in adults are shown in Table 11.1.[3–14]

Intracranial Hematoma

Primary intraventricular hemorrhage commonly causes acute hydrocephalus, although a more delayed course has been noted. Usually, the hemorrhage is massive (Fig. 11.1A, see also Chapter 14). Intraventricular introduction of a thalamic, caudate, or large lobar hematoma produces acute ventricular enlargement. Acute hemorrhage in the cerebellum, particularly when it extends to the vermis, may rapidly block the fourth ventricle, leading to obstructive hydrocephalus (Fig. 11.1B).

Hydrocephalus in intracerebral hematoma is an independent predictor of poor outcome.[15–17] In addition, one study seriously questioned the use of ventriculostomy in parenchymal supratentorial hemorrhage.[18] Ventricular drainage controlled intracranial pressure but did not consistently improve level of consciousness, suggesting direct irreversible tissue damage from hydrocephalus. Moreover, hemorrhagic dilatation of the fourth ventricle has been identified as an important indicator of poor outcome, confirming the impression that sudden massive enlargement causes damage to the periaqueductal area.[19]

Acute hydrocephalus in pontine hemorrhage is merely a consequence of its destructive hemorrhage, and ventriculostomy will not reverse coma. Extension to the mesencephalon and occasionally bilaterally to the thalamus precludes awakening. (After several unsuccessful attempts in our patients, we generally have abandoned ventriculostomy in this condition.)

Cerebellar hematoma and acute hydrocephalus can be treated by ventriculostomy when the fourth ventricle is blocked and no brain stem compression is evident on computed tomographic (CT) scans. Only in this particular clinical situa-

Table 11.1. Masses Causing Acute Obstructive Hydrocephalus

Type	CT Scan Characteristics	Treatment
Intraventricular tumors		
Colloid cyst	Rounded, anterior 3V, widened SP, collapse of posterior 3V, ID or HYP	Surgery or stereotactic aspiration
Plexus papilloma	Oval, 4V, LV, HYP	Total excision
Ependymoma	Lobulated, 4V, LV, ID	Excision and radiotherapy
Oligodendroglioma	Lobulated, LV, HYP, C	Resection
Ganglioglioma	3V, ID, HYP	Resection
Astrocytoma	LV, HD or HYP, irregular shape	Radiation, resection
Epidermoid cyst	4V, HYP, ID	Resection
Masses in pineal region		
Pineoblastoma	Lobulated, HD at peripheral rim, C	Resection, radiation
Germinoma	ID, rounded	Radiation
Teratoma	HD or HYP, C, lipid content	Resection
Vein of Galen aneurysm	HYP, rounded, triangular	Endovascular occlusion

C, calcifications; CT, computed tomography; HD, hypodense; HYP, hyperdense; ID, isodense; LV, lateral ventricle; SP, septum pellucidum; 3V, third ventricle; 4V, fourth ventricle.

tion can ventriculostomy be beneficial; in all other instances, decompression of the pons by suboccipital craniotomy is more logical.

Aneurysmal Subarachnoid Hemorrhage

CT scan evidence of acute hydrocephalus is common in aneurysmal subarachnoid hemorrhage (Fig. 11.2). Acute hydrocephalus may be caused by obstruction of CSF outflow at the level of the ambient cisterns, by clogging of the arachnoid space with subarachnoid blood, or occasionally from the mass effect of a giant aneurysm obstructing the third ventricle.[20] Commonly, the temporal horns are dilated early, typically before identifiable dilatation of the third and lateral ventricles. Ventriculostomy is certainly justified when clinical worsening in level of consciousness is clearly documented, when serial CT scans unmistakably demonstrate further enlargement, or when the third ventricle has changed into a balloon-shaped structure. One may argue that

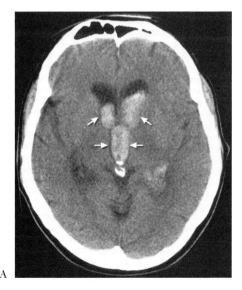
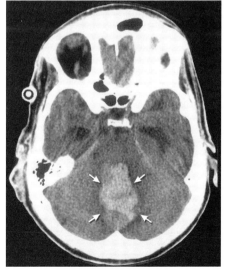

A   B

Figure 11.1 *A:* Acute hydrocephalus in intraventricular hemorrhage due to sudden arterial jet of blood (*arrows*). *B:* Acute hydrocephalus (note enlarged temporal horns) associated with cerebellar hematoma effacing the fourth ventricle (*arrows*).

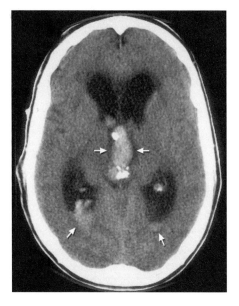

Figure 11.2 Acute hydrocephalus in subarachnoid hemorrhage with intraventricular blood (third ventricle and posterior horns, *arrows*) from ruptured anterior cerebral aneurysm.

early ventriculostomy is a safeguard against rebleeding in the first hours; but conversely, it may be argued that reducing the CSF pressure may reduce the sealing pressures of the aneurysm and thus increase the risk of bleeding. However, early

ventriculostomy did not increase rebleeding in our study with patients before they underwent early repair of the aneurysm.[21]

Bacterial Meningitis

Obstruction of the ventricular communication with the subarachnoid space by inflammatory exudate is the most likely mechanism of bacterial meningitis. Acute obstructive hydrocephalus can occur several weeks after bacterial meningitis begins and typically appears insidiously. The ventricular system, however, can be enlarged soon after the illness but usually to a minor degree and transiently (Fig. 11.3). Rarely is there a need to place a ventriculostomy tube early when hydrocephalus occurs within the first days, but late-onset hydrocephalus (10% in adult bacterial meningitis) may require placement of a drain.

Pineal Region Tumors

Pineal region tumors predominate in young adults (and children). Compression of the quadrigeminal plate depends on the size of the tumor, and compression of the cerebral aqueduct or tumor growth into the posterior third ventricle produces obstructive hydrocephalus.

Pineal parenchymal neoplasms can be divided into pineoblastoma (with histologic characteristics

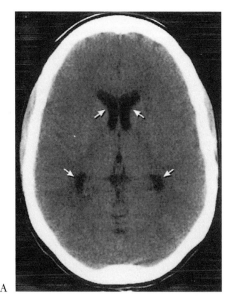

A

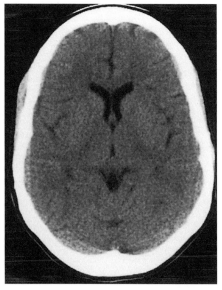

B

Figure 11.3 *A:* Acute hydrocephalus in pneumococcal meningitis (*arrows*). *B:* Resolution (particularly temporal horns) of the enlargement but also reappearance of sulci 4 days after antibiotic therapy.

nearly identical to those of medulloblastoma) and pineocytoma (characteristic rosette formation).

The outcome of pineoblastoma is poor, with survival rarely extending beyond 2 years.[6] Pineocytoma with neuronal differentiation, such as large rosette formation or ganglion cells, has a much better long-term outcome, up to three decades after diagnosis, resection, and radiotherapy. Radiosurgery may be useful as adjuvant therapy.[22] Germinomas may arise from this location, as may other germ cell tumors, such as teratomas, embryonal carcinoma, endodermal sinus tumor, and choriocarcinoma.

Germinomas are very radiosensitive, and long-term survival or cure is expected after resection. CSF should be sampled at the time of ventricular shunting. Choriocarcinoma and pineal germinoma secrete human chorionic gonadotropin. Alpha-fetoprotein is increased in endodermal sinus tumors, infiltrating teratoma, embryonal carcinoma, and choriocarcinoma.[23] CSF markers may help in differentiation. High-dose methotrexate has been suggested in patients with distant metastasis (bone and meninges).[24]

Colloid Cyst of the Third Ventricle

The incidence of colloid cyst of the third ventricle is about 0.5%–2% of all intracranial tumors. This developmental abnormality is filled with homogeneous viscous material containing cellular debris. Its location in the third ventricle causes intermittent marked enlargement of the ventricles or ventricular diverticula, and death may ensue if recurrent headaches are not sufficiently investigated.[5,25,26] Colloid cysts are a cause of sudden death in pediatric patients.[27,28] Deterioration was observed in 32% of symptomatic patients, emphasizing its not so benign presence.[29]

In the Karolinska Hospital–based series of 37 consecutive patients, five patients were admitted to the emergency department and two died despite emergency ventriculostomy.[30,31]

Full resection should be planned. Unfavorable long-term results were associated with aspiration and subtotal resection.[30] However, transcallosal microsurgery produced excellent results.[30–33]

Ependymoma

Neoplastic growth of the epithelial lining on the ventricular surface is most commonly supratento-rial in adults and more commonly intratentorial in children.[7,34] Seeding throughout the CSF occurs in some instances. These malignant tumors grow slowly, and outcome is determined by grade, with 5-year survival of 80% in patients with low-grade tumors. Anaplastic or poorly differentiated ependymoma with typical histologic features of high mitotic activity, vascular proliferation, and necrosis reduces survival to 50%.

Plexus Papilloma

Tumors of the choroid plexus often are papillary and highly vascularized. Intratumoral hemorrhage is frequent. Localization is commonly in the fourth ventricle in adults.[35,36] These tumors do not invade and are comparatively easy to resect.

Epidermoid Cysts

Epidermoid cysts are ectodermal elements displaced during embryogenesis that become symptomatic in adults.[37] Rupture of the cyst may cause aseptic ventriculitis. Predilection is for the fourth ventricle; and because of compression of the brain stem, cranial nerve palsy, ataxia, and hemiparesis may occur. Because of its slow growth and pliable nature, however, it may produce only intermittent headaches.

Neuroimaging in Acute Hydrocephalus

Different sites of obstruction in acute hydrocephalus are shown in Figure 11.4. CT scanning clearly delineates the degree of hydrocephalus and in many instances the obstructing tumor. Usually, the largest parts of the ventricular system (the anterior horns of the lateral ventricles) enlarge first, the temporal horns next, and then the third and fourth ventricles. When hydrocephalus has developed over weeks, subependymal effusions are clear evidence of increased CSF pressure. These periventricular hypodensities may occur in up to 40% of patients with acute obstructing hydrocephalus, but this capping surrounding the ventricle may also be evident in elderly patients with long-standing hypertension and diabetes but no hydrocephalus.[38]

The degree of hydrocephalus can be carefully assessed by several measuring systems. These sim-

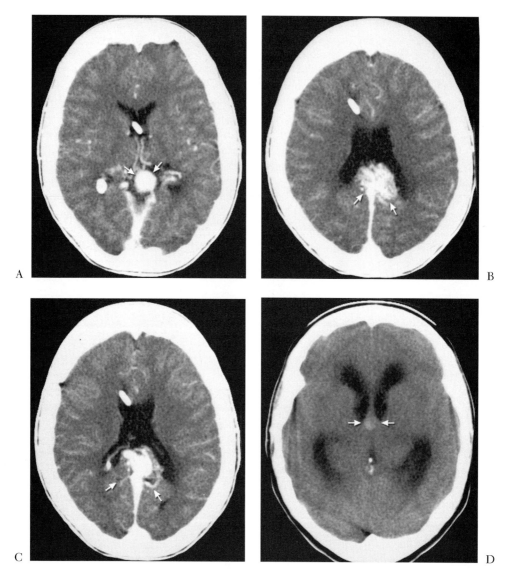

Figure 11.4 Examples of different sites of obstruction (*arrows*). *A–C:* Arteriovenous malformation with giant vein of Galen. *D,E:* Colloid cyst in third ventricle (note absence of third ventricle).

ple linear measurements not only determine the degree of hydrocephalus but also can be used to monitor change. The *ventricular size index* measures the bifrontal diameter (transverse inner diameter) and divides it by the frontal horn diameter. The *bicaudate index* might be more reliable because consistent normal values have been established. This index is determined by the width of the frontal horns at the level of the caudate nuclei divided by the maximum width of the brain at the same level (Fig. 11.5). Alternatively, ven-

tricular volume can be measured on CT or magnetic resonance imaging (MRI), outlining each slice and multiplying the area of outline by slice thickness. The total volume is the sum of these volumes including the calculated interslice gaps. In adults, there is little experience in acute neurologic disorders with this technique.[39]

The temporal horns remain sensitive indicators for hydrocephalus on CT scans. Temporal horns, usually barely visible, become large, boomerang-shaped ventricles in acute hydrocephalus. This

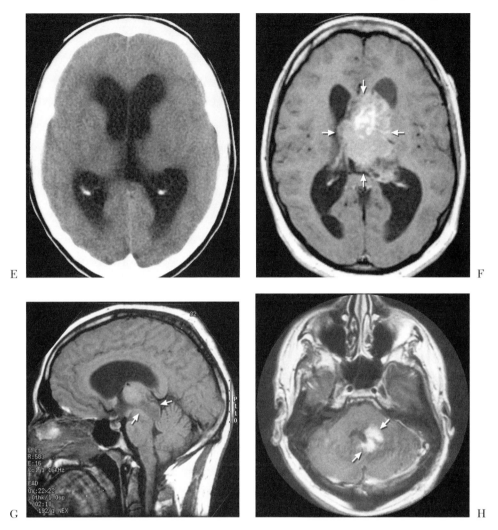

Figure 11.4 (*Continued*) Examples of different sites of obstruction (*arrows*). *F:* Neurocytoma in third ventricle. *G:* Low-grade glioma in pineal region. *H:* Central nervous system lymphoma compressing fourth ventricle.

configuration often clearly differentiates obstruction from cortical cerebral atrophy. Other features compatible with atrophy rather than hydrocephalus are widening sylvian and interhemispheric fissures, leaving marked hypodense fluid-filled spaces and prominent dilated cortical sulci.

It is important to identify tumors that may obstruct the ventricular system, particularly those located in the intraventricular compartment, which may be isodense to the brain tissue. Characteristically, colloid cysts of the third ventricle are very subtle and difficult to detect because they blend in with brain tissue. A mass should

be strongly considered if the third ventricle cannot be identified or the septum pellucidum is widened, separating the posterior medial aspects of the frontal horns. It is important to scrutinize the posterior fossa for a mass lesion that may be evident only from distortion of the fourth ventricle.

However, MRI should disclose any obstructive mass lesion.[40] MRI also is particularly important to demonstrate meningeal enhancement (e.g., in sarcoidosis or carcinomatous meningitis)[41,42] and lesions typically not well recognized on CT scanning (e.g., smaller pineal region cysts).

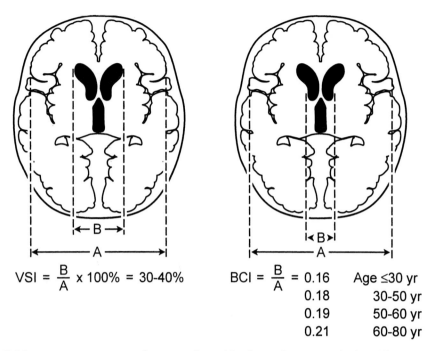

$$VSI = \frac{B}{A} \times 100\% = 30\text{-}40\%$$

$$BCI = \frac{B}{A} = 0.16 \quad \text{Age} \leq 30 \text{ yr}$$
$$0.18 \qquad 30\text{-}50 \text{ yr}$$
$$0.19 \qquad 50\text{-}60 \text{ yr}$$
$$0.21 \qquad 60\text{-}80 \text{ yr}$$

Figure 11.5 Measurement on computed tomographic scan of the ventricular system in acute hydrocephalus.

Numbers indicate normal values. The ventricular size index (VSI) is not corrected for age. BCI, bicaudate index.

Management

Untreated obstructive hydrocephalus leads to altered arousal, coma, and in some cases brain death and, thus, needs urgent neurosurgical intervention irrespective of its cause. Unfortunately, the rarity and rapid progression of acute obstructive hydrocephalus often delay diagnosis and limit the ability to treat. The emphasis in the emergency department is therefore on early intervention with ventriculostomy and identification of the trigger. Acute CSF diversion with placement of a ventriculostomy drain into the largest ventricle has priority and, if feasible, should be performed in the emergency department suite. The ventriculostomy tube is connected to a manometric CSF drainage system draining at 10–15 cm H_2O. If the CSF is bloody, drainage at 0 cm H_2O or lower should be considered, to reduce clotting in the catheter (Box 11.2). Alternative techniques, such as fenestration of the septum pellucidum or third ventriculostomy, are highly experimental.[43,44] Placement of a ventriculostomy drain in patients with aneurysmal subarachnoid hemorrhage has been linked to rebleeding when the aneurysm is

not secured with a clip or coil. We and others have found no such relationship[21,45] and believe its placement is indicated in patients with persistent stupor, vertical downgaze, pinpoint pupils, and documented enlarging size in CT. Some endovascular radiologists prefer a ventriculostomy drain in place to safeguard (see Chapter 13) the effects of rebleeding associated with placement of coils. (Its presence will allow release of ventricular blood that otherwise would massively enlarge the ventricular system.)

Ventricular clearing of blood with ventriculostomy is not optimal and may lead to obstruction of the catheter; use of intraventricular thrombolytic agents is currently under investigation. Hemoventricle with hydrocephalus from primary intraventricular hemorrhage has been treated with additional instillation of urokinase.[46] One study of 22 patients treated with intraventricular urokinase found a trend toward better outcome than that in a nearly similar control group. Clearance of the third ventricle predicted better outcome, suggesting that the focus of monitoring of these patients should perhaps be clearance of third ventricle clot.[47]

Box 11.2. Ventriculostomy

A ventricular catheter is inserted in the right (or, better, nondominant) frontal region. The patient is fully supine. In many instances, the bur hole is placed 1–2 cm anterior to the coronal suture in the midpupillary line (Fig. 11.6). The catheter is directed to the middle of the nose. The ventricular system (particularly when dilated) is reached at 5–7 cm below the skin. After insertion, the tube is subcutaneously tunneled and secured. Many neurosurgeons administer antibiotics. Complications are rare. They include ventriculitis (probably reduced with antibiotic prophylaxis and subcutaneous tunneling); epidural, subdural, or intraparenchymal hematoma (mostly in patients with severe coagulopathy); malfunctioning through blood clot obstruction; migration against the ventricular wall; and, rarely, creation of a dural arteriovenous fistula. All are reasons to replace the catheter.

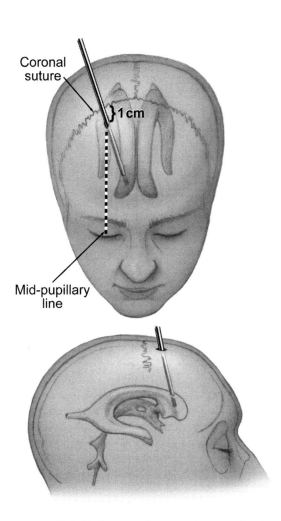

Coronal suture

1 cm

Mid-pupillary line

Figure 11.6 Technique of ventriculostomy showing landmarks and approach.

Definitive treatment of the obstructing mass warrants endoscopic removal in most cases, and some patients need permanent ventriculoperitoneal shunts or fenestration of the third ventricle, accomplished by endoscopic techniques.[48–50] The lamina terminalis, septum pellucidum, and floor of the third ventricle can all be punctured and then dilated with catheters to divert CSF. Cerebrospinal shunts usually employ valve systems draining at CSF pressures of more than 10 mm Hg. Overdrainage may lead to subdural effusions or subdural hematomas.[51]

REFERENCES

1. Maurizi CP: The puzzle of where cerebrospinal fluid is absorbed: new pieces. *Med Hypotheses* 60:102, 2003.
2. Wray SH: The neuro-ophthalmic and neurologic manifestations of pinealomas. In HH Schmidek (ed), *Pineal Tumors*. New York: Masson, 1977, p. 21.
3. Abe T, Matsumoto K, Kiyota K, et al.: Vein of Galen aneurysmal malformation in an adult: a case report. *Surg Neurol* 45:39, 1996.
4. Case Records of the Massachusetts General Hospital: Weekly clinicopathological exercises (case 35-1983). *N Engl J Med* 309:542, 1983.
5. Buttner A, Winkler PA, Eisenmenger W, et al.: Colloid cysts of the third ventricle with fatal outcome: a report of two cases and review of the literature. *Int J Legal Med* 110:260, 1997.
6. Chang SM, Lillis-Hearne PK, Larson DA, et al.: Pineoblastoma in adults. *Neurosurgery* 37:383, 1995.
7. Chiechi MV, Smirniotopoulos JG, Jones RV: Intracranial subependymomas: CT and MR imaging features in 24 cases. *AJR Am J Roentgenol* 165:1245, 1995.
8. Chiechi MV, Smirniotopoulos JG, Mena H: Pineal parenchymal tumors: CT and MR features. *J Comput Assist Tomogr* 19:509, 1995.

9. Dolinskas CA, Simeone FA: CT characteristics of intraventricular oligodendrogliomas. *AJNR Am J Neuroradiol* 8:1077, 1987.

10. Duong H, Sarazin L, Bourgouin P, et al.: Magnetic resonance imaging of lateral ventricular tumours. *Can Assoc Radiol J* 46:434, 1995.

11. Johnston IH, Whittle IR, Besser M, et al.: Vein of Galen malformation: diagnosis and management. *Neurosurgery* 20:747, 1987.

12. Lasjaunias P, Ter Brugge K, Lopez Ibor L, et al.: The role of dural anomalies in vein of Galen aneurysms: report of six cases and review of the literature. *AJNR Am J Neuroradiol* 8:185, 1987.

13. Tien RD, Barkovich AJ, Edwards MS: MR imaging of pineal tumors. *AJR Am J Roentgenol* 155:143, 1990.

14. Tomsick TA, Ernst RJ, Tew JM, et al.: Adult choroidal vein of Galen malformation. *AJNR Am J Neuroradiol* 16(Suppl):861, 1995.

15. Diringer MN, Edwards DF, Zazulia AR: Hydrocephalus: a previously unrecognized predictor of poor outcome from supratentorial intracerebral hemorrhage. *Stroke* 29:1352, 1998.

16. Liliang PC, Liang CL, Lu CH, et al.: Hypertensive caudate hemorrhage: prognostic predictor, outcome, and role of external ventricular drainage. *Stroke* 32:1195, 2001.

17. Phan TG, Koh M, Vierkant RA, et al.: Hydrocephalus is a determinant of early mortality in putaminal hemorrhage. *Stroke* 31:2157, 2000.

18. Adams RE, Diringer MN: Response to external ventricular drainage in spontaneous intracerebral hemorrhage with hydrocephalus. *Neurology* 50:519, 1998.

19. Shapiro SA, Campbell RL, Scully T: Hemorrhagic dilation of the fourth ventricle: an ominous predictor. *J Neurosurg* 80:805, 1994.

20. Smith KA, Kraus GE, Johnson BA, et al.: Giant posterior communicating artery aneurysm presenting as third ventricle mass with obstructive hydrocephalus. Case report. *J Neurosurg* 81:299, 1994.

21. McIver JI, Friedman JA, Wijdicks EFM, et al.: Preoperative ventriculostomy is not associated with increased risk of rebleeding following aneurysmal subarachnoid hemorrhage. *J Neurosurg* 97:1108, 2002.

22. Kondziolka D, Hadjipanayis CF, Flickinger JC, et al.: The role of radiosurgery for the treatment of pineal parenchymal tumors. *Neurosurgery* 51:880, 2002.

23. Allen JC, Nisselbaum J, Epstein F, et al.: Alpha-fetoprotein and human chorionic gonadotropin determination in cerebrospinal fluid. An aid to the diagnosis and management of intracranial germ-cell tumors. *J Neurosurg* 51: 368, 1979.

24. Fietz T, Thiel E, Baldus C, et al.: Successful treatment of extracranially metastasized pineal gland germinoma with high-dose methotrexate. *Ann Oncol* 13:1681, 2002.

25. Camacho A, Abernathey CD, Kelly PJ, et al.: Colloid cysts: experience with the management of 84 cases since the introduction of computed tomography. *Neurosurgery* 24: 693, 1989.

26. Jabaudon D, Charest D, Porchet F: Pathogenesis and diagnostic pitfalls of ventricular diverticula: a case report and review of the literature. *Neurosurgery* 52:209, 2003.

27. Ferrera PC, Kass LE: Third ventricle colloid cyst. *Am J Emerg Med* 15:145, 1997.

28. Opeskin K, Anderson RM, Lee KA: Colloid cyst of the 3rd ventricle as a cause of acute neurological deterioration and sudden death. *J Paediatr Child Health* 29:476, 1993.

29. de Witt Hamer PC, Verstegen MJ, De Haan RJ, et al.: High risk of acute deterioration in patients harboring symptomatic colloid cysts of the third ventricle. *J Neurosurg* 96:1041, 2002.

30. Mathiesen T, Grane P, Lindgren L, et al.: Third ventricle colloid cysts: a consecutive 12-year series. *J Neurosurg* 86:5, 1997.

31. Mathiesen T, Grane P, Lindquist C, et al.: High recurrence rate following aspiration of colloid cysts in the third ventricle. *J Neurosurg* 78:748, 1993.

32. Kondziolka D, Lunsford LD: Stereotactic management of colloid cysts: factors predicting success. *J Neurosurg* 75:45, 1991.

33. Abdou MS, Cohen AR: Endoscopic treatment of colloid cysts of the third ventricle. Technical note and review of the literature. *J Neurosurg* 89:1062, 1998.

34. Oppenheim JS, Strauss RC, Mormino J, et al.: Ependymomas of the third ventricle. *Neurosurgery* 34:350, 1994.

35. Sharma R, Rout D, Gupta AK, et al.: Choroid plexus papillomas. *Br J Neurosurg* 8:169, 1994.

36. Wolff JE, Sajedi M, Brant R, et al.: Choroid plexus tumours. *Br J Cancer* 87:1086, 2002.

37. Kendall B, Reider-Grosswasser I, Valentine A: Diagnosis of masses presenting within the ventricles on computed tomography. *Neuroradiology* 25:11, 1983.

38. Mori K, Handa H, Murata T, et al.: Periventricular lucency in computed tomography of hydrocephalus and cerebral atrophy. *J Comput Assist Tomogr* 4:204, 1980.

39. Xenos C, Sgouros S, Natarajan K: Ventricular volume change in childhood. *J Neurosurg* 97:584, 2002.

40. McConachie NS, Worthington BS, Cornford EJ, et al.: Computed tomography and magnetic resonance in the diagnosis of intraventricular cerebral masses. *Br J Radiol* 67:223, 1994.

41. Maisel JA, Lynam T: Unexpected sudden death in a young pregnant woman: unusual presentation of neurosarcoidosis. *Ann Emerg Med* 28:94, 1996.

42. Spencer N, Ross G, Helm G, et al.: Aqueductal obstruction in sarcoidosis. *Clin Neuropathol* 8:158, 1989.

43. Roux FE, Boetto S, Tremoulet M: Third ventriculocisternostomy in cerebellar hematomas. *Acta Neurochir (Wien)* 144:337, 2002.

44. Holtzman RN, Brust JC, Ainyette IG, et al.: Acute ventricular hemorrhage in adults with hydrocephalus managed by corpus callosotomy and fenestration of the septum pellucidum. Report of three cases. *J Neurosurg* 95:111, 2001.

45. Roitberg BZ, Khan N, Alp MS, et al.: Bedside external

ventricular drain placement for the treatment of acute hydrocephalus. *Br J Neurosurg* 4:324, 2001.

46. Todo T, Usui M, Takakura K: Treatment of severe intraventricular hemorrhage by intraventricular infusion of urokinase. *J Neurosurg* 74:81, 1991.

47. Coplin WM, Vinas FC, Agris JM, et al.: A cohort study of the safety and feasibility of intraventricular urokinase for nonaneurysmal spontaneous intraventricular hemorrhage. *Stroke* 29:1573, 1998.

48. Veto F, Horvath Z, Doczi T: Biportal endoscopic management of third ventricle tumors in patients with occlusive hydrocephalus: technical note. *Neurosurgery* 40:871, 1997.

49. Wisoff JH, Epstein F: Surgical management of symptomatic pineal cysts. *J Neurosurg* 77:896, 1992.

50. Hopf NJ, Grunert P, Fries G, et al.: Endoscopic third ventriculostomy: outcome analysis of 100 consecutive procedures. *Neurosurgery* 44:795, 1999.

51. Pople IK: Hydrocephalus and shunts: what the neurologist should know. *J Neurol Neurosurg Psychiatry* 73(Suppl 1): 17, 2002.

Chapter 12
Acute Spinal Cord Compression

An expedited evaluation in patients with acute spinal cord compression is paramount because reversal of tetraparesis or paraparesis is time-locked.[1] Beyond a certain interval the symptoms may remain complete, with no prospect of future ambulation or bladder control.

Patients with spinal cord compression from malignant disease often have some degree of ambulation at first evaluation. In the Memorial Sloan-Kettering series, 50% of the patients presented ambulatory, 35% paraparetic, and 15% paraplegic at the time of diagnosis.[2] In addition, it has been estimated that 30% of patients with epidural spinal cord compression from metastatic cancer become paraplegic within 1 week.[3] This observation clearly indicates a dynamic process that possibly can be halted or partly reversed. Unfortunately, unacceptable delay in diagnosis, referral, and investigation occurs in patients with spinal cord compression.[4]

Acute management of spinal cord compression and the priorities of evaluation are discussed in this chapter, but the usual considerations in patients presenting with ambulation difficulties have already been discussed in Chapter 2. Injuries severe enough to damage the spinal cord are commonly associated with head, abdominal, or chest trauma; and management of traumatic spinal cord injury is discussed in Chapter 19.

Neurologic Assessment of Acute Spinal Cord Compression

Neurologic examination should localize the lesion in patients with acute paraplegia or tetraplegia.

Sensory abnormalities localize in the vertical plane (cervical, lumbar, sacral) and, when combined with other long tract signs, point to localization in the horizontal plane (extradural, intradural, or intramedullary).[5] Clinical clues helpful in localization are found in Appendix 12.1.

The major cord syndromes are summarized in Table 12.1

All sensory modalities should be tested (pinprick, position, and vibration sense; light touch with a wisp of cotton; pressure touch; and temperature tested with a cold or hot piece of metal [e.g., warmed under running hot water]). Abnormal pinprick is usually interpreted as touch without identification of a sharp sting and is most valuable in localizing segments. When a tuning fork is unavailable to test vibration, at least position sense should be tested. Normally, movement of a few degrees in the position of the toe joints should be easily appreciated. In addition, tactile discrimination should be tested, and normally a 2- to 3-cm difference between two points should be appreciated. Normal function suggests intact posterior column tracts but also nerve root function.

Saddle anesthesia (S3–S5) is an indication of a conus medullaris lesion, which can be accurately delineated but may be missed with superficial examination in a supine patient. The sensory loss is often dissociated, with sparing of touch but loss of pinprick. Absence of dissociation suggests involvement of the cauda equina, not just the conus.

Sacral sparing of the sensory symptoms is an important sign because it implies a centrally located intramedullary lesion. (The representation of the sacral fibers is very peripheral in the cord;

Table 12.1. Major Acute Spinal Cord Syndromes

Complete

- All sensory modalities and reflexes impaired below level of severance: pinprick loss most valuable
- Flaccid, paraplegia or tetraplegia
- Fasciculations
- Urinary or rectal sphincter dysfunction
- Sweating, piloerection diminished below lesions
- Genital reflexes lost, priapism

Central

- Vest-like loss of pain and temperature
- Initial sparing of proprioception
- Sacral sensation spared
- Paraparesis or tetraparesis

Hemisection

- Loss of pain and temperature opposite to the lesion
- Sensory loss two segments below lesion
- Loss of proprioception on same side as lesion
- Light touch may be normal or minimally decreased
- Weakness on same side as lesion pain

Anterior

- Pain and temperature loss below lesion
- Proprioception spared
- Flaccid, areflexia
- Paraparesis or tetraparesis
- Fasciculations
- Urinary or rectal sphincter dysfunction
- Dysautonomia absent

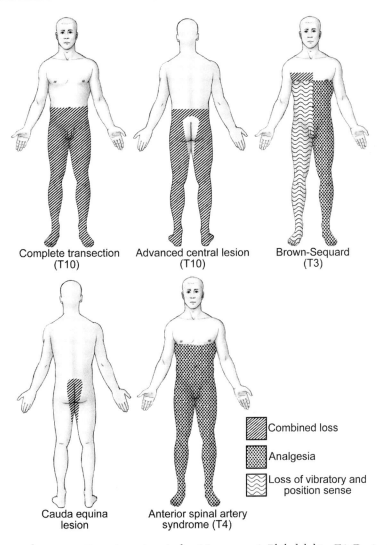

Complete transection (T10)

Advanced central lesion (T10)

Brown-Sequard (T3)

Cauda equina lesion

Anterior spinal artery syndrome (T4)

Combined loss

Analgesia

Loss of vibratory and position sense

Figure 12.1 Abnormal sensory patterns in acute spinal cord disease. (Modified from Byrne TN, Waxman SG: *Spinal Cord Compression: Diagnosis and Principles of Management.* Philadelphia: FA Davis, 1990, p. 39. By permission of the publisher.)

thus, pinprick and temperature sensation may be spared in acute central cord lesions.)

Dissociating sensory lesions may be further localized in the horizontal plane. Brown-Séquard syndrome is strongly indicative of extramedullary compression, but it may occur in patients with cancer and radiation myelopathy. Its clinical hallmark is loss of pain and temperature sensation opposite the lesion, with loss of position and vibration and more prominent leg weakness at the level of the lesion. The patient often may be puzzled by numbness in one leg and weakness in the other. Brown-Séquard syndrome is rarely uniform in presentation, but marked unilateral leg weakness with Babinski's sign and lack of position recognition of the toe should point to acute extramedullary compression. The classic patterns of sensory loss in myelopathies are depicted in Figure 12.1.

Muscle strength should be graded with the British Medical Research Council scale (Appendix 12.2) in index muscles. These are proximally iliopsoas, gluteus, quadriceps, and hamstring muscles and distally tibialis anterior and posterior, peronei, gastrocnemius, soleus, and extensor and flexor muscles of toes. Further progression of weakness can be easily assessed by this validated grading system.

Tendon, abdominal, and anal reflexes are usually unelicitable in patients with acute paraplegia from a spinal cord lesion. Abdominal reflexes involve the T7–T12 segment; however, absence of these reflexes is not particularly helpful in localization, and they are absent in most obese patients. The cremaster reflex involves the L1–L2 arc, and the anal reflexes involve the S2–S4 arc; both reflexes have localizing value in determining the segment of involvement in the spinal cord.

Immediate assessment of the bladder is warranted. Sensation of bladder distention may be lost, resulting in overflow incontinence. Detrusor areflexia can be expected with perianal anesthesia, absence of the bulbocavernosus reflex (an unpleasant but important reflex triggered when a squeeze of the glans penis is followed by contraction of the bulbocavernous muscle assessed by palpation), and poor anal tone or loss of voluntary control of the anal sphincter. Distention of the bladder should be prevented by immediate catheterization.

Pain is common in acute spinal cord compression. However, significant destructive and compressive spinal lesions may be virtually painless. Pain that is worse with lying down may signal an epidural spinal tumor and can be explained by additional traction from lengthening of the spine in the supine position.[6] Excruciating pain closely associated in time with the development of acute paraplegia or tetraplegia should suggest intramedullary, subarachnoid, or acute epidural hemorrhage, particularly in patients receiving anticoagulation. Equally important to recognize is a spinal epidural abscess, in which acute paraparesis or tetraparesis can evolve in hours. Acute chest pain followed by paraplegia may be due to aortic dissection. Pain in the lower back area may be referred from a dissecting abdominal aneurysm; it may begin in the lower lumbar spine and be followed by acute paraplegia from spinal cord infarction. In young patients, acute low back pain preceding acute paraplegia may indicate fibrocartilaginous emboli to the spinal cord from thoracic disk herniation.[7] Pain referred to the abdomen is often experienced by patients with acute spinal cord lesions, who may feel they are strapped into a corset.

Pain should be classified as local, referred, radicular, or funicular. Local spinal percussion pain (deep, boring) in the thoracolumbar spine should be evaluated by having the patient turn to the side and carefully tapping on the spinous processes with a reflex hammer. Acute radicular pain (sharp, stabbing) should be further confirmed by straight leg testing and a forceful cough or Valsalva maneuver. Funicular pain (burning, stabbing, electrical) is a less clearly characterized pain sensation of burning, jolting, and jabbing without clear localization, often occurring with sudden movements of the spine. The pain may signal intramedullary disease (e.g., tumor or demyelination).

Two neurosurgical emergencies need special mention not only because recognition may be difficult but also because presentation mimics common disorders seen in the emergency department. First, epidural spinal abscess is caused in 50% of the patients by *Staphylococcus aureus* infection. Drug use and chronic alcoholism predispose to diskitis and osteomyelitis, which may extend to the epidural space. Recognition is difficult because most confused and delirious patients have signs suggesting sepsis or acute bacterial meningitis. Local back tenderness may not be prominent, but paraparesis and loss of voluntary muscles and sphincters may rapidly become defining features in patients admitted to the emergency department. Blood cultures have a much higher yield in identifying the organism than cerebrospinal fluid (CSF) and can be isolated from blood in at least 30% of cases.[8] CSF examination in the emergency department—done to document or exclude bacterial meningitis—may also be potentially dangerous because shifts in CSF pressure that displace the spinal cord may cause sudden worsening of paraparesis. Second, epidural spinal hematoma may present with acute chest pain or pain between the shoulder blades. The pain has been described as a dagger thrust (*le coup de poignard*) and is rapidly followed by tingling, the development of a sensory demarcation, and often Brown-Séquard syndrome. This type of pain in combination with use of warfarin or tissue plasminogen activator, epidural block, or recent multilevel spine surgery should immediately point to this diagnosis.[9–13] Tetraparesis or paraparesis follows. Presentation with arm weakness and neck pain only has been reported.[13] Spontaneous spinal subarachnoid hematoma, although rare, may lead to paralysis when located dorsally in the spinal cord. A ventral type of spinal subarachnoid hematoma[12] has a much more benign presentation and resolves spontaneously. Diagnoses to consider in paraplegic patients and acute chest or lumbar pain are listed in Table 12.2.

Neuroimaging in Acute Spinal Cord Compression

A plain radiograph of the spine is useful because it quickly identifies bone destruction from metastatic disease and the consequences for stability of the spine. Plain radiographs can appear misleadingly normal in approximately 25% of patients with documented metastatic spinal cord compression; furthermore, plain radiographic abnormalities may not correspond to the location of the tumor, often showing cord compression at a much higher or lower thoracic level.

Bone scan with technetium 99m diphosphonate is occasionally used for screening and as a supplementary test,[14] but magnetic resonance imaging (MRI) of the spine, with specific attention to the level determined by clinical localization, should be considered the standard in acute spinal cord compression.[15,16] MRI of the spine can classify abnormalities as intramedullary or extramedullary, in which the lesions are often intradural. Often more than one lesion is involved, supporting a policy of MRI of the whole spine in these patients.[15]

For reference purposes, a normal MRI of the cervical, thoracic, and lumbar regions of the spine, with T_1- and T_2-weighted images, is shown in Figure 12.2. An adequate MRI study of the spine should have sagittal T_1- and T_2-weighted images with thin (4–5 mm) sections.

Several important features can be identified on MRI of the spine. On T_1-weighted images, bone marrow in the vertebral bodies produces a high intensity but a low signal of the cortical bone. T_1-weighted images may underestimate the width of the spinal canal because CSF characteristics are of low signal as well. The nerve roots may emerge on axial slices against the high-intensity signal of epidural fat and low intensity of CSF. Disks also have a low T_1 signal. The spinal cord signal is intermediate but higher than that of surrounding CSF.

On T_2-weighted images, the CSF is bright (also called "the myelographic effect"). The intravertebral disks are brighter. The nerve roots are much better appreciated on T_2 images because of the distinctive bright signal of the CSF.

Motion artifacts may produce hyperintense or hypointense bands (phantom images or harmonics) suggesting a cavity in the cord or neoplasm.

Gadolinium does not penetrate the central nervous system; therefore, if the blood–brain barrier is intact, the spine should not become enhanced. T_1-weighted images enhance the basivertebral veins, epidural venous plexus, and spinal ganglion. Necrosis in the spine appears as a high-intensity signal in T_1-weighted images after gadolinium injection. Because tumor has a high signal enhancement, gadolinium is useful in further evaluation of

Table 12.2. Acute Chest or Lumbar Pain with Paraplegia

- Aortic dissection
- Epidural (or subarachnoid) hematoma
- Epidural abscess
- Acute fibrocartilaginous emboli
- Intramedullary hematoma
- Vertebral collapse from cancer

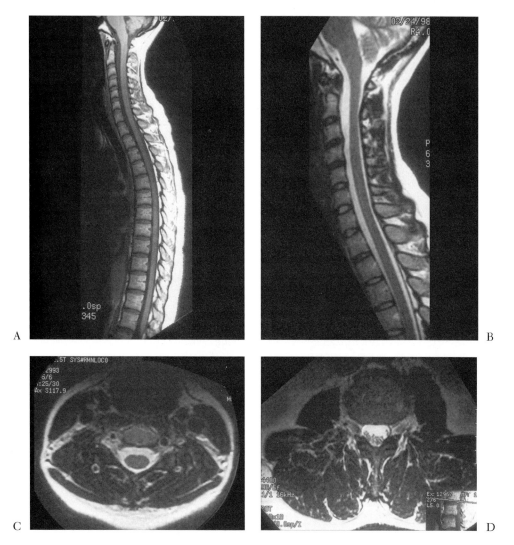

Figure 12.2 *A–D:* Normal T_1 and T_2 characteristics of sagittal and axial magnetic resonance images of the cervical, thoracic, and lumbar regions of the spine.

intramedullary, intradural, and extramedullary lesions.

Nerve root enhancement with gadolinium ordinarily does not appear unless disease is present but occasionally is observed when a dose of very high contrast is used (0.3 mmol/kg of body weight). Enhancement of the spinal nerve roots is an important finding, and several patterns have been described.[17] Diffuse enhancement of the cauda can occur in leptomeningeal metastasis, most often associated with systemic malignant disease, such as breast, lung, or skin cancer. However, diffuse enhancement can be seen in inflammatory polyradiculopathy, such as cytomegalovirus radiculopathy in acquired immunodeficiency syndrome (AIDS). Tuberculosis should be considered in persons from endemic areas and, more recently, in patients with AIDS. Epidural compression may be caused by granuloma formation, which is apparent as thickening of the nerve roots. Virtually any leptomeningeal infection can cause enhancement, including *Mycobacterium tuberculosis* infection and cysticercosis.[18] Sarcoidosis should be considered when enhancement is linear at the nerve roots.[19]

In spinal cord compression from cancer, vertebral compression fractures may not coexist with an epidural mass. Malignant lesions on MRI most often have a low-intensity signal on T_1-weighted images and a high-intensity signal on T_2-weighted images (as noted earlier, normal adult marrow has a high signal intensity on T_1 and an intermediate intensity on T_2 images). Contrast enhancement increases the sensitivity of detecting malignant lesions in further defining epidural mass effect, which may not be evident on unenhanced images.[20,21]

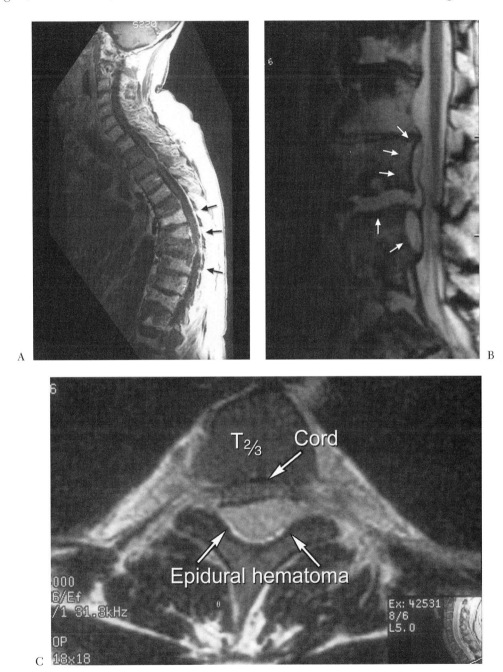

Figure 12.3 Composite magnetic resonance images of the most common causes of spinal cord compression: epidural metastasis (A), epidural abscess (B), epidural hematoma (C,D), and granulomatous disease and thickening of nerve roots (E).

The diagnosis of epidural hematoma has been greatly facilitated by MRI. A high T_2-weighted signal often identifies a hematoma that may be scattered throughout the spinal canal, with various degrees of compression at different levels. However, a hyperacute hematoma (within an hour or so) may be isointense on T_1-weighted images.[22]

MRI is the preferred test in epidural abscess, and sometimes after gadolinium enhancement, compartmentalization becomes evident.

Acute spinal cord syndromes may be caused by infarction or an arteriovenous malformation.[23,24] Arteriovenous malformation may be located in the dura and cause significant backlog

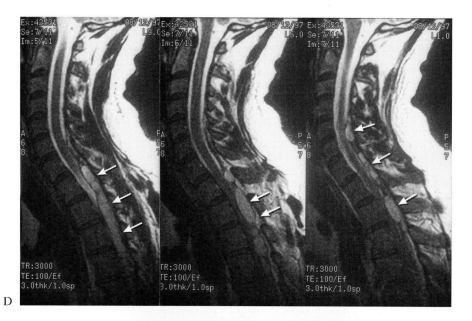

D

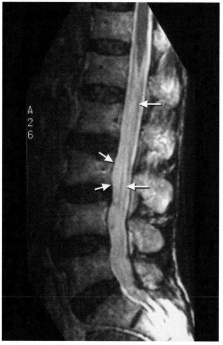

E

Figure 12.3 (*Continued*)

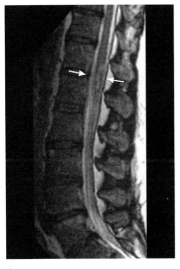
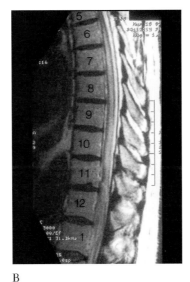
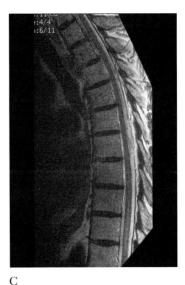

A   B   C

Figure 12.4 Common magnetic resonance images in patients with acute spinal cord syndromes but without spinal cord compression. *A:* Spinal cord infarction. *B,C:* Spinal cord swelling from dural arteriovenous malformation, with resolution after surgical extirpation.

of venous flow and a dramatic swelling of the cord.[24-26]

The characteristic MRI findings in these disorders are shown in Figures 12.3 and 12.4. Further visualization of the different compartments in the spine is demonstrated in Figure 12.5[27] for additional orientation.

Laboratory Tests

Discovery of a mass compressing the spinal cord will lead to further radiologic studies, including chest radiograph or computed tomographic (CT) mammogram, abdominal echocardiogram or CT, and any other tests, particularly positron emission tomographic (PET) scanning, focused on the disclosure of a primary tumor.

Management

The pathophysiologic mechanism of cord compression is poorly understood, but recent insights may provide an avenue of treatment (Box 12.1).

The approach to acute spinal cord compression is determined by its cause, but immediate surgical management is an established route in patients with an epidural abscess localized at a few levels, epidural hematoma, or extradural metastasis with rapidly evolving neurologic deterioration. Its ben-

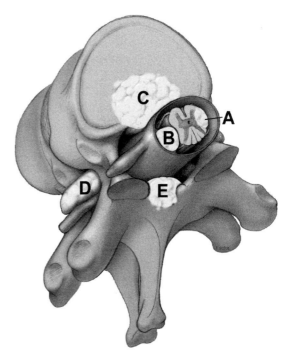

Figure 12.5 Localization of metastatic lesions in compartments inside the spinal canal: intramedullary process (*A*); leptomeningeal process (*B*); process in vertebral body extending into the epidural space (*C*); paravertebral process (*D*); and epidural process (*E*). (Modified from Byrne TN: Spinal cord compression from epidural metastases. *N Engl J Med* 1992;327:614. By permission of the Massachusetts Medical Society.)

Box 12.1. Pathophysiology of Metastatic Cord Compression

Spinal cord compression from metastatic disease may be caused by vascular congestion[28] due to venous occlusion of the paravertebral venous plexus in the epidural space. Vasogenic edema is an early feature, caused by a breakdown of the blood–spinal cord barrier. The following sequence of events after compression has been documented.[29] After 3 hours of cord compression, selective demyelination occurs without axonal damage. It evolves over 24 hours and is associated with production of prostaglandin. In experimental settings, sustained spinal cord compression for 3 hours resulted in per-

sistently absent somatosensory evoked potentials and much less chance for recovery.[30] Experimental blocking of serotonin receptors not only inhibits prostaglandin production but also delays the onset of paraplegia. Prolonged compression results in irreversible cord ischemia. If the epidural mass suddenly enlarges from hemorrhage or an extensively infiltrated vertebral body suddenly collapses, acute spinal cord compression may progress very rapidly. Further spinal cord damage may occur if the tumor mass encases radicular arteries.

Box 12.2. Radiotherapy in Spinal Canal Tumors

The radiation field is determined by the extent of involvement and includes two vertebral levels above and below the lesion. With this extended field, early local recurrence is less likely. A common radiation dose is 30 Gy in 10–20 fractions administered in 2–4 weeks. The effect is greatest in radiosensitive tumors, such as lymphoma, seminoma, myeloma, Ewing's sarcoma, and neuroblastoma, and less in breast and prostate cancers.

If paraplegia existed for approximately 1 week, recovery of ambulation can be expected 3–6 months later. Recovery is more rapid in patients with gradual onset of paraplegia over weeks. Reirradiation in relapsing patients ("infield" recurrence) frequently preserves ambulation. However, reirradiation in nonambulatory patients may result in the ability to ambulate in only a few.

Box 12.3. Corticosteroids

Dexamethasone used in patients with metastatic epidural spinal cord compression decreases water content of the spinal cord, reduces epidural swelling, and reduces tumor mass in lymphoma (it may even "disappear"). However, its most dramatic clinical effect is on pain reduction, often within hours of intravenous injection. Dexamethasone has a 4 hour half-life, and repeated doses are needed. High doses (intravenous bolus of 100 mg followed by 96 mg orally for 3 days) or high doses with gradual reduction (96 mg intravenously tapered in 14 days) may not be more effective than 10 mg intravenously fol-

lowed by 16 mg orally for 7 days and tapered in 2 weeks. There is good evidence to support the use of high-dose dexamethasone therapy in conjunction with radiotherapy.[38] Pain relief is more complete with higher doses. Corticosteroids significantly decrease gastric pH and may rapidly lead to pseudo-obstructive ileus from constipation. These side effects may be reduced by stool softeners, antacids, and H_2 blockers. Serious early side effects are psychosis, hyperglycemia, gastric ulcer bleeding, gastrointestinal perforation, and masking of clinical signs of infections.

efit lies in preservation of at least partial mobility and, equally important, complete bladder function. Outcome also depends on the ability to prevent complications and treat nonneurologic problems (lungs, skin, bladder) early.

Surgery should be the preferred approach when the primary tumor is unknown and histologic diagnosis is needed.[31–33] If vertebral collapse coincides with spinal cord compression, the chances for ambulation are lower and the potential for further deterioration after surgery is real. Spinal stabilization techniques may overcome this situation. These techniques include vertebral body resection, rod stabilization, and anterior (abdominal or thoracic) decompression. Epidural metastatic lesions often can be treated effectively only by surgery with anterior–posterior resection with instrumentation.[34] Marginal life expectancy and the degree of metastasis often preclude major surgery.

Approximately 70% of patients with malignant spinal extradural compression remain or become mobile after surgical treatment.[35] Radiotherapy is preferred in patients with known radiosensitive tumors (Box 12.2).[5] A short fractionated course, often with corticosteroids, is appropriate in most patients.[36] Single-fraction therapy should be considered when the aim of treatment is palliation of pain only. Reirradiation in patients with recurrent spinal cord compression from cancer also preserves ambulation. In one study, ambulation was achieved in two-thirds of patients but median survival was 4 months.[37] Primary chemotherapy has been advocated for lymphoma, myeloma, and germ cell tumors but in most patients is combined with radiotherapy.

Dexamethasone (Box 12.3) is given to all patients with metastatic cord compression (100 mg intravenous push followed by 16 mg orally daily in divided doses) until definitive management has been determined.

Patients with an epidural hematoma need fresh-frozen plasma and vitamin K for immediate reversal of anticoagulation to international normalized ratio (INR) levels within the normal range. Multiple doses and plasma infusions may be needed to reach an INR level of <1.5, which is satisfactory for surgical exploration. Patients with a high risk for cardioembolization (e.g., metallic heart valve) may tolerate short-term dis-

continuation of anticoagulation, but experience is limited. Reinstitution of anticoagulation is usually considered 1 week after surgery.[39] Spontaneous complete resolution of spinal epidural hematoma has been reported in approximately 7 of more than 250 cases reported in the literature, but identifying these patients and accurately predicting a benign course remain open to doubt.[40–42]

Three major factors predict favorable postoperative recovery in spontaneous epidural hematoma: incomplete cord syndrome, decompression within 36 hours in patients with complete cord syndrome, and decompression within 48 hours in patients with incomplete cord syndrome.[43] Rapid onset of paraplegia is not predictive of outcome and should not discourage surgical intervention.

REFERENCES

1. Helweg-Larsen S: Clinical outcome in metastatic spinal cord compression. A prospective study of 153 patients. *Acta Neurol Scand* 94:269, 1996.
2. Posner JB: *Neurologic Complications of Cancer*. Philadelphia: FA Davis, 1995.
3. Stark RJ, Henson RA, Evans SJ: Spinal metastases. A retrospective survey from a general hospital. *Brain* 105:189, 1982.
4. Husband DJ: Malignant spinal cord compression: prospective study of delays in referral and treatment. *BMJ* 317:18, 1998.
5. Byrne TN, Waxman SG: *Spinal Cord Compression: Diagnosis and Principles of Management*. Philadelphia: FA Davis, 1990.
6. Nicholas JJ, Christy WC: Spinal pain made worse by recumbency: a clue to spinal cord tumors. *Arch Phys Med Rehabil* 67:598, 1986.
7. Pal B, Johnson A: Paraplegia due to thoracic disc herniation. *Postgrad Med J* 73:423, 1997.
8. Tang HJ, Lin HJ, Liu YC, et al.: Spinal epidural abscess: experience with 46 patients and evaluation of prognostic factors. *J Infect* 45:76, 2002.
9. Sawin PD, Traynelis VC, Follett KA: Spinal epidural hematoma following coronary thrombolysis with tissue plasminogen activator. Report of two cases. *J Neurosurg* 83:350, 1995.
10. Stoll A, Sanchez M: Epidural hematoma after epidural block: implications for its use in pain management. *Surg Neurol* 57:235, 2002.
11. Kou J, Fischgrund J, Biddinger A, et al.: Risk factors for spinal epidural hematoma after spinal surgery. *Spine* 27:1670, 2002.
12. Komiyama M, Yasui T, Sumimoto T, et al.: Spontaneous

spinal subarachnoid hematoma of unknown pathogenesis: case reports. *Neurosurgery* 41:691, 1997.

13. Sakamoto N, Yanaka K, Matsumaru Y, et al.: Cervical epidural hematoma causing hemiparesis. *Arch Neurol* 60:783, 2003.

14. Tryciecky EW, Gottschalk A, Ludema K: Oncologic imaging: interactions of nuclear medicine with CT and MRI using the bone scan as a model. *Semin Nucl Med* 27:142, 1997.

15. Cook AM, Lau TN, Tomlinson MJ, et al.: Magnetic resonance imaging of the whole spine in suspected malignant spinal cord compression: impact on management. *Clin Oncol (R Coll Radiol)* 10:39, 1998.

16. Husband DJ, Grank KA, Romaniuk CS: MRI in the diagnosis and treatment of suspected malignant spinal cord compression. *Br J Radiol* 74:15, 2001.

17. Georgy BA, Snow RD, Hesselink JR: MR imaging of spinal nerve roots: techniques, enhancement patterns, and imaging findings. *AJR Am J Roentgenol* 166:173, 1996.

18. Zee CS, Segall HD, Boswell W, et al.: MR imaging of neurocysticercosis. *J Comput Assist Tomogr* 12:927, 1988.

19. Nesbit GM, Miller GM, Baker HL Jr, et al.: Spinal cord sarcoidosis: a new finding at MR imaging with Gd-DTPA enhancement. *Radiology* 173:839, 1989.

20. Lim V, Sobel DF, Zyroff J: Spinal cord pial metastases: MR imaging with gadopentetate dimeglumine. *AJNR Am J Neuroradiol* 11:975, 1990.

21. Sellwood RB: The radiological approach to metastatic cancer of the brain and spine. *Br J Radiol* 45:647, 1972.

22. Henderson RD, Pittock SJ, Piepgras DG, et al.: Acute spontaneous spinal epidural hematoma. *Arch Neurol* 58:1145, 2001.

23. Anderson NE, Willoughby EW: Infarction of the conus medullaris. *Ann Neurol* 21:470, 1987.

24. Criscuolo GR, Oldfield EH, Doppman JL: Reversible acute and subacute myelopathy in patients with dural arteriovenous fistulas. Foix-Alajouanine syndrome reconsidered. *J Neurosurg* 70:354, 1989.

25. Oldfield EH, Doppman JL: Spinal arteriovenous malformations. *Clin Neurosurg* 34:161, 1988.

26. Symon L, Kuyama H, Kendall B: Dural arteriovenous malformations of the spine. Clinical features and surgical results in 55 cases. *J Neurosurg* 60:238, 1984.

27. Byrne TN: Spinal cord compression from epidural metastases. *N Engl J Med* 327:614, 1992.

28. Siegal T: Spinal cord compression: from laboratory to clinic. *Eur J Cancer* 31A:1748, 1995.

29. Carlson GD, Minato Y, Okada A, et al.: Early time-dependent decompression for spinal cord injury: vascular mechanisms of recovery. *J Neurotrauma* 14:951, 1997.

30. Carlson GD, Gorden CD, Oliff HS, et al.: Sustained spinal cord compression. Part I. Time-dependent effect on long-term pathophysiology. *J Bone Joint Surg Am* 85:86, 2003.

31. Wiley RG: *Neurological Complications of Cancer.* New York: Marcel Dekker, 1995.

32. Schiff D, Batchelor T, Wen PY: Neurologic emergencies in cancer patients. *Neurol Clin* 16:449, 1998.

33. Gokaslan ZL: Spine surgery for cancer. *Curr Opin Oncol* 8:178, 1996.

34. Sundaresan N, Sachdev VP, Holland JF, et al.: Surgical treatment of spinal cord compression from epidural metastasis. *J Clin Oncol* 13:2330, 1995.

35. Huddart RA, Rajan B, Law M, et al.: Spinal cord compression in prostate cancer: treatment outcome and prognostic factors. *Radiother Oncol* 44:229, 1997.

36. Maranzano E, Latini P: Effectiveness of radiation therapy without surgery in metastatic spinal cord compression: final results from a prospective trial. *Int J Radiat Oncol Biol Phys* 32:959, 1995.

37. Schiff D, Shaw EG, Cascino TL: Outcome after spinal reirradiation for malignant epidural spinal cord compression. *Ann Neurol* 37:583, 1995.

38. Loblaw DA, Laperriere NJ: Emergency treatment of malignant extradural spinal cord compression: an evidence-based guideline. *J Clin Oncol* 16:1613, 1998.

39. Phoung LK, Wijdicks EFM, Sanan A: Spinal epidural hematoma and high thromboembolic risk: between Scylla and Charybdis. *Mayo Clin Proc* 74:147, 1999.

40. Silber SH: Complete nonsurgical resolution of a spontaneous spinal epidural hematoma. *Am J Emerg Med* 14:391, 1996.

41. Cirek B, Guven MB, Akalan N: Spontaneous spinal epidural hematoma. *Arch Phys Med Rehabil* 80:125, 1999.

42. Kumar R, Gerber C: Resolution of extensive spinal epidural haematoma with conservative treatment. *J Neurol Neurosurg Psychiatry* 65: 949, 1998.

43. Groen RJ, van Alphen HA: Operative treatment of spontaneous spinal epidural hematomas: a study of the factors determining postoperative outcome. *Neurosurgery* 39:494, 1996.

Appendix 12.1.
Localization of Spinal Cord Lesions

Foramen Magnum Syndrome and Lesions of the Upper Cervical Cord

Suboccipital pain and neck stiffness, Lhermitte's sign, occipital and fingertip paresthesias.

Sensory dissociation may be present.

Sensory findings of posterior column dysfunction may be present.

High cervical compressive findings (spastic tetraparesis, long tract sensory findings, bladder disturbance).

Lower cranial nerve palsies (CN IX–XII) may occur from regional extension of the pathologic process.

Lesions affecting the C5 segment may compromise the diaphragm.

With C5 segment lesions, biceps and brachioradialis reflexes are absent or diminished, whereas the triceps reflex and the finger flexor reflex are exaggerated (because of corticospinal tract compression at C5).

With C6 segment lesions, biceps, brachioradialis, and triceps reflexes are diminished or absent but the finger flexor reflex (C8–T1) is exaggerated.

Lesions of the Seventh Cervical Segment

Paresis involves flexors and extensors of the wrists and fingers.

Biceps and brachioradialis reflexes are preserved, and the finger flexor reflex is exaggerated.

May result in flexion of the forearm following olecranon tap. (Weakness of the triceps prevents its contraction and elbow extension, whereas muscles innervated by normal segments above the lesion are allowed to contract.)

Sensory loss at and below the third and fourth digits (including medial arm and forearm).

Lesions of the Eighth Cervical and First Thoracic Segments

Weakness that predominantly involves the small hand muscles, with associated spastic paraparesis.

With C8 lesions, the triceps reflex (C6–C8) and finger flexor reflex (C8–T1) are decreased.

With T1 lesions, the triceps reflex is preserved but the finger flexor reflex is decreased.

Possible unilateral or bilateral Horner's syndrome with C8–T1 lesions.

Sensory loss involves the fifth digit, medial forearm and arm, and rest of the body below the lesion.

Lesions of the Thoracic Segments

Root pain or paresthesias that mimic intercostal neuralgia.

Segmental lower motor neuron involvement is difficult to detect clinically.

Paraplegia, sensory loss below thoracic level, and bowel and bladder disturbances occur.

With lesions above T5, vasomotor control may be impaired.

With a cord lesion at the T10 level, upper abdominal musculature is preserved but lower abdominal muscles are weak. For example, when the head is flexed against resistance with the patient supine, the intact upper abdominal muscles pull the umbilicus upward (*Beevor's sign*).

If the lesion lies above T6, superficial abdominal reflexes are absent.

If the lesion is at or below T10, upper and middle abdominal reflexes are present.

If the lesion is below T12, all abdominal reflexes are present.

Lesions of the First Lumbar Segment

Weakness in all muscles of the lower extremities. Lower abdominal muscle paresis.

Sensory loss includes both the lower extremities up to the level of the groin and the back to a level above the buttocks.

With longstanding lesions, the patellar and ankle jerks are brisk.

Lesions of the Second Lumbar Segment

Spastic paraparesis but no weakness of abdominal musculature.

Cremasteric reflex (L2) is not elicitable, and patellar jerk may be depressed.

Ankle jerks are hyperactive.

Lesions of the Third Lumbar Segment

Some preservation of hip flexion (iliopsoas and sartorius) and leg adduction (adductor longus, pectineus, and gracilis).

Patellar jerks are decreased or not elicitable.

Ankle jerks are hyperactive.

Lesions of the Fourth Lumbar Segment

Better hip flexion and leg adduction than in L1–L3 lesions.

Knee flexion and leg extension are better performed, and the patient is able to stand by stabilizing the knees.

Patellar jerks are absent, and ankle jerks are hyperactive.

Lesions of the Fifth Lumbar Segment

Normal hip flexion and adduction and leg extension. Patient can extend legs against resistance when extremities are flexed at the hip and knee (normal quadriceps).

Patellar reflexes are present.

Ankle jerks are hyperactive.

Lesions of the First Sacral Segment

Achilles reflexes are absent, but patellar reflexes are preserved.

Complete sensory loss over the sole, heel, and outer aspect of the foot and ankle.

Anesthesia over medial calf, posterior thigh.

Conus Medullaris Lesions

Paralysis of the pelvic floor muscles and early sphincter dysfunction.

Disruption of the bladder reflex arc results in autonomous neurogenic bladder characterized by loss of voluntary initiation of micturition, increased residual urine, and absent bladder sensation.

Constipation and impaired erection and ejaculation common.

May have symmetric saddle anesthesia.

Pain may involve thighs, buttocks, and perineum.

Pain uncommon.

Cauda Equina Lesions

Early radicular pain in the distribution of the lumbosacral roots due to compression below the L3 vertebral level.

Pain may be unilateral or asymmetric and is increased by the Valsalva maneuver.

With extensive lesions, flaccid, hypotonic, areflexic paralysis develops, affecting the glutei, posterior thigh muscles, and anterolateral muscles of the leg and foot, resulting in a true peripheral type of paraplegia.

Sensory testing reveals asymmetric sensory loss in saddle region, involving anal, perineal, and genital regions and extending to the dorsal aspect of the thigh, anterolateral aspect of the leg, and outer aspect of the foot.

Achilles reflexes are absent, and patellar reflexes are variable in response.

Sphincter changes are similar to those with a conus lesion, but occurrence tends to be late in the clinical course.

Although it can be concluded that lesions of the conus result in early sphincter compromise, late pain, and symmetric sensory manifestations, whereas cauda lesions have early pain, late sphincter manifestations, and asymmetric sensory findings, this distinction is difficult to establish and is of little practical value.

Source: Data abstracted from Biller J, Brazis PW: The localization of lesions affecting the spinal cord. In Brazis PW, Masdue JC, Biller J (eds). *Localization in Clinical Neurology.* Boston: Little, Brown and Company, 1996: 63–85.

Appendix 12.2.
British Medical Research Council Scale of Muscle Strength

0	No muscular contraction
1	Muscular contraction without joint involvement
2	Muscular contraction moves joint but not against gravity
3	Muscular contraction moves joint, just overcoming gravity
4	Muscular contraction overcoming gravity and appreciable force
5	Muscular contraction not overcome by examiner

Source: Modified from *Aids to the Examination of the Peripheral Nervous System.* London: Baillière Tindall, 2000. By permission of the Guarantors of Brain.

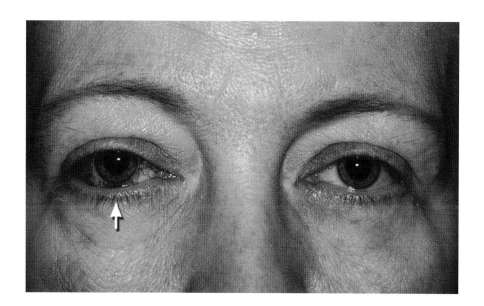

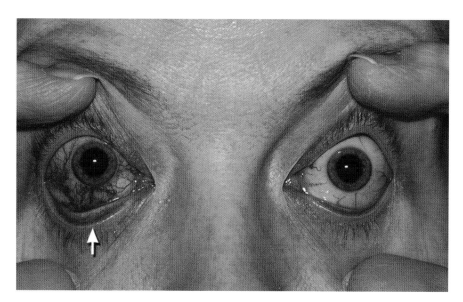

Color Figure 3.5 Exophthalmos and chemosis and red eye in traumatic carotid-cavernous fistula. The abnormality is barely seen but becomes clear with further retraction of the eyelids.

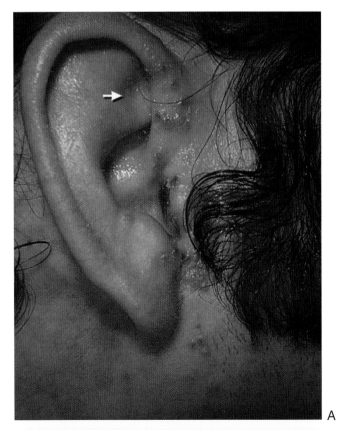

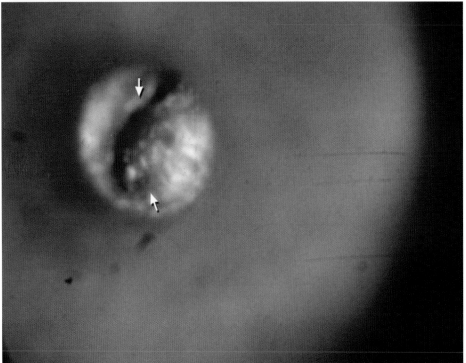

Color Figure 4.1 Vesicles in the external auditory canal (*A*) and eardrum (*B*) in a patient with herpes zoster oticus.

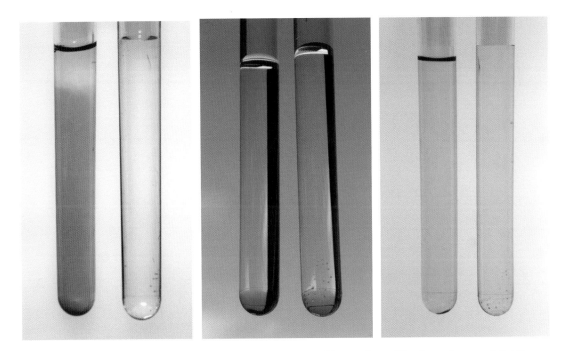

Color Figure 6.3 Tube in a patient with subarachnoid hemorrhage (bloody cerebrospinal fluid) compared with water (*left*). Note subtle xanthochromia after sedimentation, obscured by viewing in daylight (*middle*) most evident with strong light source (*right*).

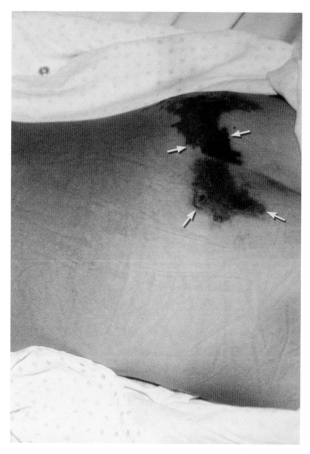

Color Figure 8.2 Excoriated coma blisters at compression points. They are found in patients with barbiturate overdose, carbon monoxide exposure, amitriptyline, theophylline, and diabetic ketoacidosis.

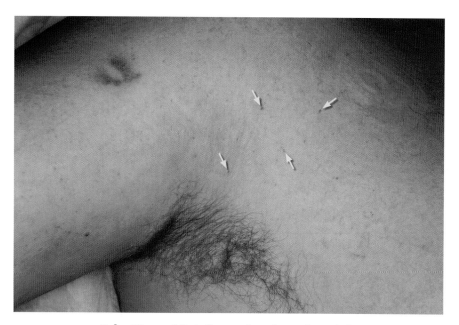

Color Figure 8.3 Axilla petechiae due to fat emboli.

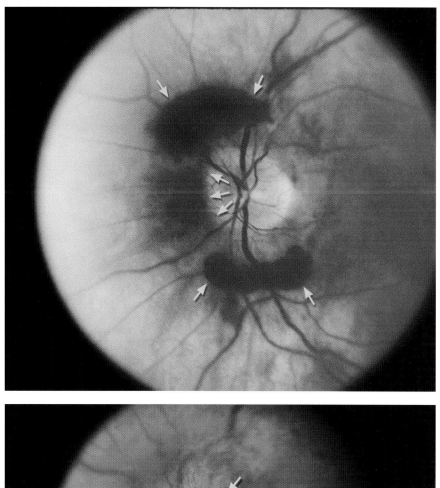

A

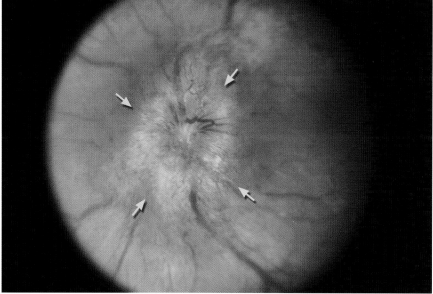

B

Color Figure 8.10 Examples of funduscopic findings. *A:* Subhyaloid hemorrhage in subarachnoid hemorrhage. *B:* Papilledema in increased intracranial pressure (typical "champagne cork" configuration).

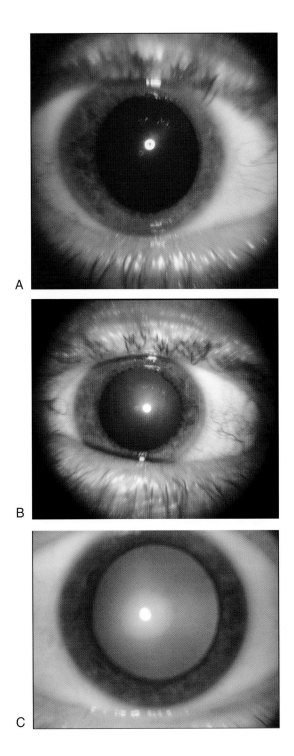

Color Figure 13.2 Terson's syndrome in aneurysmal subarachnoid hemorrhage. Funduscopy of retinal hemorrhage *A:* Absent red reflex due to vitreous hemorrhage ("black eye"). *B:* One year later, the patient had marked improvement in vision, and red reflex is beginning to reappear. After vitrectomy, vision improved considerably. *C:* Normal red reflex, shown by retroillumination with fundus camera.

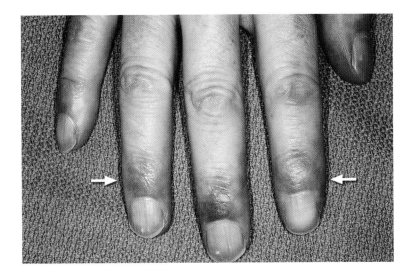

Color Figure 15.17 Blotchy fingers in antiphospholipid antibody syndrome.

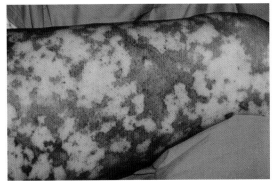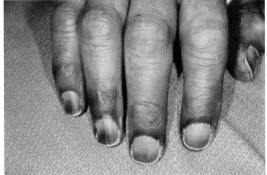

Color Figure 16.2 Purpura in meningococcal meningitis.

Chapter 13
Aneurysmal Subarachnoid Hemorrhage

Contrary to common perception, many patients with aneurysmal subarachnoid hemorrhage (SAH) come to the emergency department with headache only, alert or drowsy, and minimal neurologic findings.[1] The disastrous consequences for a patient with aneurysmal SAH thus may come later. Although the time spent in the emergency department is short, these patients need frequent neurologic assessment and close cardiopulmonary monitoring.

Recognition of SAH (Box 13.1) may seem straightforward in many cases, but errors may arise in the evaluation of patients with presumed normal findings on computed tomographic (CT) scans but typical onset of severe headache. The difficulties in assessment of patients with alleged SAH often can be traced back to misinterpretation of CT scans, failure to distinguish between bloody spinal fluid from needle trauma and true SAH, and, more simply but far more important, careless history-taking.

This chapter provides the necessary tools to appropriately assess these patients in the emergency department and transfer them to the intensive care unit.

Clinical Presentation

Fundamental in history-taking for a patient with acute headache is determination of the precise time of onset, quality of the headache, and whether the patient had similar earlier events. As described in Chapter 6, the headache in aneurysmal SAH is characteristic. A history of a severe "never experienced before," "in the middle of a sentence," "flash-like," "explosive" acute headache is very suggestive of SAH.[9] Many patients describe a brief sense of panic because they are stunned by the unexpected presentation. The often-quoted "worst headache of my life" in textbooks may not necessarily indicate acute onset or precisely define the severity of the headache (e.g., patients with chronic headaches or migraine have episodes that they commonly first classify as "the worst headache ever"). The headache usually is persistent, but resolution with the use of medication, such as nonsteroidal anti-inflammatory agents, aspirin, or even narcotics, should not be mistakenly interpreted as an argument against SAH.

When specifically asked, prior headaches may have been similar and shorter in duration. In 10%–20% of patients, an identical thunderclap headache is identified but ignored by the patient or by the consulted physician due to its rapid resolution or associated symptoms suggesting a more mundane viral infection or stress-related headache.[10–14]

Vomiting may occur several minutes into the ictus as a result of further distribution of blood throughout the subarachnoid space. It occurs in 50% of patients but is nonspecific. Profuse vomiting may override the headache and has been mistaken for a "gastric flu" by the patient or ini-

Box 13.1. Aneurysmal Rupture

What causes aneurysms to rupture is puzzling. Risk factors have included recent documented enlargement (rupture of aneurysms less than 4 mm is very rare; most ruptured aneurysms are 7–8 mm, and risk of rupture increases significantly in aneurysms 10 mm or greater), hypertension, cigarette smoking, and family history of aneurysms and SAH.[2–4] Aneurysmal rupture has been reported to have occurred during weight lifting, sexual orgasm, and brawling, events that suggest acute hypertensive stress on a thin aneurysmal wall. However, at least 50% of patients have SAH at rest.[5,6]

Intracranial pressure rises dramatically to at least the level of the diastolic blood pressure but may briefly increase to the level of the systolic blood pressure, causing a cerebral perfusion standstill.[7] The increase in intracranial pressure decreases within 15 minutes but may persist if acute hydrocephalus or shift from intracerebral hematoma has occurred. Rupture stops within 3–6 minutes after ejection of up to 15–20 mL/minute into the basal cistern[8] (Fig. 13.1).

tially consulted physician. Clinical presentations have included acute paraplegia (anterior cerebral artery rupture into frontal lobes) and severe thoracic and lumbar pain caused by meningeal irritation. These presentations obviously have resulted in a delay in cranial CT scan imaging.[1]

Clinical examination of patients with SAH includes grading of the severity of the SAH with use of the Glasgow Coma Scale and determining whether the patient has a motor deficit (World Federation of Neurological Surgeons [WFNS] scale, Table 13.1). However, stupor or coma in SAH (so-called poor-grade SAH) has many possible explanations. Impaired consciousness frequently is the result of a direct impact of the arterial jet and a massive increase in intracranial pressure, which significantly decrease cerebral perfusion pressure and thus result in global bihemispheric ischemia. Respiratory or cardiac arrest during the rupture followed by resuscitation may also result in an additional postanoxic-ischemic encephalopathy.[15] Other causes of poor-grade SAH are intracranial hematoma with brain shift and brain stem compression and acute hydrocephalus.

Neck stiffness from cervical meningeal irritation may take some time to develop and is absent in coma. Nuchal rigidity can be demonstrated by failure to flex the neck in the neutral position and failure to retroflex when both shoulders are lifted. Flat-topped retinal hemorrhages (subhyaloid hemorrhages) are characteristic of aneurysmal SAH and indicate profound SAH. These hemorrhages occur when outflow in the optic nerve venous system is suddenly obstructed by the intracranial pressure wave. Visual loss may be severe, with perception of light or hand motion only, if the hemorrhage expands and ruptures into the vit-

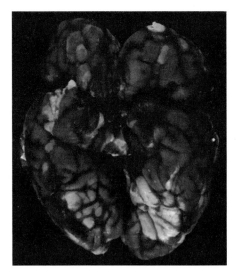

Figure 13.1 Gross pathology showing layer of subarachnoid hemorrhage at the basal part of the brain.

Table 13.1. World Federation of Neurological Surgeons (WFNS) Grading System for Subarachnoid Hemorrhage

WFNS Grade	GCS	Motor Deficit
I	15	Absent
II	14–13	Absent
III	14–13	Present
IV	12–7	Present or absent
V	6–3	Present or absent

GCS, Glasgow coma score (see Chapter 8 for full description).

reous (Terson's syndrome; *see Color Fig. 13.2 in separate color insert*).[16–18]

Neuro-ophthalmologic signs can localize the site of the aneurysm. Rupture of a posterior communicating artery or carotid artery aneurysm can produce a third nerve palsy. The pupil is dilated and unreactive to light because of compression of the exteriorly located fibers that form the light reflex. However, up to 15% of posterior communicating artery aneurysms may occur with a pupil-sparing third nerve palsy[19] (see Chapter 3). Aneurysm of the basilar artery may produce unilateral or bilateral third or sixth nerve palsy. If the basilar artery aneurysm enlarges and progressively compresses the oculomotor nuclei of the pons, horizontal gaze paralysis, skew deviation, internuclear ophthalmoplegia, and nystagmus occur, commonly in association with long tract signs such as hemiparesis and ataxia. Occlusion of the proximal posterior cerebral artery, often encased in a giant aneurysm, may occur, causing either classic Weber's syndrome (see Chapter 15) due to mesencephalon infarction (third nerve palsy with opposite hemiparesis) or homonymous hemianopia due to occipital lobe infarction.

Hemiparesis that usually involves the face, arm, and leg in SAH should point to an intracranial hematoma. An anteriorly placed intracranial hematoma in the frontal lobe may not produce motor weakness but be associated with agitation and bizarre behavior. Many patients are confused, concoct bizarre stories, or ramble nonsensically. Korsakoff's syndrome with impaired recall and fabrications has been described in ruptured anterior communicating aneurysm. Abulia, a general sense of disinterest, and lackluster attention are also features, becoming apparent days later. Temporal lobe hematoma in the dominant hemisphere may produce aphasia, but often its associated brain shift decreases the level of consciousness and word output.

Generalized tonic-clonic seizures are accompanied by aneurysmal rupture in 10% of patients or appear during rebleeding. Nonconvulsive status epilepticus or epilepsia partialis continua is very uncommon in aneurysmal SAH. It is more common in patients with additional subdural hematoma and when delayed cerebral infarction occurs.[20]

Systemic manifestations, besides vomiting, may include respiratory failure and oxygen desaturation from aspiration, pulmonary edema, or obstruction of the airway by a foreign object (e.g., pieces of teeth broken during clenching of the jaws at the time of a seizure). Cardiac arrhythmias may involve the entire spectrum of supraventricular and ventricular arrhythmias. Most of the time they are associated with electrocardiographic changes, which may simulate or indicate anterior wall or subendocardial infarction. Elevated troponin I levels may occur in approximately 25% of the cases seen on the first day and indicate left, sometimes transient, ventricular dysfunction.[21] Thus, with an incomplete medical history and no inquiry about acute headache, patients may be wrongly transferred to a medical intensive care unit (cardiac resuscitation and pulmonary edema), gastrointestinal service (vomiting), or coronary care unit (cardiac arrhythmias with new electrocardiographic changes).

The clinical state of the patient may suddenly change in the emergency department. We have seen several patients who soon after presentation had acute worsening of the headache and became significantly more drowsy, with a decrease of several points in the Glasgow coma score. Rebleeding could be demonstrated on CT scans in those instances. Other causes of further worsening in the emergency department are acute obstructive hydrocephalus and herniation from swelling surrounding a hematoma. These sequences of events should be recognized, particularly because rebleeding is highly prevalent within the first 6 hours of initial rupture.

Interpretation of Laboratory Tests

Computed Tomographic Scanning

CT scanning has a very high sensitivity and specificity for SAH.[22,23] The sensitivity of a noncontrast CT scan for SAH alone is 93% for patients seen within the first day, 84% for those seen on the second day, 50% after day 5, and 0 after day 10. The accumulation of subarachnoid blood on CT scans is characteristically diffuse, involving all basal cisterns, the interhemispheric and sylvian fissures, and the area along the convexity (Fig. 13.3). Additional lobar hematomas point to more certain localization of an aneurysm (Figs. 13.4, 13.5).[24–26]

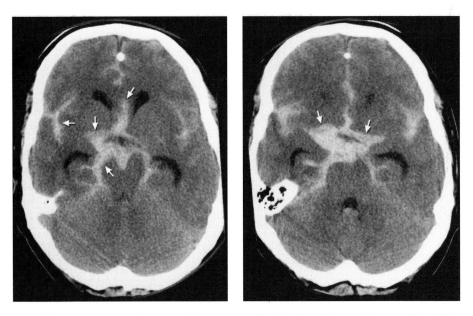

Figure 13.3 Computed tomographic patterns of subarachnoid hemorrhage. Diffuse filling of basal cistern and fissures (*arrows*) produces a hyperdense cast.

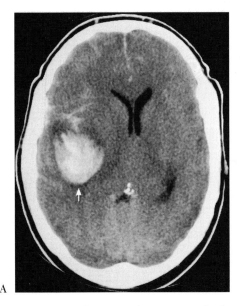

A

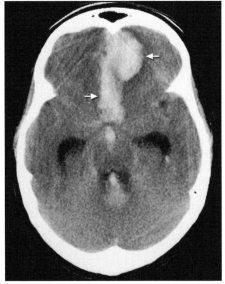

B

Figure 13.4 Computed tomographic patterns of subarachnoid hemorrhage with associated hematomas indirectly localizing ruptured aneurysms. *A:* Sylvian fissure (middle cerebral artery). *B:* Frontal hematoma (anterior cerebral artery). *C:* Hematoma in cavum septum pellucidum. *D,E:* Medial temporal lobe with subdural hematoma (carotid artery). *F:* Corpus callosum (pericallosal artery). *G–I:* Thalamic hematoma with posterior cerebral artery (P1 segment) aneurysm identified on magnetic resonance imaging. *J,K:* Premedullary hematoma with posterior inferior cerebellar artery aneurysm.

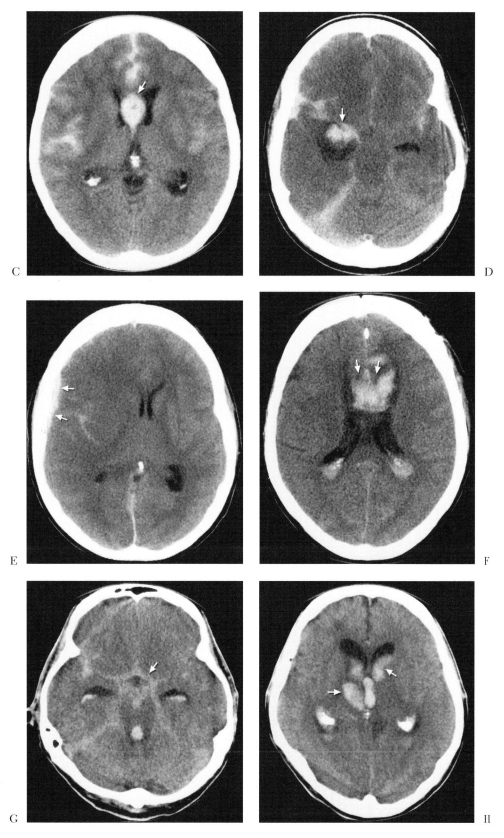

Figure 13.4 (*Continued*)

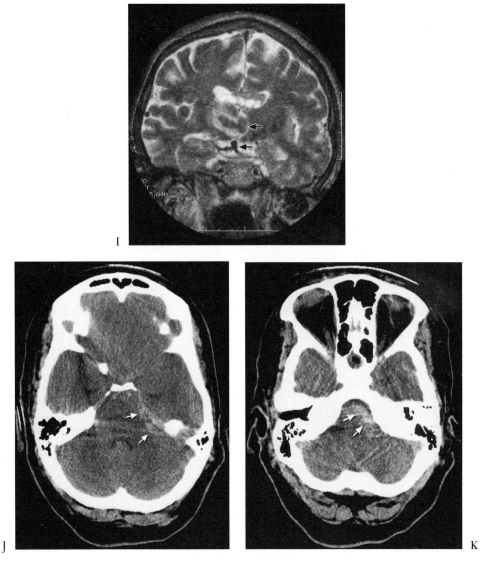

Figure 13.4 (*Continued*)

Hypodensity in both hemispheres and early loss of gray–white differentiation may develop in poor-grade SAH (Fig. 13.6). They reflect periodic acute arrest of cerebral flow caused by a very large increase in intracranial pressure at rupture. The CT scan findings are proof of early ischemic damage rather than cerebral vasospasm, which appears several days into the clinical course.

A clot in front of the brain stem with no extension beyond the suprasellar cisterns (so-called pretruncal SAH) highly predicts negative cerebral angiographic results,[27–29] but it has been estimated that in 10% of cases a posterior circulation aneurysm (most commonly, basilar caput) can be found on cerebral angiograms. The typical CT and MRI patterns of pretruncal SAH should be recognized (Box 13.2, Figs. 13.7, 13.8).

Blood can be difficult to detect on CT scans and may be very subtle, particularly in patients seen several days after the onset. The most commonly encountered false-negative CT scans are from patients with blood in the posterior horns of the ventricles (Fig. 13.9A), sylvian fissure (Fig. 13.9B), or prepontine region, in which hemorrhage may be only a small layer on the pons (Fig. 13.9C). A tiny clot (involving a few pixels) may be

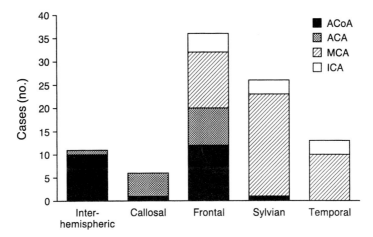

Figure 13.5 Prediction of hematoma for site of aneurysm in aneurysmal SAH. (Modified from Tokuda et al.[25] By permission of Elsevier Science.) ACA, ante- rior cerebral artery; ACoA, anterior communicating ar- tery; ICA, internal carotid artery; MCA, middle cere- bral artery.

localized in the interpeduncular cistern (Fig. 13.9D). It is easily missed, particularly if the CT scan slices through the posterior fossa and basal cisterns are 10 mm.

CT detection of aneurysms has improved with a new generation of scanners, but contrast en- hancement is needed to demonstrate an aneurysm, which is visualized only if larger than 5 mm. Larger aneurysms (>1 cm in diameter) or giant aneu- rysms (>2.5 cm) (Fig. 13.10A,B) are disclosed on

an unenhanced CT scan in most patients, although sometimes they are masked by an intracerebral hematoma. Magnetic resonance imaging (MRI) is most useful in further anatomic definition (Fig. 13.10C).

SAH may also indicate a nonaneurysmal source and has been described in central nervous system vasculitis, trauma, coagulopathy, and subacute bacterial endocarditis, but mostly with blood in sulci (Fig. 13.11).[32,33] Typical CT scan features of

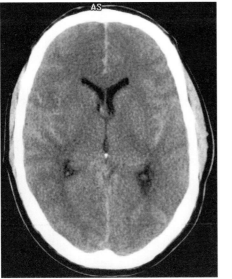
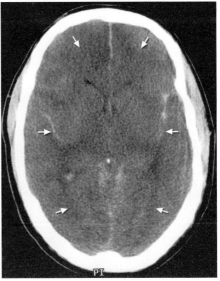

Figure 13.6 Development of bihemispheric ischemia (marked hypodensities, *arrows*) within 24 hours after subarachnoid hemorrhage.

Box 13.2. Pretruncal Nonaneurysmal Subarachnoid Hemorrhage

Pretruncal nonaneurysmal SAH (also called "perimesencephalic nonaneurysmal hemorrhage") is a benign variant of SAH. The entity is defined by blood before or surrounding the brain stem. Blood may extend to the middle of the basal part of the sylvian fissure but not to the interhemispheric fissure, convexity, or third ventricle and frontal horns of the ventricular system. True perimesencephalic hemorrhage can also be due to trauma or SAH from a superior cerebellar artery or distal posterior cerebral artery or basilar tip aneurysm. Cerebral angiographic findings are normal, although cerebral vasospasm may occur and aneurysms may be found at far distant sites. Family members may harbor aneurysms as well. Patients do very well; rebleeding and cerebral infarction do not occur. The underlying pathologic lesion is not known, although occasionally pontine capillary telangiectasias, focal dilatation of the basilar artery tip, anomalous veins, or a small bleb has been reported.[30,31] It may represent a venous hemorrhage or intramural arterial dissection.

traumatic SAH are shown in Figure 13.11C–G. It is important to consider other causes of coma and false SAH, most commonly due to anoxia and contrast for evaluation of multitrauma. False SAH in massive anoxic cerebral edema in a resuscitated patient most likely represents stagnation of flow in the dura.[34,35] Anoxic brain swelling may emerge within 1 day after cardiac resuscitation, and CT may show hyperintensity in the basal cistern, falx, and tentorium. CT scan signs of edema are usually very obvious (Fig. 13.12A,B). It is likely due to the combination of decreased attenuation from brain swelling, reduced cerebrospinal fluid (CSF) volume, and enlarged veins in the basal cisterns, all as a consequence of increased intracranial pressure. We have also noticed pseudosubarachnoid hemorrhage in bilateral subdural hematoma with obliteration of basal cisterns.[36] In addition, con-

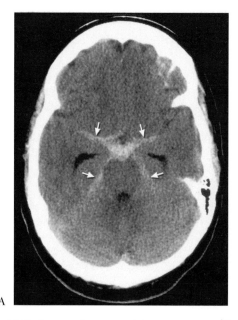
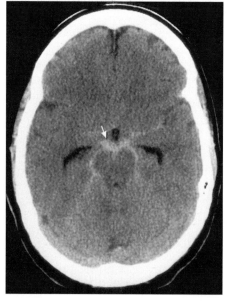

A   B

Figure 13.7 Computed tomographic scan patterns of pretruncal nonaneurysmal subarachnoid hemorrhage in different patients. The spectrum includes complete filling of suprasellar cisterns and blood on the tentorium to more restricted clots and more subtle interpeduncular hematoma. The amount of blood is not critical in its recognition. The distribution of blood is limited and should not involve the entire lateral part of the sylvian fissure or the anterior hemisphere and ventricles.

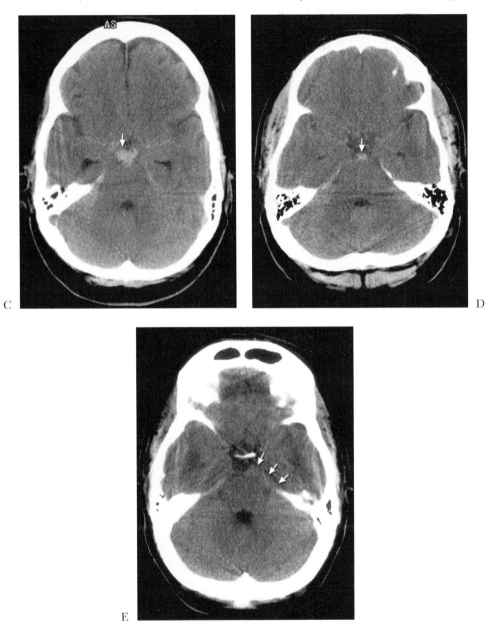

Figure 13.7 (*Continued*)

trast enhancement may significantly mimic SAH. A contrast-enhanced study may have occurred before CT scanning, and contrast material may still be visualized in patients with poor renal function or shock or both (Fig. 13.12C,D). In exceptional cases, elevated hematocrit (>20 g/dL) may cause hyperdensity if confined to the intravascular space.[37] Both situations do somewhat more superficially mimic subarachnoid hemorrhage.

Magnetic Resonance Imaging

MRI is usually not sensitive for SAH.[38,39] However, MRI may be able to show SAH when fluid attenuation inversion recovery (FLAIR) sequences are used. Recirculation of bloody CSF over the convexity is commonly seen as well (Fig. 13.13).[40] MRI may be important in demonstrating an acute SAH in the posterior fossa, which, as

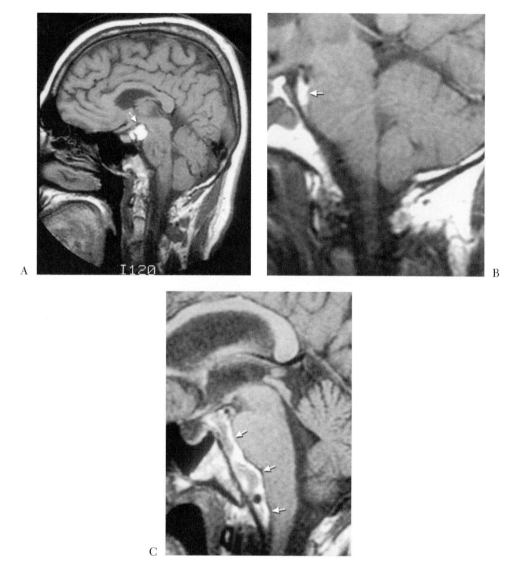

Figure 13.8 *A–C:* Magnetic resonance imaging patterns of pretruncal nonaneurysmal subarachnoid hemorrhage. Blood may involve all or part of the cisterns in front of the brain stem.

mentioned previously, may be difficult to detect on CT scan because of beam-hardening artifacts.[41,42] Often, in retrospect, CT scans showed a similar blood clot.[43] Sometimes a small deposit of blood in the sylvian fissure not visualized on CT scans can be demonstrated on MRI.

Magnetic resonance angiography (MRA) is useful in demonstrating the aneurysm,[44] and with three-dimensional time-of-flight MRA, aneurysms 3 mm in diameter and larger can be demonstrated (Fig. 13.14).[45,46] CT angiography has become a

very useful technique too. At this time, however, MRA or CT angiography is not a substitute for conventional cerebral angiography.

Cerebrospinal Fluid

As discussed in Chapter 6, the CSF should be examined for xanthochromia. If xanthochromia is found, absorption spectrophotometry could confirm oxyhemoglobin or bilirubin. This can be done hours later in stored, centrifuged CSF samples.

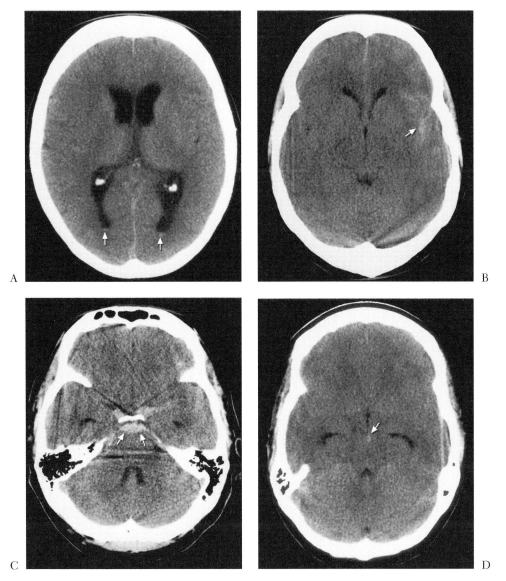

Figure 13.9 Subtle subarachnoid hemorrhage (false-negative computed tomographic scans). *A:* Dependent blood in posterior horns. *B:* Blood in sylvian fissure. *C:* Prepontine layer of blood. *D:* Small area of interpeduncular blood (see also Chapter 6).

CSF xanthochromia is detected by spectroscopy in specimens from all patients up to 2 weeks after the onset of headache. Spectrophotometry is not commonly used in the United States and is more commonplace in the United Kingdom.[47] Other tests that differentiate traumatic SAH from true SAH, such as measurements of CSF D-dimer and the sequential tube test that demonstrates the clearing of tubes tinged with blood, are all unreliable.

First Priority in Management

Stabilization of a patient with aneurysmal SAH also includes early institution of pain medication

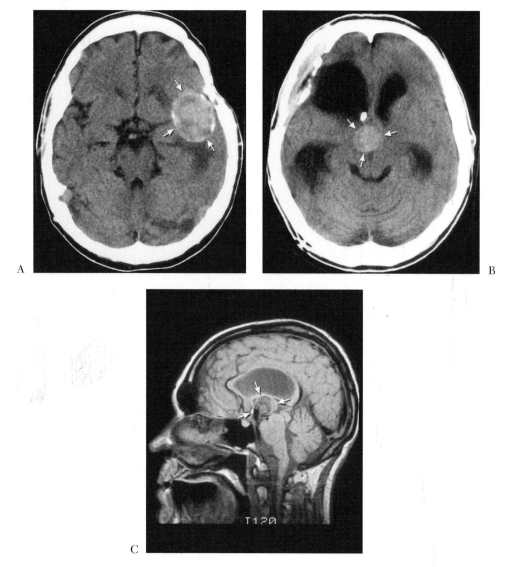

Figure 13.10 *A:* Computed tomographic scan showing giant middle cerebral artery aneurysm. *B:* Giant basilar tip aneurysm. *C:* Magnetic resonance imaging further delineates compression of the third ventricle causing obstructive hydrocephalus.

(codeine 30–60 mg every 4 hours). Management of increased blood pressure in the emergency department is a delicate balancing act. Many of the earlier studies suggesting an increased risk of rerupture with sustained hypertension should be devalued by lack of strict criteria for the diagnosis of rebleeding. Conversely, marked reduction of postrupture hypertension may precipitate a further reduction of cerebral perfusion pressure and possibly induce more ischemia. The initial management of aneurysmal SAH is shown in Table 13.2, but there are several immediate concerns that could warrant action.

Acute hydrocephalus should be treated with a ventriculostomy ideally but only when clinical deterioration can be attributed to CSF obstruction. In one recent survey, almost one in four patients received ventriculostomy, demonstrating the uncertain criteria for placement.[48] A prior perceived risk of inducing rebleeding was not found in a recent study.[49] Preoperative ventriculostomy did not increase the risk when definitive therapy fol-

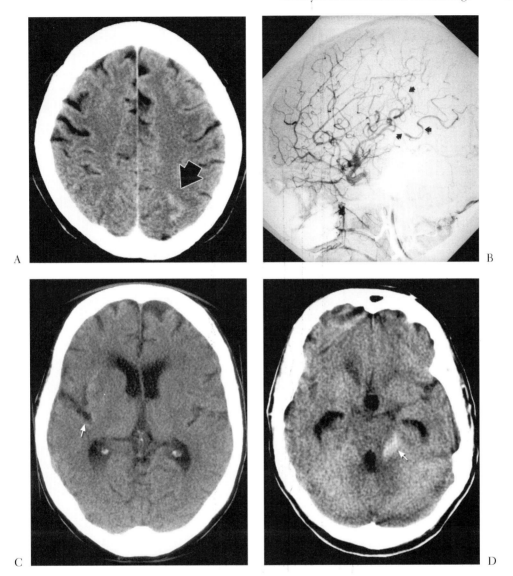

Figure 13.11 Typical nonaneurysmal locations of subarachnoid hemorrhage. *A,B:* Vasculitis. *Arrows* point to subarachnoid blood in a parietal sulcus and areas of seg-mental stenosis from vasculitis. *C–G:* Trauma (blood in fissure, cistern, and sulci or on tentorium).

lowed. Nonetheless, the level of drainage in patients with rebleeding was significantly lower than that in patients without rebleeding (mean 2.5 cm H_2O vs. 14 cm H_2O). Drainage at a level of 10–15 cm H_2O is preferred (see Chapter 11).[49]

Sudden deterioration in the emergency department often is due to rebleeding (Fig. 13.15), and emergency cerebral angiography is indicated. Placement of a platinum coil should be considered (Fig. 13.16) if the aneurysm is of sufficient size (4–10 mm). Neck size of the aneurysm should be less than 4 mm because anything larger may permit free herniation of the coil into the parent vessel, or the ratio of the largest diameter of the aneurysm to the size of its neck should be favorable; and patients should be poor surgical risks. However, the coil may become compacted after placement, increasing the risk of future rupture, in which case repeat cerebral angiography is needed in 6 weeks. A randomized study largely focused on good-grade (WFNS I or II) patients and small anterior cerebral artery and posterior

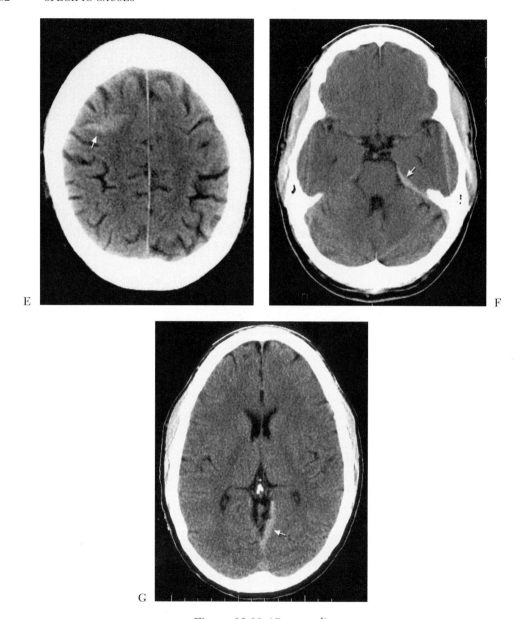

Figure 13.11 (*Continued*)

communicating artery aneurysms and found equal benefit in coiling versus clipping of the aneurysm. Results in basilar artery aneurysms are still anecdotal but very promising.[50,51] Two studies on poor-grade (WFNS V or Hunt and Hess grade 4 or 5) SAH patients found improved survival but at the expense of poor functional status.[52,53] Whether platinum coil placement equals aneurysmal clipping in future risk of rupture remains to be investigated. Data from follow-up at 1–2 years

are encouraging. However, rupture of a completely coil-occluded middle cerebral artery aneurysm after an 18-month interval has been reported.[54] Placement of coils in patients in poor neurologic state (WFNS III–IV) has been part of some aggressive protocols. Recurrent filling of the aneurysm occurred in 15% of 259 aneurysms treated by coil embolization. In some centers, annual rebleeding rates were 0.8% in the first year, 0.6% in the second year, and 2.4% in the third

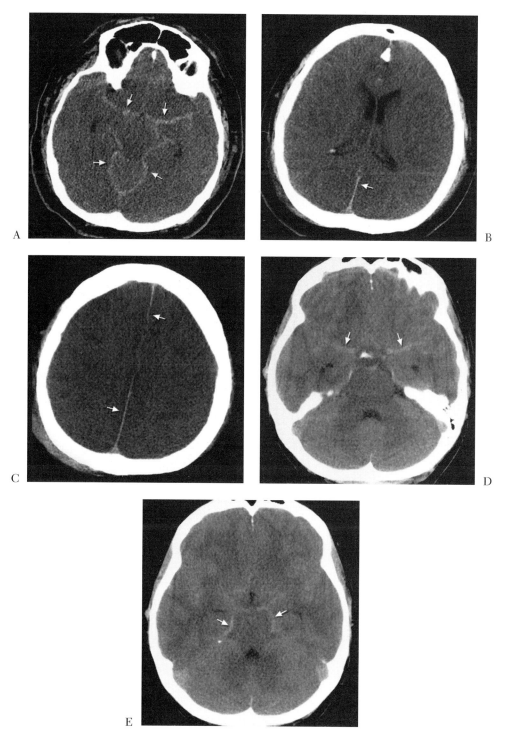

A

B

C

D

E

Figure 13.12 Pseudo–subarachnoid hemorrhage (SAH) (false-positive computed tomographic [CT] scan). *A–C:* Cerebral edema and pseudo-SAH. *D,E:* Intravascular contrast, 150 mL, from prior abdominal CT. Contrast may remain in vessels when the patient is in shock, which is often the reason for contrast CT scanning of the abdomen.

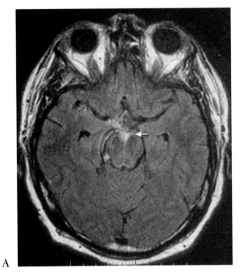 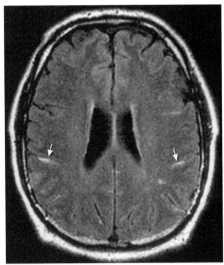

Figure 13.13 Magnetic resonance imaging with fluid attenuation inversion recovery (FLAIR) sequence: interpeduncular hemorrhage with subarachnoid blood over convexity. (From Wijdicks et al.[41] By permission of the American Heart Association.)

year after coil placement, with no rebleeding in 2 subsequent years.[55]

Early endovascular management is also indicated if SAH is caused by a dissecting vertebral aneurysm (Fig. 13.17). Rebleeding is very common, and aggressive treatment with proximal (e.g. coiling) occlusion is warranted.[56–59] Surgical management is indicated in a patient with an acute temporal lobe hematoma and early mass effect. Craniotomy with immediate clipping of the ruptured middle cerebral artery aneurysm is warranted, with deferral of cerebral angiography in most instances. Immediate surgical management of a frontal hematoma is rarely indicated. Neuro-

surgical management of most anterior cerebral artery aneurysms is more complex, requiring better definition by cerebral angiography.

Outcome Predictors

Favorable clinical and CT scan features in aneurysmal SAH are absence of syncope at the onset, full awareness at presentation,[60] lack of localizing neurologic signs, and subsequent early

Table 13.2. Initial Management of Aneurysmal Subarachnoid Hemorrhage in the Emergency Department

Endotracheal intubation in patients with GCS <8 or hypoxemia
Maintenance fluid intake of 2 L of 0.9% NaCl
Accept mean arterial blood pressure ≤120 mm Hg and systolic blood pressure <180 mm Hg; treat with esmolol 500 μg/kg IV or labetolol 20 mg (both slow IV push, 1–2 minutes)
Nimodipine, 60 mg 6 times a day
Fosphenytoin, 20 mg/kg intravenously (only with documented seizures)
Ventriculostomy in patients with acute hydrocephalus and GCS ≤10
Emergency neurosurgical evacuation in patients with progressive drowsiness and temporal lobe hematoma

GCS, Glasgow coma score.

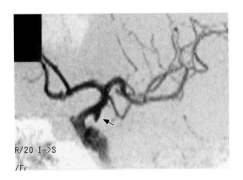

Figure 13.14 Magnetic resonance angiographic view of 6 mm aneurysm of the internal carotid artery (posterior communicating artery aneurysm).

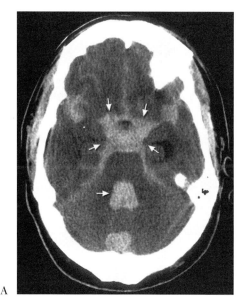

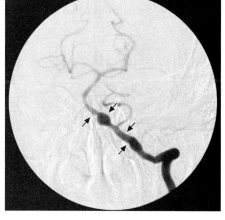

A

B

Figure 13.15 Massive subarachnoid hemorrhage with acute hydrocephalus and hemoventricle from dissect- ing vertebral aneurysm with fusiform dilatation. *A:* Com- puted tomographic scan. *B:* Cerebral angiogram.

clipping of the aneurysm. Unfavorable signs are coma at ictus, older age, major comorbidity,[61] re- bleeding, large amounts of blood on CT scan, and intraventricular hemorrhage.[60] The presence of intracerebral hematoma and retinal hemorrhage does not influence outcome. Basilar artery aneurysmal rupture has a worse outcome than rupture from other types of aneurysms.[62] Visual loss from vitreous hemorrhage has a good out- come, but recovery may take up to 3 years

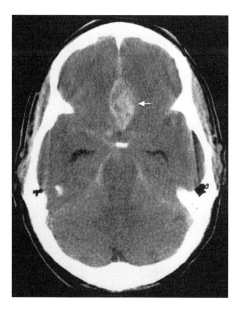

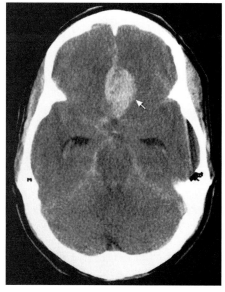

Figure 13.16 Rebleeding in the emergency department. Computed tomographic scans at 2-hour intervals *(left, right)* in a patient with new headache followed by stupor.

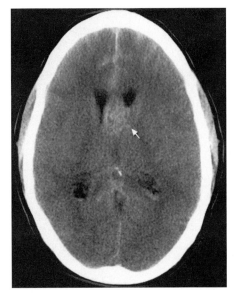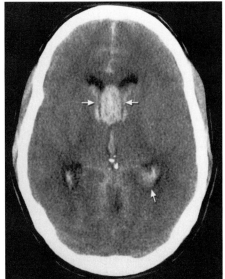

Figure 13.16 (*Continued*)

(median, 9 months).[18] Vitrectomy, at least in one eye, to remove the clot should be considered.

Triage

- Early surgical evacuation in patients with temporal lobe hematoma. Emergency coiling or clipping in any patient with CT scan–documented rebleeding and when due to a dissecting vertebral aneurysm.

- In appropriate patients (WFNS grade I and II, small [<10 mm] anterior and posterior circulation aneurysms), placement of a platinum coil should be preferred in treatment of SAH to prevent rebleeding.[63]
- Admission to a neurologic-neurosurgical intensive care unit, further observation for deterioration, and careful planning for cerebral angiography.

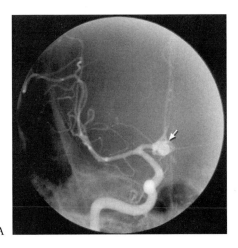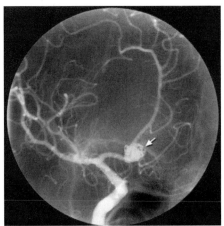

A   B

Figure 13.17 Successful endovascular coil placement in the patient in Figure 13.16. *A:* Before coil placement. *B:* After coil placement.

REFERENCES

1. Weir B: *Subarachnoid Hemorrhage: Causes and Cures.* New York: Oxford University Press, 1998.

2. Teunissen LL, Rinkel GJ, Algra A, et al.: Risk factors for subarachnoid hemorrhage: a systematic review. *Stroke* 27:544, 1996.

3. Lynch P: Ruptured cerebral aneurysm and brawling. *BMJ* 1:1793, 1979.

4. International Study of Unruptured Intracranial Aneurysms Investigators: Unruptured intracranial aneurysms—risk of rupture and risks of surgical intervention. *N Engl J Med* 339:1725, 1998.

5. Schievink WI, Karemaker JM, Hageman LM, et al.: Circumstances surrounding aneurysmal subarachnoid hemorrhage. *Surg Neurol* 32:266, 1989.

6. van der Jagt M, Hasan D, Bijvoet HW, et al.: Validity of prediction of the site of ruptured intracranial aneurysms with CT. *Neurology* 52:34, 1999.

7. Grote E, Hassler W: The critical first minutes after subarachnoid hemorrhage. *Neurosurgery* 22:654, 1988.

8. McCormick PW, McCormick J, Zabramski JM, et al.: Hemodynamics of subarachnoid hemorrhage arrest. *J Neurosurg* 80:710, 1994.

9. Lledo A, Calandre L, Martinez-Menendez B, et al.: Acute headache of recent onset and subarachnoid hemorrhage: a prospective study. *Headache* 34:172, 1994.

10. Duffy GP: The "warning leak" in spontaneous subarachnoid haemorrhage. *Med J Aust* 1:514, 1983.

11. Leblanc R: The minor leak preceding subarachnoid hemorrhage. *J Neurosurg* 66:35, 1987.

12. Leblanc R, Winfield JA: The warning leak in subarachnoid hemorrhage and the importance of its early diagnosis. *CMAJ* 131:1235, 1984.

13. Okawara SH: Warning signs prior to rupture of an intracranial aneurysm. *J Neurosurg* 38:575, 1973.

14. Waga S, Otsubo K, Handa H: Warning signs in intracranial aneurysms. *Surg Neurol* 3:15, 1975.

15. Shapiro S: Management of subarachnoid hemorrhage patients who presented with respiratory arrest resuscitated with bystander CPR. *Stroke* 27:1780, 1996.

16. Swallow CE, Tsuruda JS, Digre KB, et al.: Terson syndrome: CT evaluation in 12 patients. *AJNR Am J Neuroradiol* 19:743, 1998.

17. Lawn ND, Wijdicks EFM, Younge B: Blinding headache and two black eyes. *J Neurol Neurosurg Psychiatry* 67:246, 1999.

18. Schultz PN, Sobol WM, Weingeist TA: Long-term visual outcome in Terson syndrome. *Ophthalmology* 98:1814, 1991.

19. Nadeau SE, Trobe JD: Pupil sparing in oculomotor palsy: a brief review. *Ann Neurol* 13:143, 1983.

20. Claassen J, Peery S, Kreiter KT, et al.: Predictors and clinical impact of epilepsy after subarachnoid hemorrhage. *Neurology* 60:208, 2003.

21. Deibert E, Barzilai B, Braverman AC, et al.: Clinical significance of elevated troponin I levels in patients with non-traumatic subarachnoid hemorrhage. *J Neurosurg* 98:741, 2003.

22. Berlit P, Buhler B, Tornow K: CT findings in subarachnoidal haemorrhage (SAH). A retrospective study of 138 patients. *Neurochirurgia* (Stuttg) 31:123, 1988.

23. Sames TA, Storrow AB, Finkelstein JA, et al.: Sensitivity of new-generation computed tomography in subarachnoid hemorrhage. *Acad Emerg Med* 3:16, 1996.

24. Jackson A, Fitzgerald JB, Hartley RW, et al.: CT appearances of haematomas in the corpus callosum in patients with subarachnoid haemorrhage. *Neuroradiology* 35:420, 1993.

25. Tokuda Y, Inagawa T, Katoh Y, et al.: Intracerebral hematoma in patients with ruptured cerebral aneurysms. *Surg Neurol* 43:272, 1995.

26. Kallmes DF, Lanzino G, Dix JE, et al.: Patterns of hemorrhage with ruptured posterior inferior cerebellar artery aneurysms: CT findings in 44 cases. *AJR Am J Roentgenol* 169:1169, 1997.

27. Duong H, Melancon D, Tampieri D, et al.: The negative angiogram in subarachnoid haemorrhage. *Neuroradiology* 38:15, 1996.

28. Farrés MT, Ferraz-Leite H, Schindler E, et al.: Spontaneous subarachnoid hemorrhage with negative angiography: CT findings. *J Comput Assist Tomogr* 16:534, 1992.

29. Wijdicks EFM, Schievink WI, Miller GM: Pretruncal nonaneurysmal subarachnoid hemorrhage. *Mayo Clin Proc* 73:745, 1998.

30. Matsumaru Y, Yanak K, Muroi AI, et al.: Significance of a small bulge on the basilar artery in patients with perimesencephalic nonaneurysmal subarachnoid hemorrhage: report of two cases. *J Neurosurg* 98:426, 2003.

31. Watanabe A, Hirano K, Kamada M, et al.: Perimesencephalic nonaneurysmal subarachnoid haemorrhage and variations in the veins. *Neuroradiology* 44:319, 2002.

32. Kakarieka A: Review on traumatic subarachnoid hemorrhage. *Neurol Res* 19:230, 1997.

33. Chukwudelunzu FE, Brown RB, Wijdicks EFM, et al.: Nonaneurysmal subarachnoid hemorrhage associated with bacterial endocarditis: case report and literature review. *Eur J Neurol* 9:423, 2002.

34. Given CA, Burdette JH, Elster AD, et al.: Pseudo-subarachnoid hemorrhage: a potential imaging pitfall associated with diffuse cerebral edema. *AJNR Am J Neuroradiol* 24:254, 2003.

35. Phan T, Wijdicks EFM, Worrel G, et al.: False subarachnoid hemorrhage in anoxic encephalopathy with brain swelling. *J Neuroimaging* 10:238, 2000.

36. Rabinstein AA, Pittock SJ, Miller GM, Schindler JJ, Wijdicks EF: Pseudosubarachnoid haemorrhage in subdural haematoma. *J Neurol Neurosurg Psychiatry* 74:1131, 2003.

37. Javedan SP, Marciano F: Polycythemia mimicking subarachnoid hemorrhage in an adult athlete taking performance-enhancing drugs. *Neurology* (in press).

38. Atlas SW: MR imaging is highly sensitive for acute subarachnoid hemorrhage . . . not! *Radiology* 186:319, 1993.

39. Jenkins A, Hadley DM, Teasdale GM, et al.: Magnetic res-

onance imaging of acute subarachnoid hemorrhage. *J Neurosurg* 68:731, 1988.

40. Noguchi K, Ogawa T, Inugami A, et al.: Acute subarachnoid hemorrhage: MR imaging with fluid-attenuated inversion recovery pulse sequences. *Radiology* 196:773, 1995.

41. Wijdicks EFM, Schievink WI, Miller GM: MR imaging in pretruncal nonaneurysmal subarachnoid hemorrhage: is it worthwhile? *Stroke* 29:2514, 1998.

42. Yoon HC, Lufkin RB, Vinuela F, et al.: MR of acute subarachnoid hemorrhage. *AJNR Am J Neuroradiol* 9:404, 1988.

43. Schievink WI, Wijdicks EFM, Spetzler RH: Diffuse vasospasm after pretruncal nonaneurysmal subarachnoid hemorrhage. *AJNR Am J Neuroradiol* 21:521, 2000.

44. Curnes JT, Shogry ME, Clark DC, et al.: MR angiographic demonstration of an intracranial aneurysm not seen on conventional angiography. *AJNR Am J Neuroradiol* 14:971, 1993.

45. Ida M, Kurisu Y, Yamashita M: MR angiography of ruptured aneurysms in acute subarachnoid hemorrhage. *AJNR Am J Neuroradiol* 18:1025, 1997.

46. Vieco PT, Shuman WP, Alsofrom GF, et al.: Detection of circle of Willis aneurysms in patients with acute subarachnoid hemorrhage: a comparison of CT angiography and digital subtraction angiography. *AJR Am J Roentgenol* 165:425, 1995.

47. Allen K, Betham R, Fahie-Wilson MN, et al.: *Proposed National Guidelines for Analysis of Cerebrospinal Fluid for Bilirubin in Suspected Subarachnoid Haemorrhage.* Sheffield: UK NEQAS for Immunology and Immunochemistry, 2001.

48. Dorai Z, Hynan LS, Kopitnik TA, Samson D: Factors related to hydrocephalus after aneurysmal subarachnoid hemorrhage. *Neurosurgery* 52:763, 2003.

49. McIver JI, Friedman JA, Wijdicks EFM, et al.: Preoperative ventriculostomy and rebleeding after aneurysmal subarachnoid hemorrhage. *J Neurosurg* 97:1042, 2002.

50. International Subarachnoid Aneurysm Trial (ISAT) Collaborative Group: International Subarachnoid Aneurysm Trial (ISAT) of neurosurgical clipping versus endovascular coiling in 2143 patients with ruptured intracranial aneurysms: a randomised trial. *Lancet* 360:1267, 2002.

51. Lusseveld E, Brilstra EH, Nijssen PCG, et al.: Endovascular coiling versus neurosurgical clipping in patients with a ruptured basilar tip aneurysm. *J Neurol Neurosurg Psychiatry* 73:591, 2002.

52. Inamasu J, Nakamura Y, Saito R: Endovascular treatment for poorest-grade subarachnoid hemorrhage in the acute stage: has the outcome been improved? *Neurosurgery* 50:1199, 2002.

53. Weir RU, Marcellus ML, Do HM, et al.: Aneurysmal subarachnoid hemorrhage in patients with Hunt and Hess grade 4 or 5: treatment using the Guglielmi detachable coil system. *Am J Neuroradiol* 24:585, 2003.

54. Hodgson TJ, Carroll T, Jellinek DA: Subarachnoid hemorrhage due to late recurrence of a previously unruptured aneurysm after complete endovascular occlusion. *AJNR Am J Neuroradiol* 19:1939, 1998.

55. Byrne JV, Sohn MJ, Molyneux AJ, et al.: Five-year experience in using coil embolization for ruptured intracranial aneurysms: outcomes and incidence of late rebleeding. *J Neurosurg* 90:656, 1999.

56. Tsukahara T, Wada H, Satake K, et al.: Proximal balloon occlusion for dissecting vertebral aneurysms accompanied by subarachnoid hemorrhage. *Neurosurgery* 36:914, 1995.

57. Lylyk P, Ceratto R, Hurvitz D, et al.: Treatment of a vertebral dissecting aneurysm with stents and coils: technical case report. *Neurosurgery* 43:385, 1998.

58. Yamaura A, Watanabe Y, Saeki N: Dissecting aneurysms of the intracranial vertebral artery. *J Neurosurg* 72:183, 1990.

59. Halbach VV, Higashida RT, Dowd CF, et al.: Endovascular treatment of vertebral artery dissections and pseudoaneurysms. *J Neurosurg* 79:183, 1993.

60. Kassell NF, Torner JC, Haley EC Jr, et al.: The International Cooperative Study on the Timing of Aneurysm Surgery. I. Overall management results. II. Surgical results. *J Neurosurg* 73:18, 1990.

61. Solenski NJ, Haley EC Jr, Kassell NF, et al.: Medical complications of aneurysmal subarachnoid hemorrhage: a report of the Multicenter Cooperative Aneurysm Study. Participants of the Multicenter Cooperative Aneurysm Study. *Crit Care Med* 23:1007, 1995.

62. Schievink WI, Wijdicks EF, Piepgras DG, et al.: The poor prognosis of ruptured intracranial aneurysms of the posterior circulation. *J Neurosurg* 82:791, 1995.

63. Wijdicks EFM: Worst-case scenario: management in poor grade aneurysmal subarachnoid hemorrhage. *Cerebrovasc Dis* 5:163, 1995.

Chapter 14
Intracerebral Hematomas

By and large, intracerebral hematomas are caused by a ruptured penetrating arterial branch damaged by the effects of long-standing hypertension.[1] At one undefined moment in time, in some patients it may produce hemorrhages localized in either the caudate nucleus, putamen, thalamus, cerebellum, or pons. Hematomas involving the subcortical white matter and cortex may have different causes, including vascular malformations. This fundamental distinction is important because cerebral angiography may be urgently indicated in a lobar hematoma and of less importance in ganglionic hemorrhages in patients with known brittle hypertension.

Some types of intracerebral hematoma are surgically accessible, and early recognition of clinical and computed tomographic (CT) scan predictors of deterioration may lead to surgical evacuation. Thus, it is also important to separate cerebellar hematoma from brain stem hemorrhages. Another task is to determine at an early stage whether survival is remote or whether salvage with a reasonable opportunity for rehabilitation is possible.

In the first hours, intraparenchymal hemorrhage, in one form or another, poses significant management and triage problems.[1] Interpretation of different aspects of neuroimaging, management, stabilization, and indications for neurosurgical treatment of spontaneous intracerebral hematomas are discussed. Traumatic intracerebral hematoma is discussed in Chapter 19.

Ganglionic Hemorrhages

Location of the hemorrhage typically is in the putamen or caudate nucleus. The cause is a ruptured lateral branch of the lenticulostriate artery. Equally common are hematomas in the thalamus from ruptured thalamoperforating arteries. Many of these hemorrhages are apoplectic, creating large, destructive volumes with extension into the ventricular system.

Clinical Presentation

Supratentorial intracerebral hemorrhage may be manifested in many ways. Coma or any impaired level of consciousness can be explained by the space-occupying effect of the hematoma, causing significant shift of the brain stem; extension of the hemorrhage of the putamen into the thalamus, compressing the opposite thalamic nuclei; and rupture into the ventricular system, resulting in profound hydrocephalus. A progression to loss of many brain stem functions is not unusual.

The clinical syndromes in patients with hemorrhages into the putamen have been further divided on the basis of whether the lesion affects only the anterior part of the putamen close to the anterior limb of the internal capsule, the middle part, or the posterior part. Hemorrhage localized to the anterior part of the putamen may produce

---

Box 14.1. Growth of Parenchymal Hematoma

The volume of a hematoma may increase from continued bleeding, edema formation, and rebleeding. Continued bleeding occurs from a cascade effect. The mass exerts pressure and stretch on surrounding arteries, which subsequently rupture and build a mass in consecutive layers of fibrin. Edema in intracerebral hematoma is due to both cytotoxic and vasogenic mechanisms. It is maximal 1–3 days after the initial hemorrhage and resolves by day 5. The perilesional edematous regions contain significant clot-derived protein and expand the extracellular space, increasing the distance of white matter axons and cells from their blood supply and creating hypoxia. This may be further enhanced by systemic hypoxemia.[3] Thrombin is important in perilesional edema[4,5] because it causes inflammation, reactive gliosis, and retraction of axons and dendrites. In one experimental study, the effects of thrombin could be blocked by hirudin, which is a specific thrombin inhibitor, and edema could not be produced by other blood products.[4] Single-photon emission computed tomography suggested that edema is a form of reperfusion injury due to early ischemia after the hematoma, with flow improving significantly over time.[6] A study of regional cerebral blood flow that used radiolabeled microspheres failed to detect an ischemic penumbra in nonhypertensive animals with large-volume clots.[7]

---

purely motor hemiparesis, eye deviation to the site of the lesion, and abulia. Extension into the middle part of the putamen may additionally result in spatial neglect and decreased sensation evidenced by diminished awareness of pinprick, touch, and position. Extension of the clot into the posterior putamen leads to a more prominent left-sided neglect in right-sided lesions and fluent aphasia in left-sided lesions. Large hemorrhages in the putamen may dissect along the white matter tracts into the temporal lobe, causing a Wernicke-type aphasia, but periclot edema may also impair the function of the temporal lobe.

The neurologic deficit in a putaminal hemorrhage is commonly stable when the patient is admitted to the emergency department. However, neurologic deficits may become more pronounced, signaled by stupor instead of drowsiness or by development of a gaze preference. Progression of neurologic symptoms, indicating enlargement of the hematoma with more mass effect, is commonly noted clinically within the first 6 hours after presentation (Box 14.1).

Clinical features of a thalamic hematoma are excessive sleepiness and abulia. Stupor may ensue if the hematoma causes pressure effects on the opposite thalamus or acute hydrocephalus due to extension into the third ventricle. A thalamic hematoma with dissection into a mesencephalon causes a fluctuating level of consciousness, and episodes of stupor alternate with slow responses (see Chapter 8). Left-sided thalamic hemorrhages are associated with fluent aphasia, with nonexist-

ent phrases and poor naming but conspicuously good comprehension of spoken language. When the hematoma affects the internal capsule, hemiplegia occurs. Right-sided thalamic hematomas produce left visual neglect and hemiplegia.

Caudate hemorrhage is the least common of the classic hypertensive hemorrhages, and its clinical manifestations often can be inferred mainly from an extension to the ventricular system. More commonly, agitation, confusion, and thrashing around occur at the onset without localizing neurologic findings.[2] When the hematoma enlarges and extends from the caudate nucleus into the white matter, involving the internal capsule or putamen, level of consciousness decreases because of brain shift. Extension of the hemorrhage into the hypothalamus and diencephalon might produce complete Horner's syndrome on one side, a diagnostic clue to a large extending caudate hematoma. The clinical features are summarized in Table 14.1.

Interpretation of Diagnostic Tests

The volume in cubic centimeters can be measured on CT scan by the ellipsoid method: $[(A \times B \times C)/2)]$ (Fig. 14.1). (A is the maximum diameter, B is the diameter perpendicular to A, and C is the number of slices on which the hematoma is seen, assuming 10-mm cuts.[8] The projected grid on CT scan films is 1 cm per single step.) This approximation of hemorrhagic volume assumes that every hematoma is ellipsoidal. Nonetheless, the

Table 14.1. Ganglionic Hemorrhages

Primary Site	Extension	Telltale Signs
Caudate nucleus	Localized intraventricular hemorrhage	Headache, confusion, drowsiness–stupor, abulia
	Capsule, putamen, diencephalon	Hemiparesis, eye deviation, Horner's syndrome
Putamen	Localized	Hemiparesis, eye deviation, global aphasia
	Posterior extension	Fluent aphasia
Thalamus	Localized	Paresthesia, hemineglect, nonfluent aphasia (often preserved repetition), disorientation to place
	Mesencephalon	Slow syndrome

value obtained correlates well with a direct CT scan measurement; thus, the method is a simple, practical means of rapid volume measurement in the emergency department. In 25% of patients, enlargement of the ganglionic hematoma may appear on CT scans when reimaged within the first hours of presentation. In contrast, patients with CT scans obtained more than 6 hours after the ictus and a volume of less than 25 cm^3 are unlikely to have deterioration from further growth of the hematoma. However, anticoagulation with warfarin, despite normal international normalized ratio (INR), is a major factor in enlargement of the hematoma.

Putaminal hemorrhages are most prevalent and not infrequently massive. The volume on CT scan commonly approaches 60 cm^3, but smaller hematomas may occur without further enlargement on serial CT scans. Common types of putaminal hemorrhage are shown in Figure 14.2.

Thalamic hematomas are usually small; but because of close proximity to the ventricles, intraventricular hemorrhage may occur. Hydrocephalus may develop from obstruction of the cerebrospinal fluid (CSF) at the level of the foramen of Monro, more commonly with medially located thalamic hemorrhages (Fig. 14.3). Enlargement of the hematoma has been observed in thalamic hemorrhages, typically in conjunction with progression to coma, and markedly reduces the outlook for independent recovery (Fig. 14.4).[9] The CT scan and magnetic resonance imaging (MRI) features producing coma in patients with thalamic hematomas are shown in Figure 14.5. Caudate hemorrhage (Fig. 14.6) may be difficult to separate from intraventricular hemorrhage on CT scans, and often MRI is needed to locate the source in the caudate nucleus.

Finally, CT scan interpretation of spontaneous intracerebral hematoma may be deceiving. Some may represent hemorrhagic infarcts rather than primary intracerebral hematomas.[10] This possibility should be particularly considered in patients who have had transient ischemic attacks; who have a potential cardioembolic source for emboli, such as atrial fibrillation or left ventricular hypokinesis; and who have silent infarcts revealed on CT scans (Fig. 14.7).[9] Later, a localized putaminal hemorrhage may mimic an infarct by leaving a slit-like lesion (Fig. 14.8). This is in contrast to lobar

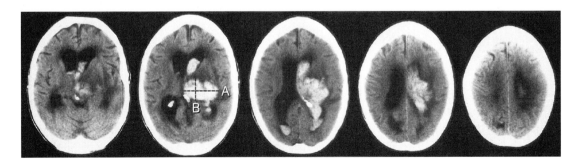

Figure 14.1 Volume of a thalamic hemorrhage as measured by the *ABC* method ($A \times B \times C \div 2$). In this example, *A* is 5 cm, *B* is 3 cm, and the number of slices (*C*) is four (hemorrhage is visible on four computed tomographic slices at 10 mm intervals). The total volume is calculated as $60 \div 2$, or 30 cm^3.

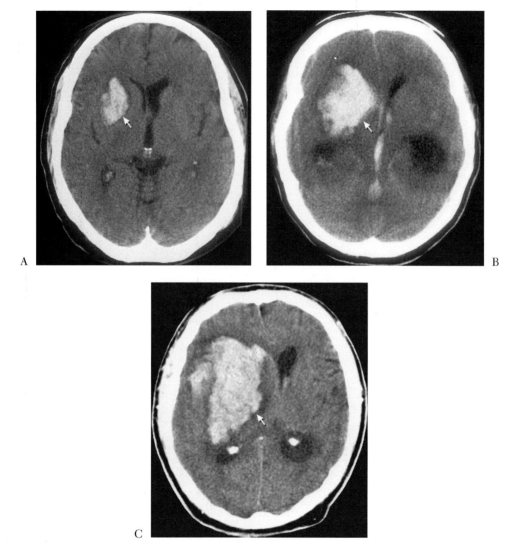

Figure 14.2 Computed tomographic scan examples of putaminal hemorrhage (*arrows*): localized (*A*), extensions to capsule and frontal lobe and intraventricular extension (*B*), and extension into the thalamus (*C*).

hematomas, which may leave a hypodensity and deformity of the ventricle.[11]

First Priority in Management

Most academic institutions in the United States and Europe manage patients with ganglionic hemorrhage medically.[12] This preference implies supportive care and monitoring of further deterioration from enlargement in volume caused by development of surrounding edema or continuous bleeding. Underlying coagulopathy should be corrected aggressively. Reversal of anticoagula-tion is essential, and fresh-frozen plasma (and vitamin K) or, if more appropriate, platelets should be infused in the emergency department.[13] In patients with a metallic heart valve or otherwise high cardioembolic risk (e.g., marked ventricular hypokinesis or atrial fibrillation and echocardiographic evidence of atrial thrombus), there is an increased risk of thromboembolization or valve thrombosis. Current data suggest that discontinuation of anticoagulation and correction to an international normalized ratio <1.5 for less than a week in these patients rarely lead to systemic embolization.[14,15]

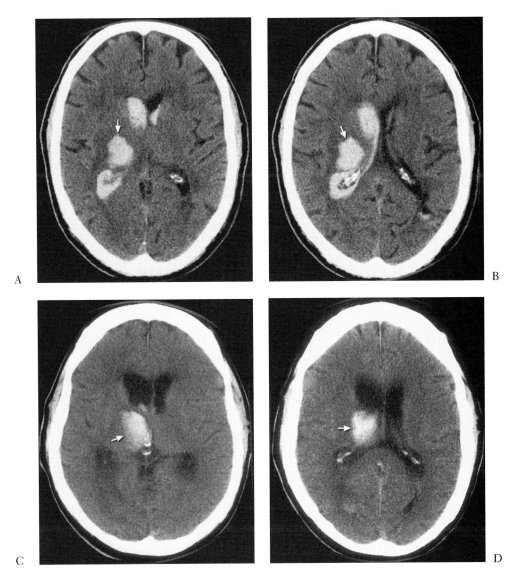

Figure 14.3 Computed tomographic scans of thalamic hemorrhage (*arrows*): lateral (*A,B*) and medial (*C,D*).

Hypertensive crisis is very common but seldom produces congestive heart failure or brief ventricular arrhythmias from a catecholamine surge. Only when blood pressure remains high (mean arterial pressure >140 mm Hg) and electrocardiographic changes or cardiac arrhythmias appear is reduction with β-blockers indicated.[16] No evidence suggests that persistent acute hypertension provokes a recurrence of bleeding in patients with a spontaneous intracranial hematoma.[17] However, vasogenic edema may develop, and persistent hypertension may contribute to an increase in in-tracranial pressure.[18] Aggressive treatment of hypertension might theoretically reduce cerebral edema in these patients, but it may increase the risk of producing further perilesional ischemia in patients with prior hypertension. The presence of an ischemic perilesional penumbra is a matter of debate.[19,20] It is generally accepted that when the mean arterial blood pressure reaches 145–150 mm Hg, the risk of enlargement of the hematoma from continuous leakage or cerebral edema is too high. Blood pressure should be reduced gradually to a mean arterial pressure of around 130 mm Hg.

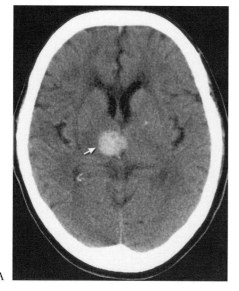
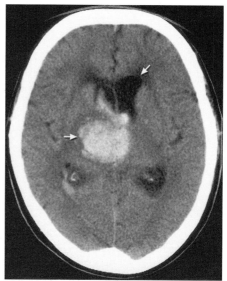

A

B

Figure 14.4 Computed tomographic images of enlargement of thalamic hemorrhage (*arrow* in *A*), intraventricular extension (*left arrow* in *B*), and hydrocephalus (*right arrow* in *B*).

Preliminary studies showed no significant change
in the periclot blood flow when antihypertensives
were administered 6 hours after onset.[21] However, this major management dilemma remains
unresolved in the first hours after the onset, particularly when blood pressures are high. The
recommended antihypertensive medication is labetalol, ≅20 mg intravenously every 10 minutes
up to 300 mg. In patients with bradycardia or
other contraindications to β-blockers, one should
consider intravenous enalaprilat 1.25 mg every 6
hours to a maximum of 5 mg.[16,22]

There is no benefit from corticosteroids,[23] and
in susceptible patients, they may increase the risk

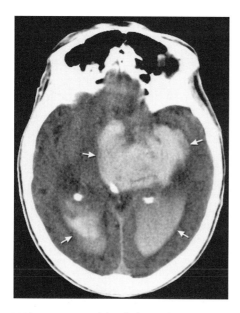
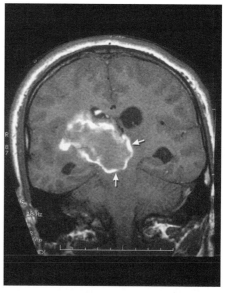

Figure 14.5 Coma caused by thalamic hemorrhage.
Left: Massive extension and enlargement of ventricles
(*arrows*). *Right:* Magnetic resonance image of the thalamic hemorrhage with extension into the midbrain.

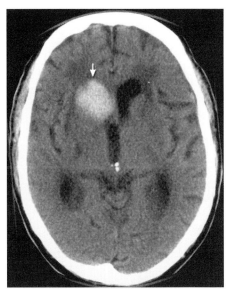 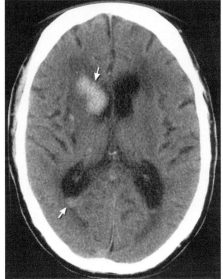

Figure 14.6 Computed tomographic images of caudate hemorrhage (*left*) and intraventricular extension (*right, arrows*).

of severe hyperglycemia or enhance pulmonary infection triggered by aspiration. The benefit of mannitol in deep ganglionic hemorrhage is not known. It is unlikely to result in improvement in outcome unless its effect on intracranial pressure and cerebral perfusion pressure is documented, nor is it known whether it may assist in the bridging period before surgical evacuation. More likely, the direct destructive effect of this type of hematoma rather than brain shift determines outcome in survivors.

Enlargement may have occurred during transport, and any further deterioration should be evaluated with a new CT scan. Enlargement 24 hours

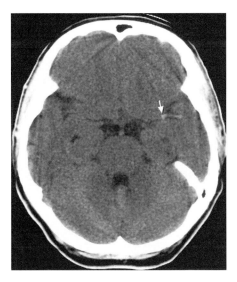 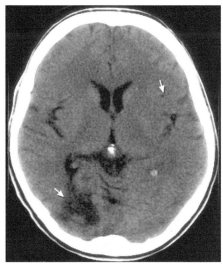

Figure 14.7 Series of computed tomographic scans in a patient with rapidly progressing neurologic deficit. There is a hyperdense middle cerebral artery sign, but, except for a dubious difference in sylvian fissure width (*arrow, left*) and an old infarct in the posterior cerebral artery territory (*arrow, right*), there is no evidence of a recent ischemic stroke by computed tomography.

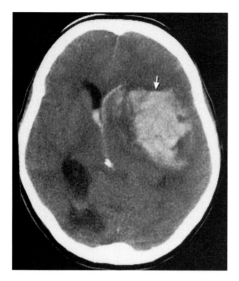 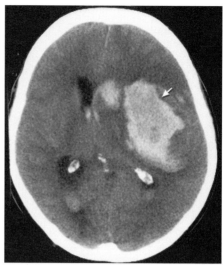

Figure 14.7 (*Continued*) Series of computed tomographic scans in a patient with rapidly progressing neurologic deficit. Several hours later, a large putaminal hemorrhage (*arrows*) represents a hemorrhagic infarct rather than a primary putaminal hemorrhage.

after onset is rare. Several systemic factors have been identified that increase the probability of enlargement, such as anticoagulation, liver disease, and poorly controlled diabetes with high systolic blood pressure (>200 mm Hg).[9]

Hemostatic therapy (aminocaproic acid, apoprotein, or activated recombinant factor VII) used within 3 hours of the ictus of intracerebral hematoma could potentially reduce growth of the hematoma, but no data are available to justify its use.[24] Its impact on outcome may be small because only 20%–30% of patients do demonstrate enlargement of the hematoma[25] and clinical deterioration is not evident in all instances.

Craniotomy in large ganglionic hemorrhages is only lifesaving. Awakening from coma rarely occurs without devastating morbidity (Box 14.2), and thus it is a questionable procedure.

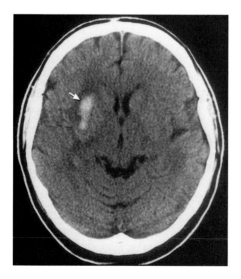 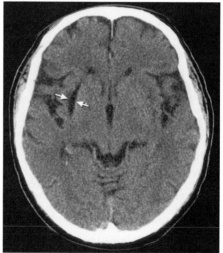

Figure 14.8 Putaminal hemorrhage (localized type) recognized 3 years later on subsequent computed tomographic scan as a slit-like lesion (*arrows, right*).

Box 14.2. Surgical Management of Ganglionic Supratentorial Hemorrhage

Most neurosurgeons prefer surgical evacuation in a deteriorating patient. Randomized surgical trials of supratentorial hemorrhage have been hampered by marginal statistical power[26–29] imbalances in baseline characteristics between groups. Surgical evacuation of a ganglionic hematoma through open craniectomy did not improve outcome. Endoscopic aspiration reduced mortality, with no improvement in morbidity in large hematomas (>50 mL) but a trend in improved outcome in smaller hematomas. Stereotactic aspiration may result in lower incidence of complications.[30] Ventriculostomy may be performed in patients with intraventricular rupture, but its effect on outcome is marginal, if any. Stereotac-

tic treatment using thrombolytics and aspiration reduced volume but not disability or mortality.[29]

A recent small randomized pilot trial, the Surgical Treatment for Intracerebral Hemorrhage (STICH) study,[31] documented reduced mortality at 1 month but not at 6 months in patients treated with surgery (median Glasgow coma score = 11, median volume = 49 mL) compared with those given medical management (median Glasgow coma score = 11, median volume = 44 mL). Future trials should analyze lobar hematomas separately from ganglionic hemorrhage and study patients at high risk of deterioration to demonstrate a possible surgical benefit.

Predictors of Outcome

A large clot (>60 cm^3 by ellipsoid volume measurement) associated with Glasgow coma score <4 intraventricular hematoma and acute hydrocephalus is likely to result in death.[32–34] A study from Sweden extrapolated that supposedly unrelated comorbidity such as preictal coronary artery disease or atrial fibrillation was an independent predictor for 30 days' mortality.[35] Extension of the hematoma into the middle putamen most likely results in persistent hemiplegia. The prognosis in thalamic hemorrhage is determined by diameter and extension to the mesencephalon. If a thalamic hematoma exceeds 2.5 cm in greatest diameter, outcome is worse. Unilateral hydrocephalus in ganglionic hemorrhage caused by trapping of the ventricular system is a CT scan sign that indicates poor outcome despite surgical evacuation or ventriculostomy.

Triage

- Observation for at least 24 hours in a neurologic–neurosurgical intensive care unit.
- Evacuation of hematoma if enlargement causes brain herniation syndromes.

Lobar Hemorrhages

In this type of intracranial hematoma, the blood dissects throughout the subcortical white matter and often involves the cortex. The clinical features are related to topography. The source of lobar hematomas is unclear in many instances. Mechanisms include a ruptured vascular malformation, cerebral amyloid angiopathy,[36] hemorrhage inside an existing brain tumor or metastatic lesion, infectious lesions (e.g., aspergillosis, toxoplasmosis), coagulation disorders, and use of sympathomimetic drugs or fibrinolytic agents.

A temporal lobe hematoma may be caused by a ruptured middle cerebral artery aneurysm.[37] Any patient with a temporal lobe hematoma, transient loss of consciousness, and a much lower level of consciousness than expected on the basis of size or brain shift should be considered to have a ruptured aneurysm of the middle cerebral artery. A CT scan should be scrutinized for basal cistern clots. A temporal lobe hematoma may indicate a hemorrhagic necrotic mass due to herpes simplex encephalitis, and febrile agitation may be the only manifestation (see Chapters 7 and 17). Multiple hematomas should point to a possible devastating sagittal sinus thrombosis with multiple hemorrhagic infarcts (see Chapter 15).

Use of thrombolytic agents has increased the frequency of intracerebral hematomas associated with thrombolysis.[38] The frequency of symptomatic intracerebral hematomas after intravenous administration of tissue-type plasminogen activator (tPA) for ischemic stroke has increased to 6%. These hemorrhages occur within 36 hours after infusion. Decrease in level of consciousness is most prevalent, but increased hemiparesis, headaches, and a surge in blood pressure have also been noted.[38] A major neurologic deficit (defined as a score of more than 20 on the National Institutes of Health Stroke Scale; see Chapter 15, Table 15.1) and early hypodensity or edema on CT scans increase the odds of later development of symptomatic intracerebral hematoma after tPA use. The risk of intracerebral hematoma after tPA for myocardial infarction is very low, but old age, dose, and history of stroke are major predisposing factors.[39]

Clinical Presentation

Frontal lobe hematomas cause abulia, contralateral arm weakness, and gaze preference toward the side of the hematoma; but when the hemorrhages are located superiorly above the frontal horn, leg weakness may be more apparent.[40] Headache is frequently present and associated with vomiting. Approximately one-third of patients have seizures within the first hours of presentation. Temporal lobe hematomas may cause Wernicke's aphasia and right-sided homonymous hemianopia. Temporal lobe hematomas in the nondominant hemisphere may produce only confusional episodes without any localizing neurologic symptoms. Parietal lobe hematoma produces prominent hemisensory symptoms, but if it extends into the posterior parietal lobe, constructional apraxia or dressing apraxia may be found if specific testing is done. Patients with an occipital lobe hematoma have a

Table 14.2. Computed Tomographic Scan Characteristics of Lobar Hematoma that Suggest the Cause

Coagulopathy	Multiple locations and compartments
	Fluid level from poor clot formation
Amyloid angiopathy	Superficially located
	Irregular border
	Recurrent hematomas
	White matter hypodensities
Tumoral hemorrhage	Central or eccentric location of hemorrhage
	Tumor mass visible
	Proportionally more white matter edema
Arteriovenous malformation	Calcification in hemorrhage mass
	Enhancement with contrast medium

sudden visual field defect, most commonly an easily identifiable homonymous hemianopia. Multiple hematomas commonly immediately involve the level of consciousness unless they are localized within one hemisphere or are small. Clinical features are determined by the largest hematoma.

Interpretation of Diagnostic Tests

Several CT scan characteristics of hematoma suggesting its origin should be recognized,[41] and they are summarized in Table 14.2. Shift of midline structures on the initial CT scan in patients with lobar hematoma admitted to the emergency department is highly predictive of further clinical de-

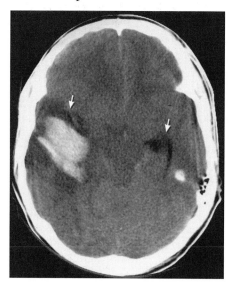
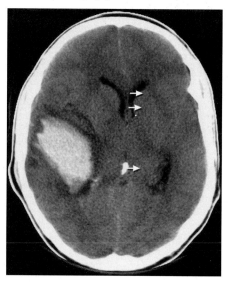

Figure 14.9 Computed tomographic scan signs predictive of deterioration in lobar hematoma (*arrow*). Note shift of septum pellucidum and pineal gland (*arrows*) and early temporal horn entrapment (*arrow, left*).[46]

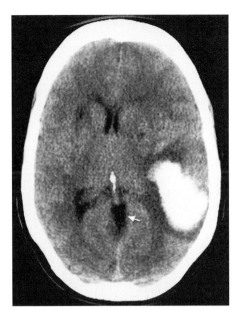
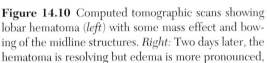
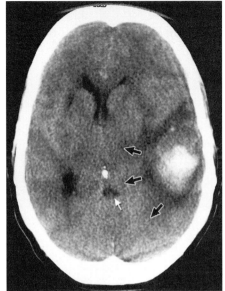

Figure 14.10 Computed tomographic scans showing lobar hematoma (*left*) with some mass effect and bowing of the midline structures. *Right:* Two days later, the hematoma is resolving but edema is more pronounced, with progressive obliteration of the supracerebellar cistern without appreciable shift of the pineal gland from edema.

terioration. The specific features are shift of the septum pellucidum, obliteration of the opposite ambient cistern, and early trapping of the temporal horn (Fig. 14.9).[35] Some of the CT scan changes may be subtle and involve effacement of the supracerebellar cistern from edema (Fig. 14.10).

Lobar hematoma may indicate an underlying metastatic lesion or primary brain tumor, and it is evident by marked fingerlike white matter edema notably out of proportion to the size of the hematoma and seldom causing brain shift (Fig. 14.11).

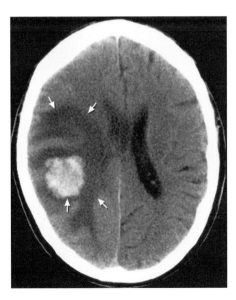
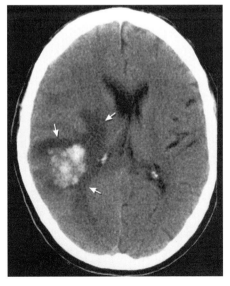

Figure 14.11 Hemorrhage in metastasis. Note the comparatively large, fingerlike edema in the white matter out of proportion to the size of the hematoma. Computed tomographic scans mask underlying metastasis, which may be more evident by magnetic resonance imaging.

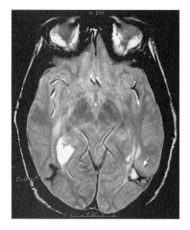 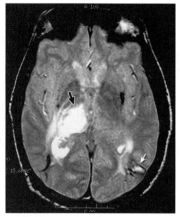 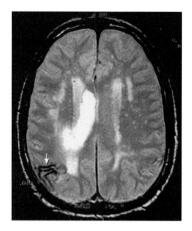

Figure 14.12 Amyloid angiopathy–associated hematoma. Magnetic resonance images show a thalamic hemorrhage (*black arrow*) and multiple areas of hemosiderin (*white arrows*), which are clues to earlier hemorrhages.

Superficially located hematomas commonly are a result of amyloid angiopathy, and MRI (preferably gradient-echo) may show earlier hemorrhages (Fig. 14.12). Coagulation-associated hematomas are commonly multiple, involving multiple compartments (Fig. 14.13).

Intracerebral hematomas after intravenous tPA for myocardial infarction characteristically are hemorrhages in multiple compartments, and fluid levels from continuing anticoagulation are evident (Fig. 14.14).

MRI is a crucial study in lobar hematoma because it may identify an underlying structural lesion. In young adults, an arteriovenous malformation is common; in older adults, earlier amyloid hemorrhages may be found, and, as alluded to, routine T_1 and T_2 MRI may initially be unrewarding and a gradient echo image may be needed.[42]

Cerebral angiography is warranted in patients with a lobar hematoma and MRI evidence of arteriovenous malformation (Fig. 14.15). Its yield in a patient with normal findings on MRI is very low.

First Priority in Management

The approach to lobar hematoma is similar to that in ganglionic hemorrhages.

Multiple intracranial lobar hematomas are often found in patients who have recently received tPA for acute myocardial infarction.[43] Fresh-frozen plasma (2 units) should be used initially. It is important to repeat a CT scan, preferably 1–3 hours after the onset, to assess the true extension and dimension of the hematomas.[38]

The decision to proceed with surgery is determined by clinical presentation. Craniotomy with evacuation of a lobar hematoma should be strongly considered in patients with evidence of brain shift on CT scan and a decrease in the Glasgow coma score because there is a high probability of further deterioration in the next hours. With expanding hematomas, emergency surgery is effective in 25% of patients if young and the hematoma is located in the parietal lobe.[44] Early surgical management is also indicated if an in-

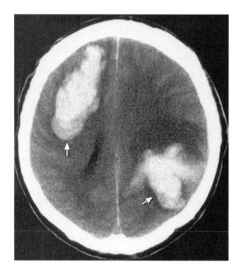

Figure 14.13 Computed tomographic scan shows multiple hemorrhages in coagulopathy.

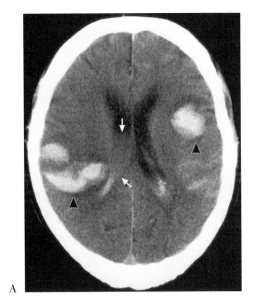

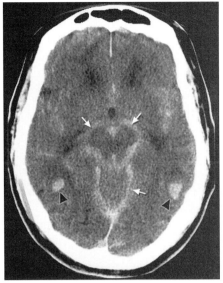

A   B

Figure 14.14 Examples of hemorrhage associated with tissue-type plasminogen activator. *A: Arrows* point to different compartments, convexity subarachnoid hemorrhage, and lobar (*arrowheads*) and intraventricular hemorrhages with fluid level. *B:* Massive subarachnoid hemorrhage and lobar hematomas.

tracerebral hematoma is associated with a ruptured middle cerebral artery aneurysm or arteriovenous malformation, but mostly after further definition by cerebral angiography.[45]

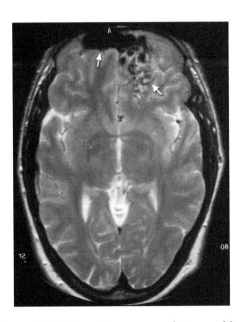

Figure 14.15 Magnetic resonance features of large arteriovenous malformation in left frontal lobe with large vein draining to the sagittal sinus.

Predictors of Outcome

Poor outcome can be expected in patients with deterioration from hematoma enlargement who need emergency surgical evacuation. Poor outcome is more common in patients with a decreased Glasgow coma score and a septum pellucidum shift of more than 6 mm.[46] Lobar hematomas associated with tPA administration are commonly fatal. Outcome is good after rehabilitation if the lobar hematoma is less than 40 cm³ on CT scan and there is no shift on CT scan in a patient seen several hours after ictus.[47] Recurrent hemorrhage has been estimated at a 2.1% annual rate, but it is tripled when anticoagulation is administered.[48] Resumption of anticoagulation in a patient with a definitive need and prior intracranial hematoma is safe for 30 days, but long-term risk is not known.

Triage

- Neurologic intensive care unit if level of consciousness is decreased and mass effect appears on CT scan.
- Smaller hematomas (<30 cm³) in alert patients can be observed in the ward if the time of ictus and presentation is beyond 6 hours.

- Surgical evacuation in patients with CT scan evidence of mass effect and documented deterioration.

Intraventricular Hemorrhage

It may be difficult clinically and by CT scan criteria to differentiate spontaneous intraventricular hemorrhage from a small thalamic or caudate nucleus hemorrhage with overwhelming filling of the lateral portion of the ventricles. In many situations, intraventricular hemorrhage is caused by a rupture of the anterior communicating aneurysm, which can dissect through the lamina terminalis to enter the third ventricle and connecting ventricles (see Chapter 13). Primary intraventricular hemorrhage may be caused by arteriovenous malformations in the proximity of the ventricular system, intraventricular tumors, and, more recently, use of thrombolytic agents. Uncommon causes are coagulopathy in patients with severe thrombocytopenia associated with a hematologic malignancy and moyamoya disease from rupture of the dilated periventricular arteries.

Clinical Presentation

Primary intraventricular hemorrhage has a clinical presentation similar to that of poor-grade aneurysmal subarachnoid hemorrhage.[49-51] Onset is acute, with immediate loss of consciousness but with ex-tensor posturing that occurs spontaneously or with any manipulation of the patient. Nonspecific shivering, myoclonic jerks, and well-characterized generalized tonic-clonic seizures are common. Many patients have rapid breathing with periods of apnea or barely audible air displacement and need to be immediately placed on a mechanical ventilator. Increased blood pressure most likely is a consequence of transmitted intracranial pressure affecting the brain stem, particularly at the flush of arterial blood through the ventricular system. Pupil reflexes may become sluggish and pupil size smaller if acute hydrocephalus develops rapidly. Any change in this direction should prompt a repeat CT scan to evaluate progression of ventricular enlargement and need for ventriculostomy.

Interpretation of Diagnostic Tests

Entire filling of all parts of the ventricular system is characteristic, with acute ballooning out of the ventricular system (Fig. 14.16). The CT scan is notoriously unreliable in demonstrating a potential cause of intraventricular hemorrhage. Thus, some patients with a thalamic or caudate hemorrhage have only a hint of parenchymal bleeding on CT scanning, and this is markedly overshadowed by the massive intraventricular hemorrhage, often filling only one ventricle. The anatomic location may indicate the origin of the hemorrhage (Table 14.3).[52,53]

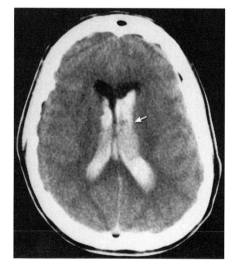 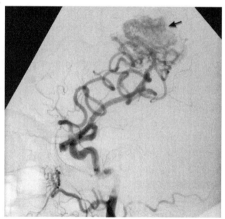

Figure 14.16 *Left:* Primary intraventricular hemorrhage. *Right:* Cerebral angiography disclosed an arteriovenous malformation.

Table 14.3. Intraventricular Hemorrhage

Intraventricular	
Unilateral ventricle	Caudate hemorrhage
	Thalamic hemorrhage
Biventricular	Arteriovenous malformation of ependymal lining or choroid plexus
	Ependymoma
	Cocaine or amphetamine
	Head injury
Cavum septum pellucidum	Anterior artery cerebral aneurysm
Fourth ventricle only	Posterior inferior cerebellar artery aneurysm

Source: Terayama et al.[17]

MRI can demonstrate hemorrhage into the thalamus or caudate nucleus and is also more sensitive to visualization of arteriovenous malformations and cavernous angiomas. Cavernous angiomas may be found at other locations inside the parenchyma, providing further clues to cavernous angioma as the main culprit in the ventricular hemorrhage. Magnetic resonance angiography should also be performed to exclude the possibility of an anterior communicating aneurysm or to document a much less common moyamoya vascular pattern. This pattern is the consequence of bilateral internal carotid artery occlusion causing dilatation to develop in the lenticulostriate, thalamoperforating, and thalamogeniculate arteries. Microaneurysms are often formed in these arteries, and they may rupture into the ventricular system.

Not only is cerebral angiography imperative to exclude an anterior communicating artery aneurysm, but the posterior circulation should also be visualized bilaterally with multiple projections because blood in the fourth ventricle might be due to a ruptured aneurysm of the distal posteroinferior cerebellar artery. One study claimed an arteriovenous malformation or an aneurysm in 50%–70% of patients, with a higher yield in patients younger than 45 years.[54]

First Priority in Management

The management of primary ventricular hemorrhage is immediate ventriculostomy in patients with a Glasgow coma score of less than 8 and marked ventricular dilatation on CT scan (see Chapter 11). A trial is under way using 3 mg of intraventricular recombinant tPA every 12 hours when no cause is found by cerebral angiography (which should then be performed immediately).[55,56] Dramatic resolution of the obstructing clot has been described, but experience with this potentially dangerous therapy is very limited and clinicoradiologic correlation has not been studied well. Recent experimental work also suggests an unwanted inflammatory response, edema of periventricular tissue and choroid plexus using tPA.[55] It should not be used in intraparenchymal hemorrhages with intraventricular extension, even if the intraventricular compartment produces most of the clot volume.[57,58]

Predictors of Outcome

Outcome remains poor (severe disability or vegetative state) in patients with primary intraventricular hemorrhage associated with acute hydrocephalus. In others, survival is common but with a severe amnesic state.[50]

Triage

- Neurologic–neurosurgical intensive care unit for monitoring of development of acute hydrocephalus or drainage with a ventriculostomy.
- Consider immediate cerebral angiography.

Cerebellar Hemorrhages

Cerebellar hemorrhages are commonly caused by rupture of a branch of the superior cerebellar artery afflicted by fibroid necrosis from long-standing hypertension. Much less frequent causes are hemorrhages associated with anticoagulation, arteriovenous malformation, or a metastatic lesion. Patients arriving in the emergency department often are initially alert but may have rapid deterioration to a lower level of consciousness and development of new brain stem signs. Features that predict clinical deterioration have been identified, as have clinical and CT scan features associated with such a poor prospect that even suboccipital craniotomy for clot evacuation may be discouraged.[59,60]

Clinical Presentation

Acute severe headache associated with vertigo and vomiting and acute gait imbalance are presenting findings. At onset, patients are unable to take a single step if standing and cry out for immediate assistance; some fall, are unable to stand up, and have to roll themselves to a telephone. Speech is slurred, and clumsiness may become apparent in one limb. A cerebellar hematoma can be further suspected if the clinical triad of ipsilateral limb ataxia, horizontal gaze palsy, and peripheral facial palsy is demonstrated, although two or fewer of these signs may be present. Other common neurologic findings are skew deviation, horizontal nystagmus, and decreased corneal reflex. In this condition, pinpoint-sized pupils indicate significant pontine compression and imply a high risk of further deterioration. Unilateral ataxia and dysarthria point to a cerebellar hemispheric hematoma. Dysautonomic features are frequent in large cerebellar hematomas, and they include episodic bradycardia and hypertension, not necessarily coupled together.

Interpretation of Diagnostic Tests

Two major types of cerebellar hemorrhage have been described. Cerebellar hemispheric hemor-

rhages are most common (Fig. 14.17A–C). For unclear reasons, vermis hematomas are more frequently seen in hemorrhages associated with acquired coagulopathy (Fig. 14.17D). Both may involve extension into the ventricle and compression of the brain stem. The typical features of brain stem compression often involve effacement of the quadrigeminal cistern, and when cerebellar tissue is herniated upward, it causes additional effacement of the supracerebellar cisterns (so-called tight posterior fossa). These CT findings should be regarded as an urgent indication for evacuation of the hematoma. CT scan features highly predictive of further deterioration are extension to the vermis and acute hydrocephalus.[57]

A cerebral angiogram can be deferred in most cases, but a ruptured posterior circulation aneurysm or arteriovenous malformation should be considered. An arteriovenous malformation should be considered in a young patient with no history of hypertension. Cerebellar hemispheric arteriovenous malformations have a characteristic bleeding pattern on CT scans and blood tracts in the direction of the cerebellar folia, particularly in the primary cerebellar fissure. The malformation may extend, rather symmetrically, into the midline as well. Blood in the quadrigeminal

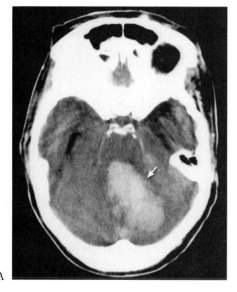

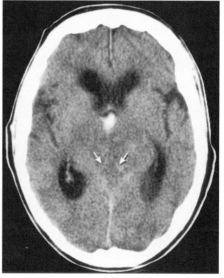

Figure 14.17 Types of cerebellar hematoma on computed tomography. *A–C:* Cerebellar hemisphere. Note effacement of the quadrigeminal cisterns, intraventricular extension, and hydrocephalus. *D:* Vermis hemi-

sphere. *E:* Cerebellar hemorrhage from arteriovenous malformation. *F:* Cerebellar hematoma with marked fluid levels (*arrows*) due to use of warfarin.

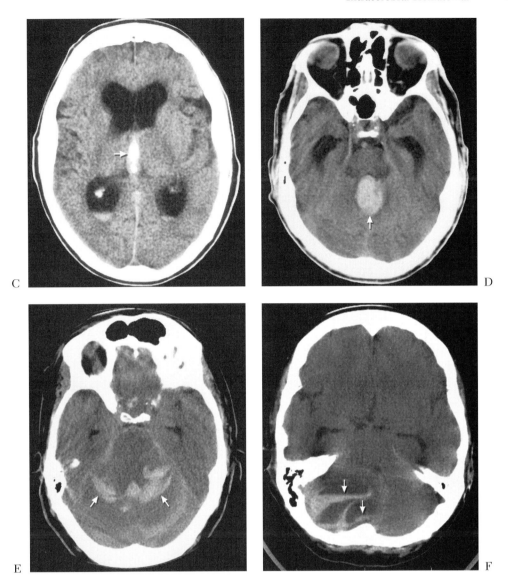

Figure 14.17 (*Continued*)

cisterns and tracts on the tentorium is characteristic (Fig. 14.17E). These cerebellar hemispheric arteriovenous malformations are unmasked by MRI and should be further defined by cerebral angiography.

First Priority in Management

Attending physicians should be primed for surgical evacuation in many patients. At our institution, clinicians usually wait for clinical deterioration before operating. Another commonly accepted precept is to remove a clot when it is 3 cm or larger in axial diameter on CT scans.[61] In patients with significant swelling, a bolus of mannitol, 1 g/kg, should be administered to bridge the time to the operating room. Administration of a corticosteroid can be considered, but valid data about its efficacy are not available.

Bradycardia may be frequently observed but should be left alone. Runs of bradycardia, however, should be treated with atropine administered intravenously (0.5 mg) if hypotension occurs.

Predictors of Outcome

Alert or minimally drowsy patients are at high risk of further deterioration when they have a midline extension of the hematoma or acute hydrocephalus. Poor outcome after surgery is very likely when acute hydrocephalus is present and corneal and doll's eye reflexes are absent. Good outcome after surgery can be expected in younger patients with intact brain stem reflexes.[59,62]

Triage

- Surgical evacuation if CT scan shows signs of tight posterior fossa.
- Observation on the ward if the hematoma is small (<3 cm) and not localized in the vermis, no deterioration has occurred, and the patient does not have an abnormal coagulation parameter.

Pontine Hemorrhage

A pontine hemorrhage is associated with high rates of death and neurologic morbidity. Hypertension is the usual cause, and arteriovenous malformation or rupture of a cavernous angioma is less common. At presentation, most patients are in a cataclysmic state and comatose with small, re-active pupils (diameter 2–3 mm), loss of horizontal gaze, and apneic spells requiring mechanical ventilation. Extension to the mesencephalon may cause significant anisocoria, which can be clinically misinterpreted as an uncal herniation syndrome (see Chapter 8). Abnormalities of eye movement have been described, such as ocular bobbing (sudden downward jerking with slow return to midcentral position), skew deviation, and abnormal horizontal conjugate gaze that is more apparent after caloric stimulation with ice water. Quadriplegia with extreme rigidity is frequent, but if the hematoma is unilaterally localized in the pons, hemiplegia may occur. Complete destruction of the mid-pons is common, and the tegmentum is seldom spared; thus, locked-in syndrome is rarely found in this condition. Dysautonomic features with marked hypertension, tachycardia, and hyperthermia (>39.5°C) may be profound.[63] In contrast, pontine hemorrhages in cavernous hemangioma are not catastrophic and are manifested by acute oculomotor abnormalities or ataxia only.[64]

Interpretation of Diagnostic Tests

The CT scan patterns are shown in Figure 14.18. Pontine hemorrhages can be divided into massive pontine hemorrhage with extension to the mid-

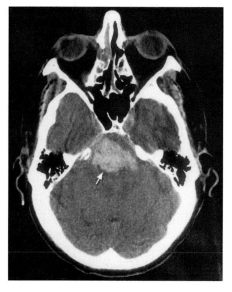
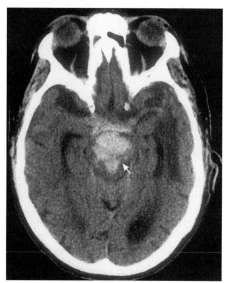

Figure 14.18 Types of pontine hemorrhage on computed tomographic images. *A–C:* Extension to midbrain and thalamus. *D:* Massive destructive hemorrhage limited to pons. *E,F:* Basal tegmental hemorrhage.

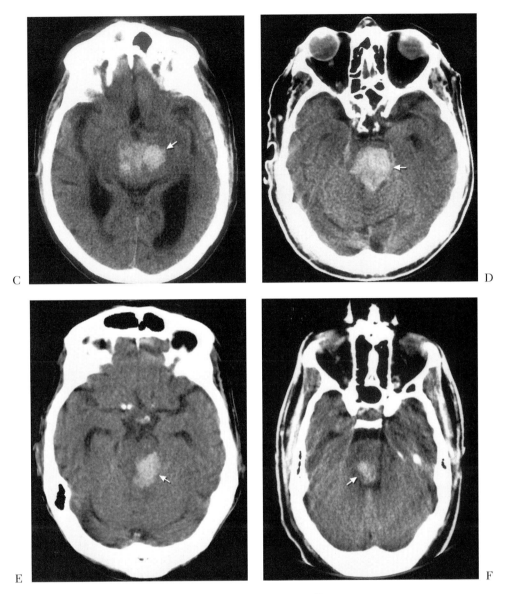

Figure 14.18 (*Continued*)

brain and thalamus, pontine hemorrhage with unilateral extension to the midbrain, and basal tegmental pontine hemorrhage. The lesion should be differentiated from a large fusiform aneurysm, which may produce identical clinical features due to basilar artery thrombosis (Fig. 14.19). Rarely, a unilateral tegmental hemorrhage is found; it is usually very circumscribed and barely involves major pontine structures. It may be caused by a cavernous hemangioma (Fig. 14.20).

First Priority in Management

Endotracheal intubation is needed in virtually all patients. Blood pressure is markedly increased, but aggressive management does not appear to have much effect on size. Blood pressure may become very high, with diastolic pressure in the range of 140–150 mm Hg. Labetalol may be needed to reduce the blood pressure to a more acceptable level. Ventriculostomy is not helpful because de-

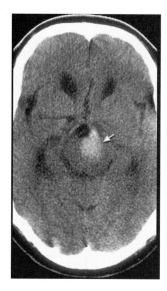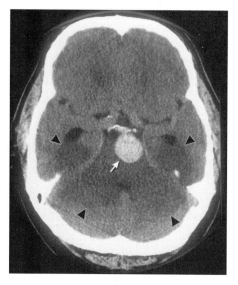

Figure 14.19 Pseudopontine hemorrhage. *Left:* Fusiform basilar aneurysm associated with acute basilar artery occlusion mimics pontine bleeding. *Right:* Note development of hypodensities on follow-up computed tomographic scan and better delineation of the aneurysm.

terioration is related to extension or evolving swelling surrounding the hematoma. Stereotactic surgical evacuation has not been shown to improve outcome, and morbidity remains substantial. The effect of corticosteroids is unknown.

Predictors of Outcome

Good recovery occurs only in patients who are alert on admission and have small unilateral pontine hemorrhages.[64] Cavernous malformations of the brain stem may continue to cause repeated hemorrhages. In one selected population of treated patients, the rate was up to 30% per person per year. Whether stereotactic radiosurgery improves outcome is uncertain, but resection should be strongly considered to prevent devastating future morbidity.[65] Clinical or CT scan features observed only in patients with a fatal outcome are a core temperature in excess of 39.8°C,

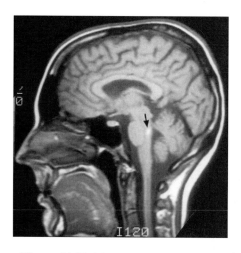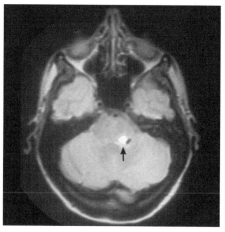

Figure 14.20 Magnetic resonance images showing limited pontine hemorrhage from cavernous hemangioma.

tachycardia defined as more than 110 beats/minute, CT evidence of extension to the midbrain and thalamus, and acute hydrocephalus on the initial CT scans.[63]

Triage

- Neurologic intensive care unit for support, observation, and, if appropriate, discussion of level of care.
- Patients with small pontine hemorrhages may be transferred to a ward for elective MRI, cerebral angiography, and surgical evacuation.

REFERENCES

1. Quershi AI, Tuhrim S, Broderick JP, et al.: Spontaneous intracerebral hemorrhage. N Engl J Med 344:1450, 2001.
2. Stein RW, Kase CS, Hier DB, et al.: Caudate hemorrhage. Neurology 34:1549, 1984.
3. Sutton LN, Barranco D, Greenberg J, et al.: Cerebral blood flow and glucose metabolism in experimental brain edema. J Neurosurg 71:868, 1989.
4. Lee KR, Colon GP, Betz AL, et al.: Edema from intracerebral hemorrhage: the role of thrombin. J Neurosurg 84:91, 1996.
5. Xi G, Wagner KR, Keep RF, et al.: Role of blood clot formation on early edema development after experimental intracerebral hemorrhage. Stroke 29:2580, 1998.
6. Mayer SA, Lignelli A, Fink ME, et al.: Perilesional blood flow and edema formation in acute intracerebral hemorrhage: a SPECT study. Stroke 29:1791, 1998.
7. Qureshi AI, Wilson DA, Hanley DF, et al.: No evidence for an ischemic penumbra in massive experimental intracerebral hemorrhage. Neurology 52:266, 1999.
8. Kothari RU, Brott T, Broderick JP, et al.: The ABCs of measuring intracerebral hemorrhage volumes. Stroke 27:1304, 1996.
9. Kazui S, Naritomi H, Yamamoto H, et al.: Enlargement of spontaneous intracerebral hemorrhage. Incidence and time course. Stroke 27:1783, 1996.
10. Bogousslavsky J, Regli F, Uske A, et al.: Early spontaneous hematoma in cerebral infarct: is primary cerebral hemorrhage overdiagnosed? Neurology 41:837, 1991.
11. Sung CY, Chu NS: Late CT manifestations in spontaneous lobar hematoma. J Comput Assist Tomogr 25:938, 2001.
12. Weir B: The clinical problem of intracerebral hematoma. Stroke 24 (Suppl 12):I93, 1993.
13. Radberg JA, Olsson JE, Radberg CT: Prognostic parameters in spontaneous intracerebral hematomas with special reference to anticoagulant treatment. Stroke 22:571, 1991.
14. Wijdicks EFM, Schievink WI, Brown RD, et al.: The dilemma of discontinuation of anticoagulation therapy for patients with intracranial hemorrhage and mechanical heart valves. Neurosurgery 42:769, 1998.
15. Phan TG, Koh M, Wijdicks EFM: Safety of discontinuation of anticoagulation in patients with intracranial hemorrhage at high thromboembolic risk. Arch Neurol 57:1710, 2000.
16. Tietjen CS, Hurn PD, Ulatowski JA, et al.: Treatment modalities for hypertensive patients with intracranial pathology: options and risks. Crit Care Med 24:311, 1996.
17. Terayama Y, Tanahashi N, Fukuuchi Y, et al.: Prognostic value of admission blood pressure in patients with intracerebral hemorrhage. Keio Cooperative Stroke Study. Stroke 28:1185, 1997.
18. Powers WJ: Acute hypertension after stroke: the scientific basis for treatment decisions. Neurology 43:461, 1993.
19. Siddique MS, Fernandes HM, Woolridge TD: Reversible ischemia around intracerebral hemorrhage: a single-photon emission computerized tomography study. J Neurosurg 96:736, 2002.
20. Qureshi AI, Wilson DA, Hanley DF, et al.: No evidence for ischemic penumbra in massive experimental intracerebral hemorrhage. Neurology 52:266, 1999.
21. Powers WJ, Zazulia AR, Videen TO, et al.: Autoregulation of cerebral blood flow surrounding acute (6 to 22 hours) intracerebral hemorrhage. Neurology 57:18, 2001.
22. Diringer MN: Intracerebral hemorrhage: pathophysiology and management. Crit Care Med 21:1591, 1993.
23. Poungvarin N, Bhoopat W, Viriyavejakul A, et al.: Effects of dexamethasone in primary supratentorial intracerebral hemorrhage. N Engl J Med 316:1229, 1987.
24. Mayer SA: Ultra-early hemostatic therapy for intracerebral hemorrhage. Stroke 34:224, 2003.
25. Brott T, Broderick J, Kothari R, et al.: Early hemorrhage growth in patients with intracerebral hemorrhage. Stroke 28:1, 1997.
26. Hankey GJ, Hon C: Surgery for primary intracerebral hemorrhage: is it safe and effective? A systematic review of case series and randomized trials. Stroke 28:2126, 1997.
27. Prasad K, Browman G, Srivastava A, et al.: Surgery in primary supratentorial intracerebral hematoma: a meta-analysis of randomized trials. Acta Neurol Scand 95:103, 1997.
28. Schaller C, Rohde V, Meyer B, et al.: Stereotactic puncture and lysis of spontaneous intracerebral hemorrhage using recombinant tissue-plasminogen activator. Neurosurgery 36:328, 1995.
29. Teernstra OPM, Evers SMAA, Lodder J, et al.: Stereotactic treatment of intracerebral hematoma by means of a plasminogen activator: A multicenter randomized controlled trial (SICHPA). Stroke 34:968, 2003.
30. Marquardt G, Wolff R, Sager A, et al.: Subacute stereotactic aspiration of haematomas within the basal ganglia reduces occurrence of complications in the course of haemorrhagic stroke in non-comatose patients. Cerebrovasc Dis 15:252, 2003.
31. Morgenstern LB, Frankowski RF, Shedden P, et al.: Surgical Treatment for Intracerebral Hemorrhage (STICH): a single-center, randomized, clinical trial. Neurology 51:1359, 1998.

32. Lampl Y, Gilad R, Eshel Y, et al.: Neurological and functional outcome in patients with supratentorial hemorrhages. A prospective study. *Stroke* 26:2249, 1995.

33. Hemphill JC III, Bonovich DC, Besmertis L, et al.: The ICH score. A simple, reliable grading scale for intracerebral hemorrhage. *Stroke* 32:891, 2001.

34. Phan TG, Koh M, Vierkant RA, et al.: Hydrocephalus is a determinant of early mortality in putaminal hemorrhage. *Stroke* 31:2157, 2000.

35. Nilsson OG, Lindgren A, Brandt L, et al.: Prediction of death in patients with primary intracerebral hemorrhage: a prospective study of a defined population. *J Neurosurg* 97:531, 2002.

36. Wakai S, Kumakura N, Nagai M: Lobar intracerebral hemorrhage. A clinical, radiographic, and pathological study of 29 consecutive operated cases with negative angiography. *J Neurosurg* 76:231, 1992.

37. Tokuda Y, Inagawa T, Katoh Y, et al.: Intracerebral hematoma in patients with ruptured cerebral aneurysms. *Surg Neurol* 43:272, 1995.

38. Hart RG, Boop BS, Anderson DC: Oral anticoagulants and intracranial hemorrhage. Facts and hypotheses. *Stroke* 26:1471, 1995.

39. Gurwitz JH, Gore JM, Goldberg RJ, et al.: Risk for intracranial hemorrhage after tissue plasminogen activator treatment for acute myocardial infarction. *Ann Intern Med* 129:597, 1998.

40. Ropper AH, Davis KR: Lobar cerebral hemorrhages: acute clinical syndromes in 26 cases. *Ann Neurol* 8:141, 1980.

41. Weisberg LA: Subcortical lobar intracerebral haemorrhage: clinical–computed tomographic correlations. *J Neurol Neurosurg Psychiatry* 48:1078, 1985.

42. Aguirre GK, Ellenbogen JM, Pollar J, et al.: Amyloid angiopathy. *Neurology* 59:1656, 2002.

43. Kaufman HH, McAllister P, Taylor H, et al.: Intracerebral hematoma related to thrombolysis for myocardial infarction. *Neurosurgery* 33:898, 1993.

44. Rabinstein AA, Atkinson JL, Wijdicks EF: Emergency craniotomy in patients worsening due to expanded cerebral hematoma: to what purpose? *Neurology* 58:1367, 2002.

45. Griffiths PD, Beveridge CJ, Gholkar A: Angiography in non-traumatic brain hematoma. An analysis of 100 cases. *Acta Radiol* 38:797, 1997.

46. Flemming K, Wijdicks EFM, Li H: Can we predict poor outcome at presentation in patients with lobar hemorrhage? *Cerebrovasc Dis* 11:183, 2001.

47. Flemming KD, Wijdicks EFM, St Louis EK, et al.: Predicting deterioration in patients with lobar hemorrhages. *J Neurol Neurosurg Psychiatry* 66:600, 1999.

48. Vermeer SE, Algra A, Franke CL, et al.: Long-term prognosis after recovery from primary intracerebral hemorrhage. *Neurology* 58:205, 2002.

49. Gates PC, Barnett HJ, Vinters HV, et al.: Primary intraventricular hemorrhage in adults. *Stroke* 17:872, 1986.

50. Darby DG, Donnan GA, Saling MA, et al.: Primary intraventricular hemorrhage: clinical and neuropsychological findings in a prospective stroke series. *Neurology* 38:68, 1988.

51. Findlay JM, Grace MG, Weir BK: Treatment of intraventricular hemorrhage with tissue plasminogen activator. *Neurosurgery* 32:941, 1993.

52. Naff NJ, Tuhrim S: Intraventricular hemorrhage in adults: complications and treatment. *New Horiz* 5:359, 1997.

53. Yeh HS, Tomsick TA, Tew JM Jr: Intraventricular hemorrhage due to aneurysms of the distal posterior inferior cerebellar artery. Report of three cases. *J Neurosurg* 62:772, 1985.

54. Chang DS, Lin CL, Howng SL: Primary intraventricular hemorrhage in adult—an analysis of 24 cases. *Kaohsiung J Med Sci* 14:633, 1998.

55. Carhuapoma JR: Thrombolytic therapy after intraventricular hemorrhage: do we know enough? *J Neurol Sci* 202:1, 2002.

56. Wang YCH, Lin CW, Shen CC, et al.: Tissue plasminogen activator for the treatment of intraventricular hematoma: the dose–effect relationship. *J Neurol Sci* 202:35, 2002.

57. Schwarz S, Schwab S, Steiner HH, et al.: Secondary hemorrhage after intraventricular fibrinolysis: a cautionary note: a report of two cases. *Neurosurgery* 42:659, 1998.

58. Coplin WM, Vinas FC, Agris JM, et al.: A cohort study of the safety and feasibility of intraventricular urokinase for nonaneurysmal spontaneous intraventricular hemorrhage. *Stroke* 29:1573, 1998.

59. St Louis EK, Wijdicks EFM, Li H, et al.: Predictors of poor outcome in patients with spontaneous cerebellar hematoma. *Can J Neurol Sci* 27:32, 2000.

60. St Louis EK, Wijdicks EFM, Li H: Predicting neurologic deterioration in patients with cerebellar hematomas. *Neurology* 51:1364, 1998.

61. Wijdicks EFM, St Louis EK, Atkinson JD, et al.: Clinicians' biases toward surgery in cerebellar hematomas: an analysis of decision-making in 94 patients. *Cerebrovasc Dis* 10:93, 2000.

62. Donauer E, Loew F, Faubert C, et al.: Prognostic factors in the treatment of cerebellar haemorrhage. *Acta Neurochir* (Wien) 131:59, 1994.

63. Wijdicks EFM, St Louis E: Clinical profiles predictive of outcome in pontine hemorrhage. *Neurology* 49:1342, 1997.

64. Rabinstein AA, Tisch D, McClelland RL, et al.: Cause is the main predictor of outcome in patients with pontine hemorrhage. *Cereb Dis* 17:66–71, 2004.

65. Porter RW, Detwiler PW, Spetzler RF, et al.: Cavernous malformations of the brainstem: experience with 100 patients. *J Neurosurg* 90:50, 1999.

Chapter 15
Major Ischemic Stroke Syndromes

The causes of ischemic stroke are numerous, but only a few are common. The benefits of therapy in most instances so far are small. Treatment of acute ischemic stroke with thrombolytics has become a staple of care in the emergency department. However, clot retrieval and thrombus obliteration devices have come into existence.[1] Controversies and uncertainties remain about the use of thrombolytic agents, and some skeptics do not take the results at face value, alleging baseline imbalances in trials and comparatively small numbers of patients.[2–5] In addition, many patients still do not qualify for intravenous or intra-arterial thrombolysis, mostly due to prehospital delay time[6,7] (in one study, only 0.06% of all stroke admissions in 16 Connecticut hospitals[8]). In addition, the time window for intravenous administration of tissue-type plasminogen activator (tPA) remains within 3 hours and cannot be extended to 6 hours.[3,9–11] To complicate matters further, there is also documented evidence of increased mortality partly due to increased hemorrhage risk in routine practice outside the rigor of clinical trials.[8]

Patients with an ischemic stroke and candidates for such aggressive management usually present with a major neurologic deficit, often involving the entire function of an arm and a leg, speech, perception of the left side of the body, and, if the lesion is localized in the brain stem or cerebellum, stance, swallowing, and vision. These deficits can be quantified by use of the National Institutes of Health (NIH) Stroke Scale (Table 15.1),[12,13] and grading is practical when interventional therapies are under consideration.

This chapter discusses the most commonly encountered clinical presentations and the difficulties in management of major ischemic stroke syndromes. Some of the less frequently encountered disorders are mentioned, particularly when different therapies are recommended. The approach to this vast diagnostic field is by the arterial system.

Large Vessel Occlusions

Ischemic stroke embodies a diverse group of patients with different modes of onset, progression, and outcome. Over time, more complete evaluation of ischemic stroke has resulted in a better definition of its mechanism.

Clinical Presentation

Characteristic clinical presentations should be familiar to any physician managing acute stroke, but the fine points can be addressed by neurologists. The essence is combining the clinical features found through neurologic evaluation with findings of neuroimaging studies to allow quick triage. The role of the emergency physician in this respect has become substantial and reduces unnecessary delays.[14]

Table 15.1. Stroke Scale of the National Institutes of Health and National Institute of Neurological Disorders and Stroke (the NIH Stroke Scale)°

Level of consciousness			Motor, right leg	
Alert	0		No drift	0
Drowsy	1		Drift	1
Stuporous	2		Cannot resist gravity	2
Coma	3		No effort against gravity	3
Level of consciousness, questions			No movement	4
Answers both correctly	0		Motor, left leg	
Answers one correctly	1		No drift	0
Incorrect	2		Drift	1
Level of consciousness, commands			Cannot resist gravity	2
Obeys both correctly	0		No effort against gravity	3
Obeys one correctly	1		No movement	4
Incorrect	2		Limb ataxia	
Gaze			Absent	0
Normal	0		Present in either upper or lower	1
Partial gaze palsy	1		Present in both upper and lower	2
Forced deviation	2		Sensory	
Visual			Normal	0
No loss	0		Partial loss	1
Partial hemianopsia	1		Dense loss	2
Complete hemianopsia	2		Neglect	
Bilateral hemianopsia	3		No neglect	0
Facial palsy			Partial neglect	1
Normal	0		Complete neglect	2
Minor	1		Dysarthria	
Partial	2		Normal articulation	0
Complete	3		Mild to moderate dysarthria	1
Motor, right arm			Nearly unintelligible or worse	2
No drift	0		Language	
Drift	1		No aphasia	0
Cannot resist gravity	2		Mild to moderate aphasia	1
No effort against gravity	3		Severe aphasia	2
No movement	4		Mute	3
Motor, left arm				
No drift	0			
Drift	1			
Cannot resist gravity	2			
No effort against gravity	3			
No movement	4			

° A sum score of 10 or greater is strongly indicative of a large vessel occlusion, predominantly in the middle cerebral artery. Examination may take only 5 minutes.

Source: Modified from Brott T, Adams HP Jr, Olinger CP, et al.: Measurements of acute cerebral infarctions: a clinical examination scale. *Stroke* 20:864, 1989. By permission of the American Heart Association.

Middle Cerebral Artery Occlusion

Catastrophic cerebral infarction often is caused by an occlusion of the middle cerebral artery (MCA). Its arterial system can be occluded at the M1 segment (proximal MCA), proximal to the lateral lenticulostriatal arteries, and at the M2 segment. The M2 segment is further divided by the superior and inferior trunks, which supply the perisylvian area of the frontal and temporal lobes, respectively. The M2 MCA segment then is divided into the M3, or operculum, segment and the M4, or cortical, branches.

The most devastating MCA occlusion is at M1 or the stem, with a thrombus possibly extending into the carotid artery. Occlusion at the origin of the MCA may lead to gaze preference, hemianopsia, and flaccid hemiplegia of the arm, with some sparing of movement in the leg. Global aphasia and speech apraxia occur if the left MCA is involved and left body neglect, aprosodia (lack of affection or pitch in speech), and bilateral ptosis (see Chapter 3) if the right MCA is involved. Hemisensory loss with no grimacing or withdrawal to pinprick is typical. A multimodulary speech deficit is common in left MCA occlusion. The patient has eyes open and may look about but is unable to follow any command or does so in an inappropriate manner. There is an inability to move the lips and tongue and to blow out the cheeks. Speech may be characterized by repetitive stopping and starting and fumbling words.[15] Other patients are mute. Occlusion of the superior trunk of the left MCA produces exactly the same characteristics and therefore cannot be differentiated clinically. However, occlusion of the inferior trunk of the left MCA produces a Wernicke-type aphasia and a superior homonymous quadrantanopsia ("pie in the sky").

An infarct may preferentially involve the perforating arteries of the MCA (lenticulostriate arteries) when the collateral supply from the anterior circulation and posterior cerebral artery (PCA) is sufficient to protect the remainder of the hemisphere from infarction. A comma-shaped infarct, or so-called striatocapsular infarct, occurs with hemiplegia equally severe in the arm and leg and with fairly mild sensory symptoms.

In many patients, the defect may further evolve or fluctuate and, in some, surprisingly, may disappear. Decrease in deficit may occur in patients with large territorial MCA occlusions ("spectacular shrinking deficit").[16] It is explained by fragmentation of the obstructing clot. In 13% of patients, deterioration occurs after initial dramatic improvement and is attributed to reocclusion.[17,18]

Anterior Cerebral Artery Occlusion

Most anterior cerebral artery (ACA) distribution infarctions are caused by a cardioembolic source or by artery-to-artery embolization from internal carotid artery stenosis with a diameter reduction of more than 70%.[19] The clinical symptoms of acute ACA occlusion are complex and may not be obvious. Usually, occlusion involves severe weakness of the leg in combination with other frontal lobe symptoms, such as abulia, loss of vitality, and incontinence. Transcortical motor and sensory aphasia, characterized by lack of spontaneous speech and comprehension but the ability to repeat phrases, has been reported in an infarction involving the ACA territory. Apraxia of the left

arm with normal use of the right arm is typical, and this dissociation can be explained by corpus callosum infarction interrupting connecting fibers and can occur irrespective of occlusion of the right or left ACA. The disorder is revealed when patients can name objects placed in the right hand but are unable to recognize and name objects in the left hand.

An important artery that may become occluded is the recurrent artery of Heubner. Infarction of this territory produces weakness in the contralateral arm and side of the face, with dysarthria and hemichorea. If bilateral occlusions occur, a syndrome of akinetic mutism may evolve.

Vertebrobasilar Artery Occlusion

The basilar artery contributes several paramedian vessels to the pons, as well as short circumference vessels, and two major cerebellar arteries, the proximal anterior inferior cerebellar artery (AICA) and, more distally, the superior cerebellar artery (SCA). The basilar artery divides into both posterior cerebellar arteries. Occlusions are possible at several levels, most often from artery-to-artery embolization. Occlusion of the basilar artery or its branches may produce several ischemic syndromes. Lodging of an embolus at the tip of the basilar artery results in infarction of the brain stem, thalamus, and occipital and medial temporal lobes. Cerebellar infarction may involve each or all of the feeding arteries to the cerebellum with propagation of clot to the cerebral artery (posterior inferior cerebellar artery [PICA], AICA, and SCA). Less dramatic syndromes of brain stem infarction, many carrying French eponyms, are shown in Table 15.2 for easy reference, but they are rarely complete at presentation. (These syndromes are interesting exercises in localization and, thus, are favorites of neurologists.)

Occlusion of the basilar artery results in a profound neurologic deficit but may start with any of these brain stem syndromes. However, a study of patients with basilar artery occlusion and thromboembolization found that sudden disturbance of consciousness was a predominant clinical symptom and was followed by brain stem signs without a clear unifying syndrome. In many patients, ophthalmoparesis and bulbar weakness develop early after onset.[20] Sudden vertigo, dysarthria, and quadriparesis are presenting features. Intranuclear ophthalmoplegia is common, explained by

Table 15.2. The Classic Brain Stem Syndromes

Eponym	Lesion	Features
Midbrain		
Weber	Cerebral peduncle	Ipsilateral III nerve palsy
		Contralateral hemiparesis
Benedikt	Tegmentum red nucleus	Ipsilateral III nerve palsy
		Contralateral tremor, chorea
Parinaud	Quadrigeminal plate	Paralysis of upward gaze
Chiray-Foix-Nicolesco	Lateral	Hemiataxia
		Hemichorea
		Decreased vibration and proprioception
		Arm and leg weakness with or without facial weakness
Pons		
Raymond	Paramedian area	Ipsilateral lateral rectus muscle paresis, contralateral hemiplegia
Millard-Gubler	Medial lower	Ipsilateral facial palsy with contralateral hemiplegia (often also VI palsy)
Foville	Medial lower	Ipsilateral VII
		Ipsilateral paralysis of lateral gaze
		Contralateral hemiparesis
Raymond-Céstan	Medial	Quadriplegia
		Anesthesia
		Nystagmus
Brissaud	Ventral	Ipsilateral facial spasm
		Contralateral hemiparesis
Medulla Oblongata		
Wallenberg	Lateral	Horner syndrome (ipsilateral), IX, X palsy
		Crossed hemianesthesia
Avellis	Nucleus ambiguus tractus solitarius	X, XI palsy (ipsilateral face, contralateral body)
	Spinothalamic tract	Contralateral dissociated hemianesthesia
Schmidt	Vagal nuclei	X, XI
	Bulbar and spinal nuclei of accessory fibers	
Jackson	Nuclear vagus, accessory, hypoglossus nerve	X, XI, XII
Tapia	Motor nuclei vagus and hypoglossus	X, XII

interruption of the intranuclear connections through the medial lemniscus fasciculus; cold water irrigation may bring this on in a comatose patient (see Chapter 8). Patients may have hemiparesis mimicking a hemispheric lesion. Brief rhythmical shaking movements, most likely a forme fruste of extensor posturing, can be observed and are commonly misinterpreted as seizures, again leading to false localization in the hemisphere. An occluding embolus at the junction of the basilar artery and PCA may further interrupt the thalamic perforating artery and result in infarction of the thalamus bilaterally, midbrain,

and occipital lobes. Vertical gaze palsy, abnormal convergence, skew deviation, behavioral disturbances, and visual hallucinations are common combinations and have been named "top-of-the-basilar syndrome." Cortical blindness or *polyopia* (multiple images stacked up) due to bilateral occipital lobe ischemia may be a prominent presenting feature.

Many patients have progression to coma, with quadriplegia and pathologic withdrawal or extensor motor responses to pain. In our series of 25 patients with basilar artery occlusion who required mechanical ventilation, one-third lost most brain stem reflexes within the first 24 hours.[21] Failure to trigger the ventilator does occur and may remain the only intact clinical sign.

Locked-in syndrome is the result of occlusion of the perforating arteries of the paramedian basilar artery, leading to dysfunction of the corticospinal tract, corticobulbar tract, and exiting sixth nerve fibers. The level of consciousness is normal, and the patient can communicate only with vertical eye movements and blinking (see Chapter 8). Thalamic involvement or extension to the dorsal mesencephalon, thus affecting the reticular formation, may cause intermittent drowsiness and failure to consistently answer questions.

Cerebellar infarctions may involve the PICA, SCA, and, much less commonly, AICA. PICA occlusions may have different clinical presentations depending on the area of involvement, which may include the lateral medulla. Mainly, these occlusions are manifested by acute headache, vertigo, ataxia of gait, or limb ataxia, but isolated vertigo due to involvement of the vestibular portion of the vermis may be seen.

SCA occlusions may be the most frequent cerebellar infarct, and acute dysarthria and ipsilateral dysmetria may be very prominent. This type of occlusion may closely mimic dysarthria-clumsy hand-lacunar syndrome. Vertigo is much less apparent.

AICA occlusions are manifested by a characteristic acute deafness or profound unilateral hearing loss, but facial paralysis, Horner's syndrome, facial numbness, and loss of sensitivity to pain and temperature may occur as well.

Evolving cerebellar swelling may displace the pons or compress the medulla from tonsillar herniation (see Chapter 8). Impairment of consciousness occurs after a delay of 2–4 days, but patients may have cerebellar swelling at the time of admission to the emergency department.

Posterior Cerebral Artery

The PCA produces characteristic neurobehavioral syndromes that can be easily recognized in the emergency department. A proximal PCA occlusion involving the dominant hemisphere (most often the left side) leads to alexia without agraphia. This dissociation syndrome is caused by an infarction of the splenium of the corpus callosum; patients are unable to read, but the ability to write is preserved because of intact language centers.

Color agnosia may accompany a dominant hemispheric lesion. This color-naming disturbance should be tested in patients with right homonymous hemianopsia. Infarction of the dominant angular gyrus results in Gerstmann's syndrome, which involves *finger agnosia* (inability to name the fingers), inability to calculate, right–left disorientation, and agraphia. Right nondominant PCA occlusion may lead to *prosopagnosia* (inability to recognize familiar faces, such as those of family members or celebrities), in addition to a visual field defect.

Bilateral PCA occlusion can lead to two relatively rare syndromes, such as cortical blindness, in which patients may not recognize that they are blind and may relate vivid descriptions of the emergency room and persons surrounding them, all untrue, and Balint's syndrome, with bilateral involvement in the border zone areas between ACA and PCA territories, often occurring after an episode of severe hypotension. Patients complain of "blindness," are unable to describe a full scene, and cannot describe more than two components of a visual field at the same time (*simultanagnosia*). In this syndrome, ocular apraxia may be observed, that is, lack of quick focusing on a new stimulus, previously called *spasm of fixation.* When a stimulus is entering a visual field and even when told this is occurring, patients are not immediately alert to the stimulus. In addition, there is *optic ataxia*, referring to difficulty pointing accurately at a target under visual guidance. This can be brought about with the simple finger-pointing test. Distal occlusion of the PCA produces only a visual defect, usually with sparing of the macula due to collateral supply from the MCA.

Interpretation of Diagnostic Tests

Computed Tomographic Scanning and Magnetic Resonance Imaging

Before third-generation computed tomographic (CT) scanners, CT scanning in a patient with possible ischemic stroke was performed only to "exclude a hemorrhage." The definition of brain structures has improved with the newer generation of CT scanners, and the signs of early ischemia can be recognized. The vascular territories should be known when one views CT scans (Fig. 15.1). If no obvious hypodensity is present, the

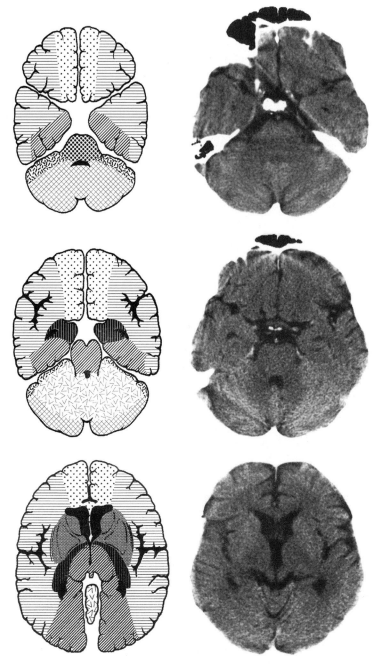

Figure 15.1 Vascular territories of the brain (computed tomographic scans and corresponding arterial territories). ACA, anterior cerebral artery; AChA, anterior choroidal artery; AICA, anterior inferior cerebellar artery; BA, basilar artery; LSA, lenticulostriate artery; MCA, middle cerebral artery; PCA, posterior cerebral artery; PICA, posterior inferior cerebellar artery; SCA, superior cerebellar artery.

CT scan should be carefully scrutinized for early signs of cerebral infarction: sulci effacement and an obscured outline of the lentiform nucleus or decrease in tissue attenuation (Fig. 15.2). The subtle differences between gray and white matter are more easily detected when several CT window settings are used. Obscuration of the lentiform nucleus is the most frequent earliest sign[22]

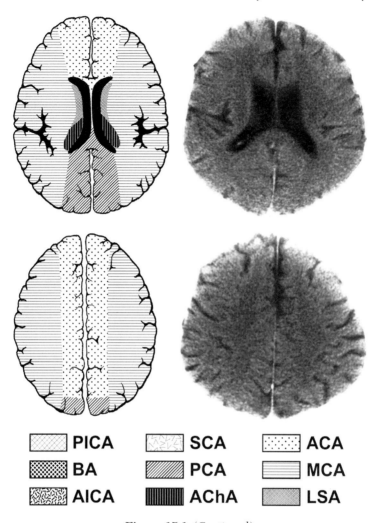

PICA	SCA	ACA
BA	PCA	MCA
AICA	AChA	LSA

Figure 15.1 (*Continued*)

and may appear within the first hour of infarction (Fig. 15.2A). In a small study of 25 patients, it appeared in one of two patients within an hour of the ictus, in seven of eight patients in the second hour, in all three patients in the third hour, in seven of eight patients in the fourth hour, and in all four patients scanned thereafter.[22] Early abnormalities on the CT scan also involve the parenchyma, with loss of the precise delineation between gray and white matter and, particularly, loss of the insular ribbon.[23] The insular segment of the MCA supplies the insular ribbon, and with complete occlusion of the MCA, the insular region becomes a watershed arterial zone.[24] In addition, the insular cortex is the region most distant from the collateral flow from the ACA and PCA (Fig. 15.2B).

In some patients, the extent of the ischemic territory is noted by eye deviation on CT (Fig. 15.3).[25] Hypodensity may involve the entire MCA territory (Fig. 15.4A) but is usually evident days after onset. Hypodensity on CT scans may involve only the M2 territory (Fig. 15.4B) or the lenticulostriate arteries (Fig. 15.4C). A hypodensity can be seen within hours after MCA trunk occlusion.[26] Transferred patients seen several hours after onset who had CT scanning during previous hospitalization at the time of the ictus should have a repeat CT scan, which may show a developing hypodensity.

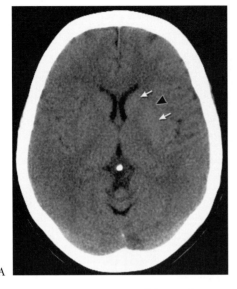
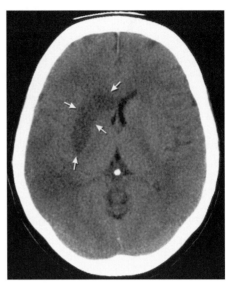

A   B

Figure 15.2 *A:* Normal definition of the caudate nucleus, lentiform nucleus (*arrows*), and insular ribbon (*arrowhead*) in the left hemisphere has disappeared in the right hemisphere. *B:* One day later, a CT scan shows a hypodensity in that area (*arrows*).

A hyperdense MCA sign[27] actually indicates the clot in the MCA and has been recognized as a prognostic feature. In our studies, a hyperdense MCA together with early swelling (sulci efface-

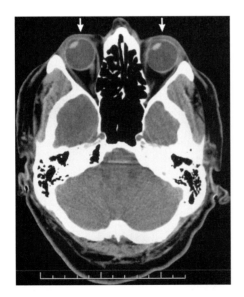

Figure 15.3 Note eye deviation on computed tomographic (CT) exam.

ment) predicted deterioration from further brain swelling.[28–30] In other reports, hemorrhagic transformation was deemed more likely in patients who had a hyperdense MCA sign.[27,31,32] When the clot fragments and breaks up, the hyperdense MCA sign disappears, often spontaneously or, at times, after intravenous administration of tPA (Fig. 15.5A,B).[33] Swelling from MCA infarction often involves shift of the septum pellucidum followed by early trapping of the temporal horn. Involvement of the ACA circulation indicates a carotid occlusion (Fig. 15.6).

Cerebral infarction is better visualized on magnetic resonance imaging (MRI) than on CT scanning.[34] Additional findings on MRI include lack of normal flow voids, representing the occluded vessel.[35] Arterial enhancement of the T_1-weighted images in the ischemic zone after administration of gadolinium contrast material is caused by slow flow in an otherwise high-flow arterial system distal to the obstructing lesion.[36] This finding is seen in approximately 50% of patients with acute cortical infarcts.[35]

Newer MRI techniques using diffusion-weighted imaging (DWI) or fluid-attenuated inversion recovery (FLAIR) are extremely sensitive

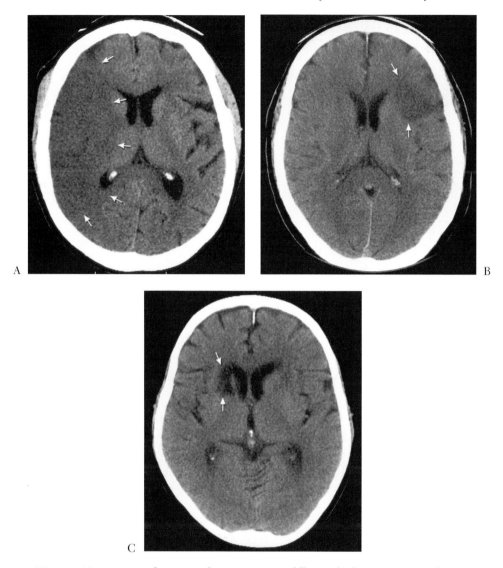

Figure 15.4 Computed tomographic scans. *A:* Middle cerebral artery stem occlusion. *B:* Superior division occlusion. *C:* Striatocapsular infarct.

for early infarction.[37] In DWI, areas of hyperintensity (bright areas) indicate decreased movement of water,[38,39] and the study is superior within 6 hours of presentation when compared with CT or MRI alone (Fig. 15.7*A* and *B*).[40] Several studies have shown that early infarction underlies the high signal intensity. It most likely reflects failure of water movement in tissue in this zone of infarction. When these areas of restricted diffusion are quantified using the apparent diffusion coefficient, they are seen as a hypodense area (Fig.

15.8). The size of the lesion with this abnormality predicts future outcome; however, the critical size for possible improvement is not known, and DWI cannot distinguish which lesions may be reversible after specific treatment (particularly thrombolytic therapy). Practical use of DWI in acute situations remains undefined, and most currently published studies on these MR sequences represent a fraction of the admitted patients with acute stroke. FLAIR sequences are also superior to routine MR sequences, and a recent study com-

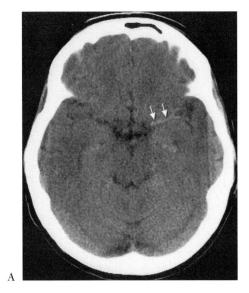
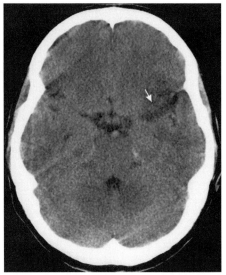

A   B

Figure 15.5 *A,B:* Hyperdense middle cerebral artery sign. The sign disappeared after administration of tissue-type plasminogen activator, but infarction developed.

paring multimodality MR techniques found a sensitivity of 98% for DWI and 91% for FLAIR for detecting ischemic brain lesions within hours of the ictus.[41] The accuracy of DWI for subcortical

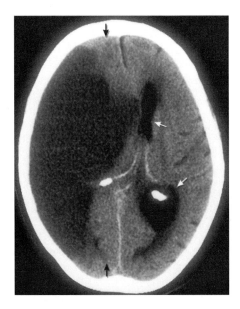

Figure 15.6 Signs of late swelling of middle cerebral artery infarct on computed tomography. Note sparing of the anterior cerebral artery and posterior cerebral artery territories (*black arrows*), shift, and contralateral hydrocephalus (*white arrows*).

infarcts is 95%.[42] An important recent development is the potential value of MRI diffusion (DWI) and perfusion (PWI) to assess salvageability of tissue when considering thrombolysis. It seems from preliminary studies that a mismatch between DWI and PWI (hypoperfusion lesion more than diffusion lesion) may be present in a considerable proportion of patients and could suggest the presence of a reversible penumbra after thrombolysis.[43] These evolving but not established techniques could be used to assess patients who may be eligible outside the accepted clinical windows, assuming that DWI abnormalities would indicate cell injury.[44]

Currently, CT scanning remains the most important initial study and, in most institutions without immediate 24-hour MRI services, is not likely to be replaced soon by these more sensitive, and undoubtedly superb, tests for the diagnosis of ischemic stroke. Until then, it is therefore of utmost importance that physicians treating ischemic stroke be familiar with the early signs on high-definition CT scans.[45]

Using MRI and MRA, vertebrobasilar artery occlusion is diagnostic in virtually all cases, although the extent of the infarction may take some time to mature (Fig. 15.9). A marked discrepancy between the initial CT scan (which may show only a hyperdense basilar artery sign) and the MRIs

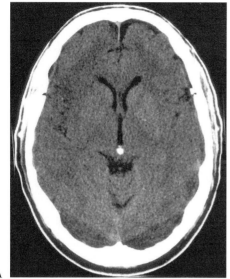

A   B

Figure 15.7 *A,B:* Fluid-attenuated inversion recovery (FLAIR) image of evolving right middle cerebral artery stroke compared with virtually normal computed tomographic scan.

may be seen. CT scanning of cerebellar infarcts may be characterized by only a faintly developed hypodensity and distortion of the fourth ventricle. MRI is also the preferred test in cerebellar infarcts because it defines the degree of compression and herniation (Fig. 15.10).

Computed Tomographic Scan Angiography
CT scan angiography with a high dose of contrast medium is beginning to replace MR angiographic studies.[46] It immediately provides the site of arterial occlusion and an estimate of the capacity of the collaterals. However, the introduction of a

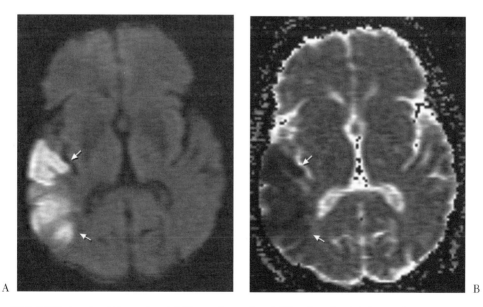

A   B

Figure 15.8 DWI showing (*A*) restricted diffusion (*arrow*) and (*B*) reduced ADC (*arrows*). ADC, apparent diffusion coefficient.

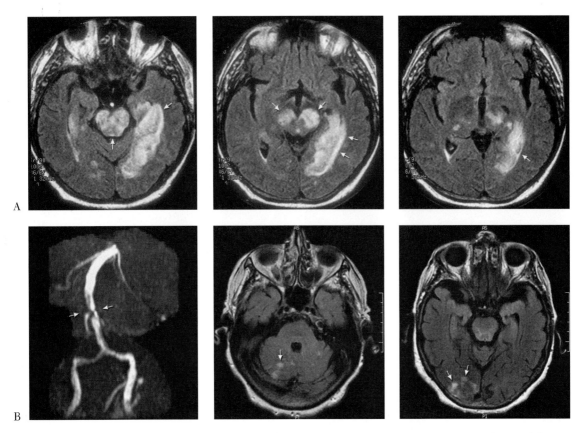

Figure 15.9 Examples of vertebrobasilar occlusive disease on magnetic resonance imaging. *A:* Study with fluid attenuation inversion recovery shows infarction in temporal lobe, pons–mesencephalon, thalamus, and occipital lobe very consistent with occlusion of the top of the basilar artery. *B:* Midbasilar stenosis on magnetic resonance angiography and cerebellar and occipital infarct (*arrows*).

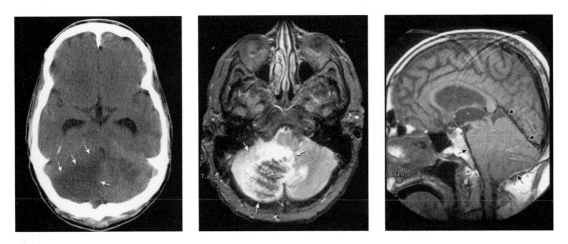

Figure 15.10 Cerebellar stroke with swelling and early hydrocephalus (*left*) from fourth ventricle obstruction on computed tomographic scan and magnetic resonance imaging (*middle, right*).

large amount of contrast material remains of concern in patients with increased serum creatinine levels, and the additional acquisition time may have an effect on the first 3-hour period in which intravenous tPA is used, particularly in institutions not yet equipped for the study.[47,48] In addition, observer agreement among neuroradiologists may be marginal in acute occlusion of the MCA, particularly in the assessment of symmetrical arterial enhancement.[49] Thus, the study may be less practical when used to assess vascular occlusion before the use of intravenous tPA.[47,48]

The role of CT scan angiography in basilar artery occlusion has not been determined, but the study may be useful in patients with fluctuating symptoms, to assess whether occlusion is imminent, a finding that only then may lead to conventional cerebral angiography. It may also resolve problems with localization in patients with predominant hemiplegia.

Cerebral Angiography

Cerebral angiography remains the standard means of determining the extent of occlusion and collateral circulation. Its use in acute situations is defined by whether intra-arterial thrombolysis is considered and thus requires a certified interventional neuroradiologist. However, in approximately one-third of patients, cerebral angiography done immediately after an ischemic stroke yields normal findings or shows a distal branch occlusion or a carotid occlusion unsuitable for thrombolysis.

First Priority in Management

Initial management should involve supportive stabilizing measures and consideration of thrombolysis. The contraindications for thrombolysis are shown in Table 15.3. Although CT scan findings should be normal, it is not known whether very early signs of infarction (effacement of the lentiform nucleus) preclude the use of tPA; but current practice is to accept early changes and only defer thrombolysis with large hypodensity (more than one-third of the territory), sulci effacement, and other signs of brain swelling. These signs may reduce the chance of recovery (are indicators of permanent ischemia) or perhaps increase the risk of intracerebral hematoma.

There is concern about possible unnecessary exclusion of patients eligible for intravenous tPA.

Table 15.3. Eligibility Criteria for Using Intravenous Recombinant Tissue-type Plasminogen Activator for the Treatment of Acute Ischemic Stroke

Clinical indication
    Ischemic stroke within 3 hours of onset of symptoms (the last time patient was noted to be at baseline neurologic status before the stroke)
Clinical contraindications
    Any history of intracranial hemorrhage
    Pretreatment of systolic blood pressure >185 mm Hg
    Diastolic blood pressure >110 mm Hg
    Mild neurologic signs (e.g., isolated sensory deficit)
    Symptoms suggesting subarachnoid hemorrhage
    Stroke or serious head trauma within the preceding 3 months
    Gastrointestinal or urinary hemorrhage within the preceding 21 days
    Major surgery within the preceding 14 days
    Arterial puncture at a noncompressible site within the preceding 7 days
    Seizure at the onset of stroke
    Taking oral anticoagulants
    Received heparin within previous 48 hours
Radiographic contraindications
    Evidence of intracranial hemorrhage on computed tomography of the brain
Laboratory contraindications
    Prothrombin time >15 seconds (international normalized ratio >1.7)
    Platelet count < 100 × 10^9/L
    Elevated partial thromboplastin time
    Blood glucose level <50 mg/dL

tPA has been inappropriately deferred in patients with "mild deficits," prior use of aspirin, prior strokes, or old age. In some instances, the physician allows a few more minutes to observe improvement, followed by deferral of tPA after crossing the 3-hour limit.[50] The exclusion criteria of seizure onset are debatable, as is "major surgery preceding 14 days." When surgery involves body areas that can be amenable to homeostasis, thrombolysis should not be automatically deferred. Cervical arterial dissection is not an absolute contraindication.[51]

Intravenous thrombolysis with tPA can be started if symptoms have not abated within 3 hours after onset. A reasonable, albeit arbitrary, guideline is an NIH Stroke Scale score of more than 4. This could reduce the chance of significantly worsening a minimal deficit with an intracerebral hematoma. The ictus should be pre-

Box 15.1. Recombinant Tissue-type Plasminogen Activator (tPA)

Currently used fibrinolytic agents are plasminogen activators. tPA catalyzes plasmin formation from plasminogen. Plasmin degrades circulatory fibrinogen and the fibrin lattice of thrombi into soluble end products. Heparin enhances plasmin generation and, thus, enhances the tPA effect, which has a biologic half-life of 3–8 minutes. The major source of tPA is vascular endothelium; tPA has a high affinity for fibrin-bound plasminogen. It results in a less severe systemic thrombolytic state than that seen with urokinase. In clinical use, tPA causes a marked decrease in or depletion of measurable circulating plasminogen and fibrinogen, resulting in prolongation of the partial thromboplastin time.

cisely known and not estimated. It is typically not known when patients have awakened from a night's sleep. Administration of tPA is intravenous, in a dose of 0.9 mg/kg (maximum 90 mg), with 10% of the total dose given in a 1- to 2-minute bolus and 90% in a 1-hour infusion (Box 15.1).[52]

When patients are seen between 3 and 6 hours after onset, intra-arterial administration of tPA should be considered.[53,54] This requires expertise available in tertiary centers. A randomized study showed efficacy of clot lysis in patients eligible for this procedure.[55,56]

Fluctuation often occurs in patients with an MCA (M1) occlusion, and some improvement may be related to improved collateral flow and partial dissolution of the thrombus. Cerebral angiography, however, should not be deferred for that reason; and in many patients, an occluding thrombus is present that is suitable for thrombolysis. Combined "bridging" therapy is cerebral angiography after a reduced (usually half) dose of intravenous tPA and no improvement clinically. This is followed by intra-arterial lysis of the clot, if still present. This approach has been studied in a very small series of patients, but no improved outcome was observed.[57] Intravenous heparin is not used 24 hours after intravenous tPA but is recommended after intra-arterial tPA. A summary of current practice recommendations for thrombolysis (intra-arterial or intravenous) is shown in Figure 15.11. Deviation from this protocol may be considered in extreme circumstances. For example, the presence of a hyperdense MCA sign in an elderly patient (>80 years) with a high NIH Stroke Scale score may indicate a poor outcome and a comparatively high rate of hemorrhagic conversion. In young patients (arbitrarily defined as less than 40 years), we believe a cerebral angiogram is warranted to define the occlusion. Be-

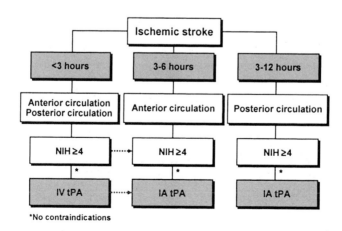

Figure 15.11 Algorithm for use of intravenous (IV) or intra-arterial (IA) thrombolysis. tPA, tissue plasminogen activator; NIH, National Institutes of Health.

Table 15.4. Initial Management of Acute
Ischemic Stroke in Anterior Circulation

Protect airway, endotracheal intubation if desaturation is
  noted on pulse oximeter
No antihypertensive medication, accept mean arterial
  pressure of ≤130 mm Hg, use of 5 mg of labetalol
  intravenously if pressure is continuously elevated and no
  other cause is apparent
Rehydrate with 0.9% NaCl, 2 L/24 hours
Correct hyperglycemia (glucose 100–150 mg/dL) with
  insulin
Correct hyperthermia with a cooling blanket
If computed tomographic scans show swelling and coma is
  rapidly deepening, give mannitol 20%–25%, 1 g/kg, and
  consider decompressive hemicraniectomy

cause many of these occlusions represent less or-
ganized venous clots due to a high prevalence of
patent foramen ovale in this population, we consider mechanical disruption first before proceed-
ing with intra-arterial tPA.[58,59]

Management of a massive ischemic stroke remains complex. Many therapeutic measures are
unproved. The initial guidelines for stabilization
are shown in Table 15.4. Options are intravenous
heparin, blood pressure augmentation, and rehydration. The use of intravenous heparin is an unresolved issue and has many opponents. Propo-
nents use intravenous heparin in patients with
large artery occlusions due to a cardiogenic
source.[60] It should not be used in patients with a
large territorial infarction to reduce the chance of
early significant hemorrhagic conditions. It is important not to aggressively manage hypertension
because cerebral perfusion is marginal in the area
of infarction. We discontinue any antihypertensive agent and accept any mean arterial blood
pressure less than 130 mm Hg in the first 24
hours. Patients should remain normovolemic,
normoglycemic,[61] and normothermic. Mannitol
can be considered when swelling leads to clinical
deterioration, but decompressive hemicraniectomy to relieve intracranial pressure and reduce
brain stem shift may be indicated (Box 15.2). The
procedure may still result in profound disability.[63–65] Early preemptive decompressive hemicraniectomy in patients at risk is not justified.
Some patients with mass effect on CT scan recover spontaneously.[65]

The outcome of untreated basilar artery occlusion is poor. Many series without the use of intra-

arterial thrombolysis have reported 80%–90%
mortality or poor outcome. The management of
basilar artery occlusion has been revolutionized by
the use of intra-arterial thrombolysis within 12
hours of presentation.[54,66] MRI abnormalities
showing early infarction in the cerebellum and
pons probably should not preclude the use of intra-arterial thrombolysis because they may indicate ischemia rather than permanent infarction.[54]
Recanalization can be demonstrated in approximately 60% of patients, with clinical improvement
in a similar proportion. However, the selection of
patients potentially eligible for intra-arterial
thrombolysis is not well defined. (Some centers
have used thrombolysis in patients 14–79 hours after onset of symptoms, but most of these patients
had fluctuating clinical courses interrupted by a
sudden, more severe deficit.[66]) Initial stabilization
of acute stroke in the posterior circulation is shown
in Table 15.5.

Predictors of Outcome

Large hemispheric infarcts have a worse prognosis when early swelling and mass effect are evident on CT scans. Overall, mortality is 50%, but
if clinical signs of herniation occur, mortality approaches 80%. Indicators of poor prognosis are
use of mechanical ventilation to protect the airway and coma. Basilar artery occlusion is associated with major fluctuations in neurologic findings; thus, outcome remains difficult to predict
early in the clinical course, certainly in the emergency department. The involvement of the thalamus in top-of-the-basilar artery occlusions can
cause a devastating loss of memory despite frequent recovery from ataxia. Locked-in syndrome
at presentation or coma virtually never is associated with a functional outcome, but an incomplete
clinical picture may improve substantially. Outcome in patients with acute basilar artery occlusion who have apnea is poor, and we and others
rarely have found survivors.[21] However, dramatic
reversals of coma and locked-in syndrome have
been reported after urokinase injected intra-arterially but only within an ictus and treatment interval of 12–15 hours.[54]

The cerebral angiogram has important prognostic features in basilar artery occlusion. Occlusion of a short restricted portion of the basilar artery has a higher probability of recanalization after

Box 15.2. Decompressive Hemicraniectomy

Large hemispheric infarcts may be caused by carotid artery or MCA occlusion. Swelling may occur after an interval of several days and cause a herniation syndrome.[62] Supportive therapies, such as hyperventilation and administration of mannitol, glycerol, barbiturates, and corticosteroids, have been unsuccessful. A large craniectomy with duraplasty to allow swelling outside the skull may be considered. There is some anecdotal evidence that this procedure has increased survival and resulted in 30%–50% functional outcome. The surgical procedure should be offered to patients irrespective of the involved hemisphere. Alternative therapies, such as moderate hypothermia (32°C or 33°C) or combined hypothermia and decompressive surgery, have appeared successful. Large randomized trials are needed to resolve many uncertainties about the outcome in patients with these interventions.[63]

intra-arterial thrombolysis than that of longer segments. In addition, collateral circulation has predicted a better outcome after recanalization.[66]

Cerebellar infarcts may cause sudden deterioration from swelling and pontine compression. Outcome remains good, including in patients who have emergency surgical evacuation. Many patients of all ages may be able to ambulate with minimal assistance. Early withdrawal of care is not appropriate.

Triage

- If intra-arterial administration of tPA is considered, cerebral angiography suite.
- Neurologic intensive care unit for monitoring brain swelling, hemorrhagic conversion, and possibly intracranial pressure.
- Patients with cerebellar infarcts who have normal Glasgow coma scores and early CT scan findings may not necessarily have to be admitted to the intensive care unit, but a repeat CT scan is needed within 12 hours to monitor early swelling.

Table 15.5. Initial Management of Acute Ischemic Stroke in Posterior Circulation

Protect airway and intubate early if patient has marked bulbar symptoms
Maintain flat body position to optimize blood pressure
Perform immediate cerebral angiography of posterior circulation if intra-arterial administration of tissue plasminogen activator is possible (<12 hours from onset)
Consider ventriculostomy or suboccipital craniectomy with cerebellar swelling from infarction

- Operating room for suboccipital craniectomy or ventriculostomy, or both, in cerebellar infarcts when brain stem compression causes upward-gaze palsy, deteriorating motor responses, and pupillary changes.

Arterial Dissection

A tear in the intima permits blood to dissect its way more distally into the muscular arterial wall and create a double lumen into the artery.[67,68] It occurs most commonly in the supraclinoid segment of the internal carotid artery.[69,70] The vast majority of vertebral artery dissections are at the level of the C1 and C2 vertebral bodies or at the intradural segment. The clot may dissect under the intima (subintimal) or throughout the media (subadventitial), causing distention of the vessel wall inward, producing occlusion, or outward, creating a pseudoaneurysm (Fig. 15.12).[68] A false luminal channel can be created when intramural hemorrhage exits at a more distal site, but this is uncommon. Intracranial dissections may perforate the thin media and adventitia, causing subarachnoid hemorrhage, with CT scan patterns similar to those of aneurysmal subarachnoid hemorrhage (Chapter 13).[71] A pseudoaneurysm does not rupture but may become a nidus for emboli and thus may need surgical therapy if antiplatelet agents are ineffective.

Dissection of the internal carotid vertebral artery is mostly spontaneous and may represent 10%–25% of ischemic strokes in adults aged 35–50.[69,70] Predisposing factors have been reported, and they may be more common in vertebral ar-

gesting a primary arteriopathy that increased the vulnerability of the arteries to trauma.[77]

Clinical Presentation

Headache or neck pain is present in approximately 60% of patients. The headache can be sudden but infrequently is a typical "thunderclap headache" (see Chapter 6). Thunderclap headache should suggest subarachnoid hemorrhage from dissection through the entire wall in the intracranial portion. Headache may precede an ischemic stroke by several days and may not be clearly remembered or vocalized by the patient. The character of the headache is dull and seldom throbbing. Retro-orbital headache of sudden onset should point to carotid artery dissection. Carotid artery dissection might be associated with a new presentation of Horner's syndrome, pulsatile tinnitus, and lower cranial nerve involvement, particularly the twelfth cranial nerve, causing weakness of the tongue. Other lower cranial nerves can become compressed in the cervical parapharyngeal space.[69] The ninth to twelfth cranial nerves are in close proximity to the internal carotid artery and alone or in combination can become involved, producing dysarthria, dysphasia, dysphonia, and dysgeusia (metallic or bad taste). Less common are a decreased sensation of the frontal division of the trigeminal nerve, oculomotor palsy, and abducens palsy.[78] Carotid dissection may be almost completely without any clinical neurologic deficits except for a new carotid bruit. This finding in a young patient with sudden facial or occipital headache should point to a dissection and prompt immediate neuroimaging studies.

Cerebral infarction involves MCA branch occlusions from propagated emboli. The interval between dissection and cerebral infarction varies widely, from minutes to 1 month, but is less than a week in most patients.[79] Low-flow ("misery") infarction involving watershed areas is an uncommon mechanism[80,81] despite trickle flow with poor collateral compensation in some patients. Carotid occlusion may result in a malignant infarct with massive swelling involving the ACA and MCA territories.

Dissection of the extracranial vertebral artery is manifested almost immediately by signs of an ischemic stroke in the cerebellum involving, as expected, the territory of the PICA. Severe ver-

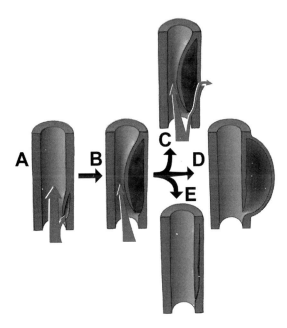

Figure 15.12 Process of arterial dissection (A) leading to occlusion (B), rupture (C), and pseudoaneurysm (D) or healing (E).

tery dissection than in carotid artery dissection. The dissection can be the result of a direct force to the artery, possibly triggered by strenuous activity, head turning, or chiropractic maneuvers but also by seemingly trivial insults, such as a brief Valsalva maneuver.[67] There is a seasonal predilection for autumn.[72] An increased incidence of upper respiratory infection during this period may suggest an inflammatory cause or insults from repeated coughing. Dissections have been associated with congenital abnormalities of the wall of the artery, such as cystic medial necrosis, fibromuscular dysplasia,[73] Marfan's syndrome, Ehlers-Danlos syndrome type IV, α_1-antitrypsin deficiency, autosomal-dominant polycystic kidney disease, and familial lentiginosis.[74] In a prospective study of dissections at the Mayo Clinic, joint and skin laxity and facial stigmata of an underlying vasculopathy were found but could not be characterized as typical arteriopathy.[75]

Dissection of the carotid or vertebral artery may be associated with head injury,[76] but in a report on five patients with traumatic dissections of the internal carotid arteries, cystic medial necrosis and marked lack of elastic fibers were found, sug-

tigo, vomiting, and appendicular ataxia might be presenting symptoms. In patients with vertebral artery dissection, the lateral medulla may become involved, causing typical Wallenberg's syndrome (see Table 15.2).[82] Swelling of the infarcted cerebellar tissue might cause considerable mass effect, displacement of the pons, and obstructive hydrocephalus.

Interpretation of Diagnostic Tests

Magnetic Resonance Imaging and Magnetic Resonance Angiography

MRI may replace conventional cerebral angiography as the first diagnostic test because it provides a definitive diagnosis in a large proportion of cases. Magnetic resonance angiography (MRA) is highly sensitive and specific in the diagnosis of internal carotid artery dissection but much less sensitive for a diagnosis of vertebral artery dissection.[83,84] Combined MRI and MRA compared with conventional arteriography has a sensitivity of 84% and a specificity of 99% for the diagnosis of carotid dissection.[85] MRI also may show the typical dense "crescent" or "double-lumen" sign, which reflects an intramural thrombus, often found at lower slices (Fig. 15.13).

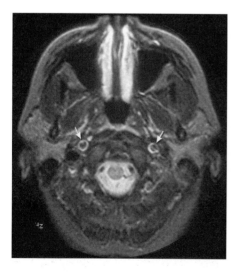

Figure 15.13 Magnetic resonance image showing double-lumen sign (*arrows*) in bilateral carotid dissections.

Cerebral Angiography

Cerebral angiography remains the standard procedure. The most typical angiographic finding is relatively smooth, irregularly tapered luminal narrowing, often producing a very high stenosis (string sign) (Fig. 15.15).[84] Dissections may occur in both vertebral arteries, in the carotid and vertebral arteries, or in all four arteries at the same time. A pseudoaneurysm might be found later, with typical fusiform appearance.

First Priority in Management

Carotid dissections might resolve within 6 weeks but reconstitution to a normal lumen after 6 months is uncommon (Fig. 15.14). Many physicians favor anticoagulation with intravenous heparin followed by warfarin (aiming at an international normalized ratio between 2 and 3) until MRI and MRA show recanalization, but this is deferred if the dissection involves the intracranial portion because of the risk of causing subarachnoid hemorrhage (although very low [10%] in patients with intracranial dissection).[86] Antithrombotic therapy with aspirin 325 mg daily or clopidogrel 75 mg daily can be continued for another 3 months, but this period is arbitrary. Aneurysmal dilatation also may disappear spontaneously. However, it might become a source of recurrent transient ischemic attacks. If embolization occurs despite antiplatelet therapy, aneurysmal dilatation warrants surgical therapy or coil embolization of the artery with stenting of the occluded artery.[87] Endovascular treatment may be considered in patients with intracranial vertebral artery dissections and possibly tailored to those with large or growing aneurysmal dilations and certainly when associated with subarachnoid hemorrhage (see Chapter 13).[88]

Predictors of Outcome

Permanent stenosis of the carotid artery remains associated with a low incidence of recurrent stroke (0.7%), and ischemic strokes have occurred despite aspirin or warfarin.[89] Dissection may recur in 1% per year (2% in the first month).[90] Patients with associated hereditary disorders do not have a higher incidence of recurrence of dissection, and a history of dissection in a family member does

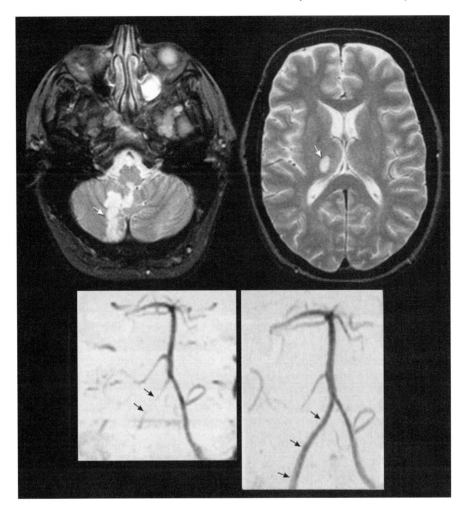

Figure 15.14 Magnetic resonance angiography shows a right vertebral artery dissection and cerebellar and thalamic infarcts (*arrows*). Recanalization of the right vertebral artery occurred in 3 months.

increase the incidence of recurrence. Outcome from infarction due to dissection appears more favorable in younger patients than in older patients with similar infarcts; the explanation is not known. Massive swelling may occur because of involvement of the anterior circulation; mortality is high without decompressive craniectomy.

Triage

- Admission to the ward for intravenous administration of heparin in patients with extracranial dissections.
- Admission to the neurologic–neurosurgical intensive care unit when early hemispheric brain swelling is evident on CT scans.
- Admission to the neurologic–neurosurgical intensive care unit for patients who have vertebral artery dissections with cerebellar infarct.

Multiple Small Vessel Occlusions

Multiple cerebral infarctions represent a separate entity but with different causes. The differential diagnosis is particularly complex in younger persons, and extensive evaluation of underlying coagulopathies or intrinsic vasculopathies is needed.

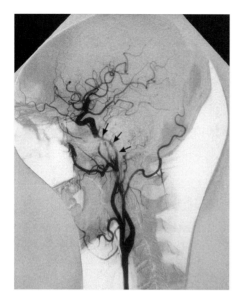

Figure 15.15 Cerebral angiogram of distal carotid artery dissection (*arrows*).

The diagnostic considerations in these patients seen in the emergency department are shown in Table 15.6. Only the disorders that are clinically the most relevant are discussed here.

Vasculitis of the Central Nervous System

Granulomatous vasculitis or isolated angiitis of the central nervous system (CNS) is an emergency and may rapidly lead to permanent devastating ischemic strokes or, less commonly, to intracranial hematomas or subarachnoid hemorrhage.[91,92] Progressive or recurrent neurologic symptoms are common, but because of the infrequent occurrence of this disorder, they may not be recognized as typical features of CNS vasculitis until the destruction is permanent. Delay in diagnosis has been established as an unfortunate fact.[93]

The presentation of CNS vasculitis as subarachnoid hemorrhage is mentioned in Chapter 13 and as a consequence of herpes zoster encephalitis in Chapter 17.

Clinical Presentation
Two-thirds of patients present with severe, persistent headache overriding any other symptom. Profound aphasia, apraxia, or hemiparesis may occur, but acute confusion and, most typically, emotional lability with crying or bizarre hysterical or childish behavior are more common. Some patients become dull and abulic, particularly with preferential involvement of the anterior cerebral

Table 15.6. Diagnostic Considerations in Patients with Multiple Cerebral Infarctions

Cerebral angiitis	Primary isolated angiitis (granulomatous) of the central nervous system
	Giant cell arteritis
	Associated systemic or collagen vascular disease (sarcoidosis, Behçet's disease, polyarteritis nodosa, Wegener's granulomatosis, systemic lupus erythematosus, Sneddon's syndrome)
	Associated infections (herpes zoster, cytomegalovirus, neurosyphilis)
	Drug-induced (amphetamines, heroin)
Vasculopathy	Malignant angioendotheliomatosis (intravascular lymphomatosis)
	Moyamoya disease
	Hereditary endotheliopathies
	Nonatherosclerotic vasculopathy with skin abnormalities (e.g., Fabry's disease, Degos' disease)
Endocarditis	Subacute bacterial infections
	Nonbacterial thrombotic (marantic) in advanced cancer
Coagulopathies	Protein C deficiency
	Antiphospholipid antibody syndrome
	Protein S deficiencies
	Antithrombin III deficiencies
Hemoglobin disorders	Sickle-cell syndromes
Platelet disorders	Thrombotic thrombocytopenic purpura
	Antiphospholipid antibody syndrome
	Hemolytic-uremic syndrome

circulation. Multifocal neurologic findings can be expected because the pattern involves scattered inflammation of the medium- and small-sized arteries.[93]

CNS vasculitis may be secondary to a systemic illness or drug abuse. Skin lesions, joint swelling, or additional evidence of mononeuritis multiplex or progressive polyneuropathy may point to a connective tissue disorder or systemic vasculitis. The use of an amphetamine often can be inferred only from a careful history of drug use, which is not volunteered by most patients with strokes.[94–96]

Infectious causes can produce CNS vasculitis, but other localizations should be evident (e.g., retina for cytomegalovirus, painful crusty skin lesions for herpes zoster, pulmonary manifestations associated with *Histoplasma* or *Coccidioides immitis*, or systemic manifestations of human immunodeficiency virus infection). Finally, lymphoproliferative disorders (Hodgkin's lymphoma) may be associated with vasculitis.[97]

Moore's criteria for the diagnosis of isolated angiitis of the CNS are (*1*) recent severe onset of headaches, confusion, or multifocal neurologic deficits that are recurrent or progressive; (*2*) typical angiographic findings; (*3*) exclusion of systemic disease or infection; and (*4*) leptomeningeal and parenchymal biopsy findings that confirm vascular inflammation and exclude infection, neoplasia, and noninflammatory vascular disease.[92,98,99]

Interpretation of Diagnostic Tests

COMPUTED TOMOGRAPHIC SCANNING AND MAGNETIC RESONANCE IMAGING. The sensitivity of CT scanning in isolated angiitis is low, but occasionally subarachnoid hemorrhage due to rupture of involved sulcal arteries can be found (see Chapter 13).[100] CT scanning may help diagnose Wegener's granulomatosis, characterized by bone thickening and focal erosive changes of the nasal septum and soft tissue masses in the sinuses. MRI abnormalities should reveal infarction involving several vascular territories, producing effacement of sulci and hyperintense signals following the gyri (Fig. 15.16). In some patients, the initial predilection sites are the parieto-occipital lobes, mimicking reversible posterior leukoencephalopathy.[101] Lesions deep in the white matter that spare the overlying cortex are less common.[102] Conversely,

it can be generally stated that normal MRI findings, certainly with FLAIR sequences, virtually exclude widespread CNS vasculitis.[103] MRA may be useful as an initial screening test; but it overestimates narrowing, may not visualize abnormalities in medium-sized or smaller arteries due to current poor resolution, and therefore does not match cerebral angiography.

CEREBRAL ANGIOGRAPHY. The sensitivity of cerebral angiography in CNS vasculitis is high, approximately 95%–99%. A cerebral angiogram with negative findings has been described in biopsy-proven CNS vasculitis. Suggestive findings are changed vessel caliber, with constriction, occlusion ("cutoffs"), irregularities, and dilatation showing a characteristic beading pattern (Fig. 15.16*D*). Alternative explanations for the angiographic findings include cerebral vasospasm (very unusual on the day of onset of hemorrhage), advanced atherosclerosis (proximal carotid artery abnormalities or irregularities in the proximal vertebrobasilar system may be suggestive of atheromatous disease), and radiation-induced occlusive vasculopathy (abnormalities inside the radiation field).[104,105] The inflammatory changes in the wall eventually lead to fibrosis and may lead to fixed angiographic narrowing.[106]

BLOOD AND SEROLOGY. It is important to exclude a connective tissue disorder by measurement of antinuclear antibody, rheumatoid factor, antineutrophil cytoplasmic antibodies, sedimentation rate, and serology against human immunodeficiency virus, herpes zoster virus, cytomegalovirus, syphilis, and *Toxoplasma*. It is also important to obtain a urine sample for amphetamines.

CEREBROSPINAL FLUID. A profound inflammatory response is usually absent, including in patients with progressive disease. Mildly increased protein may be the only sign. Mild pleocytosis ($\leq$20 lymphocytes/mm^3) has been found in fewer than 50% of cases.[107]

BRAIN BIOPSY. Biopsy should involve the area that is abnormal on MRI, and available series claim 70% sensitivity. Random brain biopsy has a very low yield and probably should be deferred if angiographic findings are diagnostic and the cere-

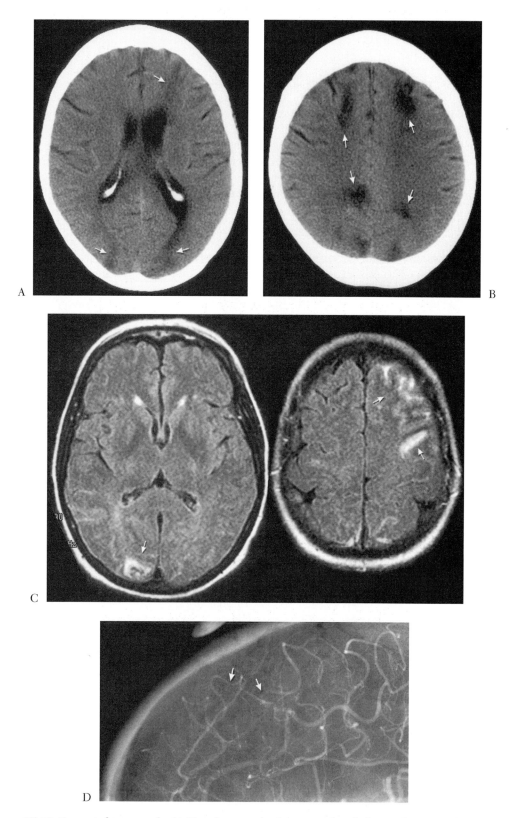

Figure 15.16 Computed tomography (*A,B*) and magnetic resonance imaging (*C*) show multiple infarcts associated with central nervous system vasculitis. *D:* Cerebral angiographic findings of segmental stenosis and beading are typical.

212

brospinal fluid is normal. The biopsy specimen, which should include the dura, leptomeninges, cortex, and white matter, is fixed in 10% buffered formalin for light microscopy.[108] Tissue samples should be frozen or stored with dry ice for later interpretation by electron microscopy. The pathologic hallmark is an infiltrate consisting of lymphocytes, histiocytes, and plasma cells involving the intima or media, with occasional necrosis of both leptomeningeal and intracerebral vessels.[109] Giant cells may be seen in areas of fragmented internal elastic lamina. Prominent necrosis should suggest polyarteritis nodosa. (Unfortunately, less characteristic or ambiguous pathologic findings may be the only result after a brain biopsy.)

First Priority in Management

Administration of corticosteroids in patients with presumed clinical CNS vasculitis is advised, and it should begin if no other causes are evident and if the patient is known to have collagen vascular disease. Brain biopsy within days in corticosteroid-treated patients should not mask inflammation and certainly not necrosis. Methylprednisolone 1 gram for 3 days and cyclophosphamide 15 mg/kg using slow infusion should be started with active disease, and there is a reasonable consensus among experts that only such an aggressive treatment can reverse CNS inflammation. It is followed by corticosteroids 1.5 mg/kg daily, and cyclophosphamide 2 mg/kg daily orally. Corticosteroid administration can be tapered to a lower dose after 4 weeks, but cyclophosphamide, which has very low side effects with this dose, should be given for 1 year. The patient should be familiar with a 20% risk of infertility from cyclophosphamide, and egg or sperm harvesting should be offered. Proton pump inhibitors should be added for stomach ulcer protection and possibly cotrimoxazole for *Pneumocystis carinii* pneumonia prophylaxis. Adequate hydration with intravenous fluids and frequent monitoring of the white blood cell count are needed to reduce the risk of hemorrhagic cystitis, and one should change the dose in case of neutropenia.

Predictors of Outcome

Recurrence is more common when patients are treated with corticosteroids alone. Outcome can be very good after aggressive combination therapy with administration of cyclophosphamide for

at least 1 year (the estimated relapse rate then is <10%). Corticosteroid doses can be tapered after 6 months. Mortality is uncommon, but functional outcome can be quite severely impacted when cerebral infarcts are widespread or located in both frontal lobes.

Triage

- Urgent cerebral angiography and neurosurgical consultation for possible cerebral biopsy
- Neurology ward

Hematologic Disorders

Albeit unusual, disorders of coagulation, disorders of the structure of red blood cells, and platelet dysfunction may cause multiple cerebral infarcts in rapid succession.[110,111] These disorders may not be apparent with routine automated laboratory evaluation in the emergency department, which measures only white blood cell count, platelet count, and sedimentation rate. Both small and large arteries may become occluded, and neurologic deficits may vary. Noteworthy clinical features of these hematologic disorders are discussed in this section.

Clinical Presentation

RED BLOOD CELL DISORDERS. Sickle-cell syndromes are rather prevalent, in most instances caused by a single amino acid substitution in the globin β chains (valine instead of glutamic acid). Sickle-cell disease or sickle-cell trait (heterozygotic state) is more prevalent in African-American patients, often manifested after a hypoxemic trigger, cold, or excessive alcohol consumption. Sickled masses of red blood cells occlude the arterial and venous systems, but other mechanisms, such as vasculopathy or fat embolization from infarcted bone marrow, may be operative. Stroke as a first presentation of sickle-cell disease has rarely been documented, but earlier ischemic strokes, predominantly those localized in the subcortical white matter, may be silent. One should inquire about previous episodes of *Streptococcus pneumoniae* infections, osteomyelitis by *Salmonella* species, painless hematuria, painful priapism, retinal–vitreous hemorrhage, or crises resulting in chest and abdominal pain.

Polycythemia vera, a more complex disorder of

increased erythrocytes and platelets, causes increased viscosity. It should be considered in patients with generalized pruritus, splenomegaly, headaches, and paresthesias. With a prevalence of five cases per one million persons, it is very uncommon.

Polycythemia may occur as a consequence of hypoxemia with cyanotic heart disease or obstructive pulmonary disease, but its association with ischemic stroke is less evident also, because precise understanding of the mechanism is lacking.

PLATELET DISORDERS. Thrombotic thrombocytopenic purpura should be considered in multiple strokes of undetermined cause when patients present with a documented gradual decrease in platelet count. Middle-aged women are predominantly affected. Characteristic additional clinical signs are hematuria, myalgia, bloody diarrhea, fever, and, in some patients, rapidly developing renal failure. These symptoms, caused by platelet microthrombi, may not appear in 25% of cases, and ischemic stroke may be the defining illness. Seizures are comparatively frequent, and nonconvulsive status epilepticus may be a presenting feature. Headache, acute confusional episodes, and hemiparesis may progress to coma if not aggressively treated with plasma exchange.

Thrombocytosis may occur in many underlying disorders, often chronic myeloid leukemia and myelofibrosis, or as a myeloproliferative disorder itself. Cerebrovascular manifestations, although recognized as a complication of myeloproliferative disorders, are not well characterized.

ANTIPHOSPHOLIPID ANTIBODY SYNDROME. This increasingly recognized syndrome associated with antiphospholipid antibodies is a common manifestation in younger patients.[112–115] Both anticardiolipin antibodies and lupus anticoagulants can be demonstrated, but they may not be linked to each other. Evidence of arterial occlusions (ocular, peripheral artery, pulmonary, or mesenteric artery) or venous occlusions (deep venous thrombosis or jugular venous thrombosis[113]), miscarriages, and prior unexplained pulmonary hypertension are clues to the diagnosis. In 20% of patients, ischemic stroke is part of this syndrome. Inappropriate treatment results in a high rate of recurrence of cerebral infarction.[112,113,116] Clinical features may include cardiac bruit (from associated mitral valve lesions or, possibly, Libman-Sacks endocarditis) and livedo reticularis.[116] Blotchy hands and feet should point to the diagnosis (see Color Fig. 15.17 in separate color insert). Multiorgan failure may be a presenting feature.[117]

Interpretations of Laboratory Tests

BLOOD AND SERUM. Hemoglobin electrophoresis yields the diagnosis in sickle cell disease. Associated findings are increased leukocyte count, recent decrease in hemoglobin concentration (hemolytic anemia), and hyperbilirubinemia.

Polycythemia vera is diagnosed by increases in hematocrit and white cell count and, at later stages, bone marrow metaplasia. Laboratory criteria (minor criteria) are platelets $>400,000/\mu L$, leukocytes $>12,000/\mu L$, leukocyte alkaline phosphatase score >100, and vitamin B_{12} >900 pg/mL.

Thrombotic thrombocytopenic purpura is considered when the following laboratory findings are present: fragmented red blood cells (schistocytes, or helmet cells), increased reticulocytes, unconjugated bilirubinemia with normal prothrombin time and partial thromboplastin time, and normal fibrin degradation products (differentiating it from disseminated intravascular coagulation and antiphospholipid antibody syndrome.) Lactate dehydrogenase is greatly increased. Haptoglobin should be low or even unmeasurable.

Anticardiolipin antibodies can be determined, but only a high titer of immunoglobulin G (IgG) is diagnostic[117,118] (many laboratories define high titer as 20–100 IgG phospholipid units or more). IgM titers may vary significantly and can be increased by nonspecific stimuli, such as fever, infection, and pharmaceutical agents. Activated partial thromboplastin time (PTT) is a good screening test. Prolonged PTT may occur in one-third of patients with antiphospholipid antibody syndrome.

MAGNETIC RESONANCE IMAGING. Multiple cerebral infarcts, often involving branches of the ACA and MCA territory, are nonspecific but can be visualized on MRI with much higher sensitivity. The study is particularly diagnostic in thrombotic thrombocytopenic purpura and antiphospholipid antibody syndrome (Fig. 15.18).

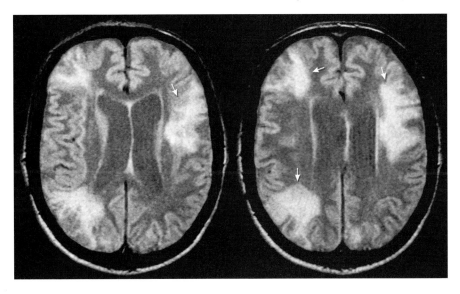

Figure 15.18 Magnetic resonance images showing multiple ischemic infarcts (*arrows*) in antiphospholipid antibody syndrome.

First Priority in Management

The recommended management options for specific hematologic disorders are summarized in Table 15.7. Specific treatment in these disorders is seldom started immediately in the emergency department because of the necessary delay for diagnostic tests.

Predictors of Outcome

Outcome is difficult to predict because of the rarity of the disorders; thus, general rules apply. Multiple small vessel occlusions may result in full recovery. Untreated, the disorders may lead to multi-infarct dementia, disabling hemiplegia, and speech and language disorders.

Triage

- Neurology ward.
- Intensive care unit in life-threatening thrombotic thrombocytopenic purpura, sickle-cell crises, and evidence of other sites of vascular occlusion.
- Concomitant medical illnesses may warrant admission to a medical or surgical intensive care unit.
- Hematology consultation and consideration of bone marrow biopsy.

Table 15.7. Management of Stroke in Unusual Hematologic Disorders

Disorder	Management
Sickle-cell disease	Exchange transfusion
	Oral folate
Polycythemia vera	Phlebotomy, 500 mL (aim at hematocrit ≤42%)
	Hydroxyurea, 500 mg twice daily
Thrombotic thrombocytopenic purpura	Plasma exchange (up to three exchanges)
	Prednisone, 60 mg
	Alternatively, intravenous immunoglobulin (e.g., Gammagard S/D), 1 g/kg
Thrombocytosis (any cause)	Plateletpheresis
	Avoid anticoagulation
Antiphospholipid antibody syndrome	Heparin and long-term warfarin (international normalized ratio 3 or 4)
	Cyclophosphamide (when associated with systemic lupus erythematosus)

Cerebral Venous Sinus Thrombosis

Cerebral venous sinus thrombosis is rare, equally distributed in males and females; however, the incidence rises steeply in the second and third decades in women because of its association with the use of oral contraceptives. The clinical spectrum of cerebral venous sinus thrombosis varies from a mild headache to progressive papilledema with rapidly deteriorating multiple hemorrhagic infarcts. The disorder is an acute neurologic emergency that may have a catastrophic outcome if not timely treated with intravenous heparin and, if available, endovascular lysis of the propagating thrombus within the cerebral venous system. Many conditions can be associated with cerebral venous thrombosis; however, despite extensive laboratory tests and increasingly sophisticated evaluation of coagulopathies, up to one-third of cases remain entirely unexplained. Causes associated with cerebral venous thrombosis are oral contraceptive use, pregnancy, the puerperium, antiphospholipid antibody syndrome and lupus anticoagulant, congenital coagulopathies, and damage to the jugular vein associated with surgical trauma or sacrifice, or due to direct cannulation. Infectious causes, such as acute sinusitis, mastoiditis, infections involving the facial skin, and dental abscesses, need immediate recognition and treatment.

Clinical Presentation

The common early feature is headache refractory to commonly prescribed pain medication. The headache is related to increased intracranial pressure, which in turn is associated with venous hypertension. Venous hypertension reduces the reabsorption of cerebrospinal fluid and results in papilledema. The progression of headache, seizures, and focal neurologic deficits is rapid, in days; but in approximately one-third of patients, the course may be protracted.[119] Cerebral infarction is typically hemorrhagic and may involve multiple territories. When multiple cerebral infarcts cause substantial swelling, herniation can occur.[120] A large intracranial temporal hematoma may progress to uncal herniation syndrome. Involvement of a cortical vein alone is rare. Commonly, the vein of Labbé is involved in these types of cortical infarct, which are located in the parietotemporal region. (This is the largest superficial vein and mostly drains the posterior temporal region.) Cortical vein thrombosis may be manifested by focal or generalized seizures evolving into focal neurologic findings such as aphasia and hemiparesis.[121]

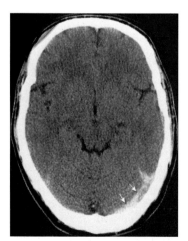 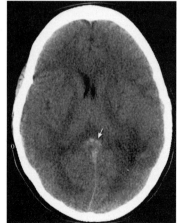 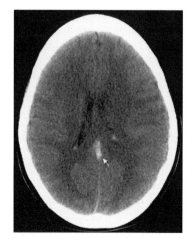

Figure 15.19 Computed tomographic scan with "string sign" (transverse sinus). Note hyperdensity in sigmoid sinus (*left*), transverse sinus (*middle*), and vein of Galen and straight sinus (*right, arrows*).

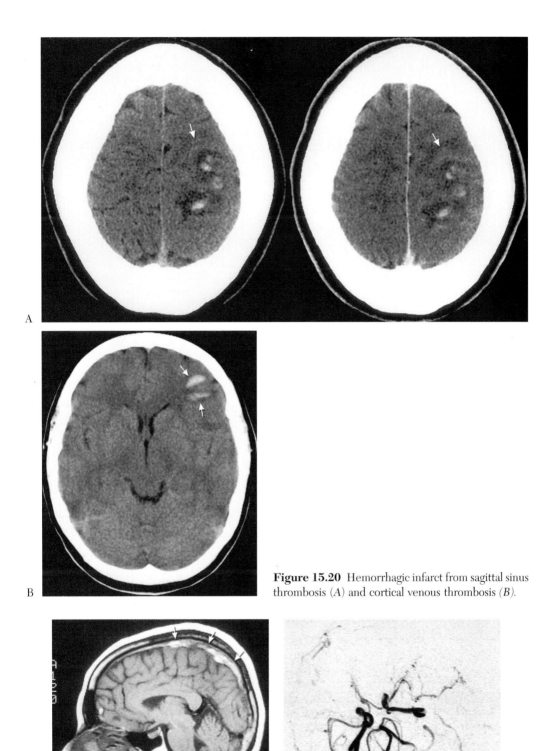

Figure 15.20 Hemorrhagic infarct from sagittal sinus thrombosis (A) and cortical venous thrombosis (B).

Figure 15.21 Magnetic resonance imaging and magnetic resonance angiography diagnosis of sagittal sinus (A) and left transverse sinus (B) thrombosis.

Interpretation of Diagnostic Tests

Neuroimaging

A typical CT scan feature is the cord or string sign, representing clot in the transverse sinus (Fig. 15.19). CT scanning may show multiple hemorrhagic infarcts with early swelling (Fig. 15.20). MRI and MRA usually are diagnostic and reveal the extent of venous thrombosis. Flow void is absent, and thrombus appears hyperintense on T_1-weighted and hypointense on T_2-weighted images (Fig. 15.21).[122,123] In a study of transcranial Doppler ultrasonography, increased flow velocities or asymmetries in venous flow velocities were noted;[124] however, the practical value of the technique in the emergency department is not known, and extent can be better defined by MRI and magnetic resonance venography.[125]

Serum

A propensity toward thrombosis should be examined by measuring antithrombin III, protein C and protein S for deficiencies[126] and lupus anticoagulant or antiphospholipid antibodies. Factor V Leiden and the recently discovered 20210A allele mutation of the prothrombin gene may increase the risk of cerebral venous thrombosis.[119,127,128]

First Priority in Management

Currently, there is a shift in the management of cerebral venous thrombosis. Intravenous heparin has substantially reduced morbidity and mortality, even in patients with already developed hemorrhagic infarcts.[129] Low-molecular-weight heparin was not more effective in a randomized trial.[130] Nonetheless, thrombosis may progress despite adequate anticoagulation. Recanalization with thrombolytic agents through a catheter in the thrombosed vein has been successful in some case series.[131]

Predictors of Outcome

In a large group of patients, 86% had good recovery and those with involvement of only a portion of the venous system had even better recovery.[119] Absence of associated cancer, common in many published series, is a predictor of good outcome.[132] However, coma at presentation, seizures, and intracerebral hematomas do not predict poor outcome. A major discrepancy exists between the devastation seen on MRI and the outcome, and neuroimaging should not be a major factor in deciding on future care. Blindness from papilledema or seizures may become persistent sequelae.

Triage

- Patients receiving intravenous heparin who have progression: to the neurointerventional suite for endovascular lysis of the clot
- Neurosurgical intensive care unit to consider evacuation of hemorrhagic mass.
- Treatment of increased intracranial pressure if multiple hemorrhagic infarcts and edema occur.

REFERENCES

1. Leary MC, Saver JL, Gobin YP, et al.: Beyond tissue plasminogen activator: mechanical intervention in acute stroke. Ann Emerg Med 41:838, 2003.
2. Yaeger EP, Morris DL, Rosamond WD, et al.: Use of the National Institutes of Health Stroke Scale in the emergency department setting. Ann Emerg Med 35:628, 2000.
3. Wardlaw JM, Warlow CP, Counsell C: Systematic review of evidence on thrombolytic therapy for acute ischaemic stroke. Lancet 350:607, 1997.
4. Wardlaw JM, Lindley RI, Lewis S: Thrombolysis for acute ischemic stroke: still a treatment for the few by the few. West J Med 176:198, 2002.
5. Sandercock P, Berge E, Dennis M, et al.: A systematic review of the effectiveness, cost-effectiveness and barriers to implementation of thrombolytic and neuroprotective therapy for acute ischaemic stroke in the NHS. Health Technol Assess 6:iii, 2002.
6. Caplan LR, Mohr JP, Kistler JP, et al.: Should thrombolytic therapy be the first-line treatment for acute ischemic stroke? Thrombolysis—not a panacea for ischemic stroke. N Engl J Med 337:1309, 1997.
7. Morris DL, Rosamond W, Madden K, et al.: Prehospital and emergency department delays after acute stroke: the Genentech Stroke Presentation Survey. Stroke 31:2585, 2000.
8. Bravata DM, Kim N, Concato J, et al.: Thrombolysis for acute stroke in routine clinical practice. Arch Intern Med 162:1994, 2002.
9. Hacke W, Kaste M, Fieschi C, et al.: Randomised double-blind placebo-controlled trial of thrombolytic therapy with intravenous alteplase in acute ischaemic stroke (ECASS II). Lancet 352:1245, 1998.

10. Hankey GJ: Thrombolytic therapy in acute ischaemic stroke: the jury needs more evidence. *Med J Aust* 166: 419, 1997.

11. Meschia JF, Miller DA, Brott TG: Thrombolytic treatment of acute ischemic stroke. *Mayo Clin Proc* 77:542, 2002.

12. Brott T, Adams HP Jr, Olinger CP, et al.: Measurements of acute cerebral infarctions: a clinical examination scale. *Stroke* 20:864, 1989.

13. Powers DW: Assessment of the stroke patient using the NIH stroke scale. *Emerg Med Serv* 30:52, 2001.

14. Lewandowski C, Barsan W: Treatment of acute ischemic stroke. *Ann Emerg Med* 37:202, 2001.

15. Saito I, Segawa H, Shiokawa Y, et al.: Middle cerebral artery occlusion: correlation of computed tomography and angiography with clinical outcome. *Stroke* 18:863, 1987.

16. Minematsu K, Yamaguchi T, Omae T: "Spectacular shrinking deficit": rapid recovery from a major hemispheric syndrome by migration of an embolus. *Neurology* 42:157, 1992.

17. Alexandrov AV, Grotta JC: Arterial reocclusion in stroke patients treated with intravenous tissue plasminogen activator. *Neurology* 59:862, 2002.

18. Grotta JC, Welch KM, Fagan SC, et al.: Clinical deterioration following improvement in the NINDS rtPA Stroke Trial. *Stroke* 32:661, 2001.

19. Bogousslavsky J, Regli F: Anterior cerebral artery territory infarction in the Lausanne Stroke Registry. Clinical and etiologic patterns. *Arch Neurol* 47:144, 1990.

20. Schwarz S, Egelhof T, Schwab S, et al.: Basilar artery embolism. Clinical syndrome and neuroradiologic patterns in patients without permanent occlusion of the basilar artery. *Neurology* 49:1346, 1997.

21. Wijdicks EFM, Scott JP: Outcome in patients with acute basilar artery occlusion requiring mechanical ventilation. *Stroke* 27:1301, 1996.

22. Tomura N, Uemura K, Inugami A, et al.: Early CT finding in cerebral infarction: obscuration of the lentiform nucleus. *Radiology* 168:463, 1988.

23. Russell EJ: Diagnosis of hyperacute ischemic infarct with CT: key to improved clinical outcome after intravenous thrombolysis? *Radiology* 205:315, 1997.

24. Truwit CL, Barkovich AJ, Gean-Marton A, et al.: Loss of the insular ribbon: another early CT sign of acute middle cerebral artery infarction. *Radiology* 176:801, 1990.

25. Simon JE, Morgan JEW, Pexman JHW, et al.: CT assessment of conjugate eye deviation in acute stroke. *Neurology* 60:135, 2003.

26. von Kummer R, Nolte PN, Schnittger H, et al.: Detectability of cerebral hemisphere ischaemic infarcts by CT within 6 h of stroke. *Neuroradiology* 38:31, 1996.

27. Koo CK, Teasdale E, Muir KW: What constitutes a true hyperdense middle cerebral artery sign? *Cerebrovasc Dis* 10:419, 2000.

28. von Kummer R, Allen KL, Holle R, et al.: Acute stroke: usefulness of early CT findings before thrombolytic therapy. *Radiology* 205:327, 1997.

29. Wijdicks EFM, Diringer MN: Middle cerebral artery territory infarction and early brain swelling: progression and effect of age on outcome. *Mayo Clin Proc* 73:829, 1998.

30. Manno EM, Nichols DA, Fulgham JR, et al.: Computed tomography determinants of neurologic deterioration in patients with large middle cerebral artery infarctions. *Mayo Clin Proc* 78:156, 2003.

31. Motto C, Aritzu E, Boccardi E, et al.: Reliability of hemorrhagic transformation diagnosis in acute ischemic stroke. *Stroke* 28:302, 1997.

32. Tomsick T, Brott T, Barsan W, et al.: Prognostic value of the hyperdense middle cerebral artery sign and stroke scale score before ultra early thrombolytic therapy. *AJNR Am J Neuroradiol* 17:79, 1996.

33. Wildenhain SL, Jungreis CA, Barr J, et al.: CT after intracranial intraarterial thrombolysis for acute stroke. *AJNR Am J Neuroradiol* 15:487, 1994.

34. Kertesz A, Black SE, Nicholson L, et al.: The sensitivity and specificity of MRI in stroke. *Neurology* 37:1580, 1987.

35. Bryan RN, Levy LM, Whitlow WD, et al.: Diagnosis of acute cerebral infarction: comparison of CT and MR imaging. *AJNR Am J Neuroradiol* 12:611, 1991.

36. Katz BH, Quencer RM, Kaplan JO, et al.: MR imaging of intracranial carotid occlusion. *AJR Am J Roentgenol* 152:1271, 1989.

37. Fisher M, Prichard JW, Warach S: New magnetic resonance techniques for acute ischemic stroke. *JAMA* 274: 908, 1995.

38. Lutsep HL, Albers GW, DeCrespigny A, et al.: Clinical utility of diffusion-weighted magnetic resonance imaging in the assessment of ischemic stroke. *Ann Neurol* 41:574, 1997.

39. Zivin JA: Diffusion-weighted MRI for diagnosis and treatment of ischemic stroke. *Ann Neurol* 41:567, 1997.

40. Mullins ME, Schaefer PW, Sorensen AG, et al.: CT and conventional and diffusion-weighted MR imaging in acute stroke: study in 691 patients at presentation to the emergency department. *Radiology* 224:353, 2002.

41. van Everdingen KJ, van der Grond J, Kappelle LJ, et al.: Diffusion-weighted magnetic resonance imaging in acute stroke. *Stroke* 29:1783, 1998.

42. Singer MB, Chong J, Lu D, et al.: Diffusion-weighted MRI in acute subcortical infarction. *Stroke* 29:133, 1998.

43. Uno M, Harada M, Yoneda K, et al.: Can diffusion- and perfusion-weighted magnetic resonance imaging evaluate the efficacy of acute thrombolysis in patients with internal carotid artery or middle cerebral artery occlusion. *Neurosurgery* 50:28, 2002.

44. Warach S: Stroke neuroimaging. *Stroke* 34:345, 2003.

45. Bahn MM, Oser AB, Cross DT III: CT and MRI of stroke. *J Magn Reson Imaging* 6:833, 1996.

46. Shrier DA, Tanaka H, Numaguchi Y, et al.: CT angiography in the evaluation of acute stroke. *AJNR Am J Neuroradiol* 18:1011, 1997.

47. Brant-Zawadzki M: CT angiography in acute ischemic stroke: the right tool for the job? *AJNR Am J Neuroradiol* 18:1021, 1997.

48. Knauth M, von Kummer R, Jansen O, et al.: Potential of

CT angiography in acute ischemic stroke. *AJNR Am J Neuroradiol* 18:1001, 1997.

49. Na DG, Byun HS, Lee KH, et al.: Acute occlusion of the middle cerebral artery: early evaluation with triphasic helical CT—preliminary results. *Radiology* 207:113, 1998.

50. Barber PA, Zhang J, Demchuk AM, et al.: Why are stroke patients excluded from TPA therapy? An analysis of patient eligibility. *Neurology* 56:1015, 2001.

51. Arnold M, Nedeltchev K, Sturzenegger M, et al.: Thrombolysis in patients with acute stroke caused by cervical artery dissections. Analysis of 9 patients and review of the literature. *Arch Neurol* 59:549, 2002.

52. National Institute of Neurological Disorders and Stroke rt-PA Stroke Study Group: Tissue plasminogen activator for acute ischemic stroke. *N Engl J Med* 333:1581, 1995.

53. Gönner F, Remonda L, Mattle H, et al.: Local intra-arterial thrombolysis in acute ischemic stroke. *Stroke* 29:1894, 1998.

54. Wijdicks EFM, Nichols DA, Thielen KR, et al.: Intra-arterial thrombolysis in acute basilar artery thromboembolism: the initial Mayo Clinic experience. *Mayo Clin Proc* 72:1005, 1997.

55. del Zoppo GJ, Higashida RT, Furlan AJ, et al.: PROACT: a phase II randomized trial of recombinant prourokinase by direct arterial delivery in acute middle cerebral artery stroke. *Stroke* 29:4, 1998.

56. Saver JL: Intra-arterial thrombolysis. *Neurology* 57:S58, 2001.

57. Lewandowski CA, Frankel M, Tomsick TA, et al.: Combined intravenous and intra-arterial r-TPA versus intra-arterial therapy of acute ischemic stroke: Emergency Management of Stroke (EMS) Bridging Trial. *Stroke* 30:2598, 1999.

58. Rabinstein AA, Wijdicks EFM, Nichols DA: Complete recovery after early intraarterial recombinant tissue plasminogen activator thrombolysis of carotid T occlusion. *AJNR Am J Neuroradiol* 23:1596, 2002.

59. Tomsick T, Brott T, Barsan W, et al.: Prognostic value of hyperdense middle cerebral artery sign and stroke scale score before ultra-early thrombolytic therapy. *AJNR Am J Neuroradiol* 17:79, 1996.

60. Caplan LR: Resolved: heparin may be useful in selected patients with brain ischemia. *Stroke* 34:230, 2003.

61. Scott JF, Robinson GM, French JM, et al.: Prevalence of admission hyperglycaemia across clinical subtypes of acute stroke. *Lancet* 353:376, 1999.

62. Hacke W, Schwab S, Horn M, et al.: "Malignant" middle cerebral artery territory infarction: clinical course and prognostic signs. *Arch Neurol* 53:309, 1996.

63. Hofmeijer J, van der Worp B, Kappelle J: Treatment of space-occupying cerebral infarction. *Crit Care Med* 31:617, 2003.

64. Wijdicks EFM: Management of massive hemispheric cerebral infarct. is there a ray of hope? *Mayo Clin Proc* 75:945, 2000.

65. Wijdicks EFM: Hemicraniotomy in massive hemispheric stroke: a stark perspective on a radical procedure. *Can J Neurol Sci* 27:271, 2000.

66. Cross DT III, Moran CJ, Akins PT, et al.: Relationship between clot location and outcome after basilar artery thrombolysis. *AJNR Am J Neuroradiol* 18:1221, 1997.

67. Caplan LR, Baquis GD, Pessin MS, et al.: Dissection of the intracranial vertebral artery. *Neurology* 38:868, 1988.

68. Fisher CM, Ojemann RG, Roberson GH: Spontaneous dissection of cervico-cerebral arteries. *Can J Neurol Sci* 5:9, 1978.

69. Mokri B, Houser OW, Sandok BA, et al.: Spontaneous dissections of the vertebral arteries. *Neurology* 38:880, 1988.

70. Mokri B, Sundt TM Jr, Houser OW, et al.: Spontaneous dissection of the cervical internal carotid artery. *Ann Neurol* 19:126, 1986.

71. Mizutani T, Aruga T, Kirino T, et al.: Recurrent subarachnoid hemorrhage from untreated ruptured vertebrobasilar dissecting aneurysms. *Neurosurgery* 36:905, 1995.

72. Schievink WI, Wijdicks EFM, Kuiper JD: Seasonal pattern of spontaneous cervical artery dissection. *J Neurosurg* 89:101, 1998.

73. Houser OW, Baker HL Jr: Fibromuscular dysplasia and other uncommon diseases of the cervical carotid artery: angiographic aspects. *Am J Roentgenol Radium Ther Nucl Med* 104:201, 1968.

74. Schievink WI, Michels VV, Mokri B, et al.: A familial syndrome of arterial dissections with lentiginosis. *N Engl J Med* 332:576, 1995.

75. Schievink WI, Wijdicks EFM, Michels VV, et al.: Heritable connective tissue disorders in cervical artery dissections: a prospective study. *Neurology* 50:1166, 1998.

76. Mokri B, Piepgras DG, Houser OW: Traumatic dissections of the extracranial internal carotid artery. *J Neurosurg* 68:189, 1988.

77. Mokri B, Meyer FB, Piepgras DG: Primary arteriopathy in traumatic cervicocephalic arterial dissections [abstract]. *Ann Neurol* 42:433, 1997.

78. Schievink WI, Mokri B, Garrity JA, et al.: Ocular motor nerve palsies in spontaneous dissections of the cervical internal carotid artery. *Neurology* 43:1938, 1993.

79. Biousse V, D'Anglejan-Chatillon J, Touboul PJ, et al.: Time course of symptoms in extracranial carotid artery dissections. A series of 80 patients. *Stroke* 26:235, 1995.

80. Steinke W, Schwartz A, Hennerici M: Topography of cerebral infarction associated with carotid artery dissection. *J Neurol* 243:323, 1996.

81. Lucas C, Moulin T, Deplanque D, et al.: Stroke patterns of internal carotid artery dissection in 40 patients. *Stroke* 29:2646, 1998.

82. Yamaura A, Watanabe Y, Saeki N: Dissecting aneurysms of the intracranial vertebral artery. *J Neurosurg* 72:183, 1990.

83. Kitanaka C, Tanaka J, Kuwahara M, et al.: Magnetic resonance imaging study of intracranial vertebrobasilar artery dissections. *Stroke* 25:571, 1994.

84. Provenzale JM: Dissection of the internal carotid and vertebral arteries: imaging features. *AJR Am J Roentgenol* 165:1099, 1995.

85. Levy C, Laissy JP, Raveau V, et al.: Carotid and vertebral artery dissections: three-dimensional time-of-flight MR angiography and MR imaging versus conventional angiography. *Radiology* 190:97, 1994.

86. Hosoya T, Adachi M, Yamaguchi K, et al.: Clinical and neuroradiological features of intracranial vertebrobasilar artery dissection. *Stroke* 30:1083, 1999.

87. Schievink WI, Piepgras DG, McCaffrey TV, et al.: Surgical treatment of extracranial internal carotid artery dissecting aneurysms. *Neurosurgery* 35:809, 1994.

88. Naito I, Iwai T, Sasaki T: Management of intracranial vertebral artery dissections initially presenting without subarachnoid hemorrhage. *Neurosurgery* 51:930, 2002.

89. Kremer C, Mosso M, Georgiadis D, et al.: Carotid dissection with permanent and transient occlusion or severe stenosis. *Neurology* 60:271, 2003.

90. Schievink WI, Mokri B, O'Fallon WM: Recurrent spontaneous cervical-artery dissection. *N Engl J Med* 330:393, 1994.

91. Biller J, Loftus CM, Moore SA, et al.: Isolated central nervous system angiitis first presenting as spontaneous intracranial hemorrhage. *Neurosurgery* 20:310, 1987.

92. Calabrese LH, Duna GF: Evaluation and treatment of central nervous system vasculitis. *Curr Opin Rheumatol* 7:37, 1995.

93. Hankey GJ: Isolated angiitis/angiopathy of the central nervous system. *Cerebrovasc Dis* 1:2, 1991.

94. Citron BP, Halpern M, McCarron M, et al: Necrotizing angiitis associated with drug abuse. *N Engl J Med* 283:1003, 1970.

95. Martin K, Rogers T, Kavanaugh A: Central nervous system angiopathy associated with cocaine abuse. *J Rheumatol* 22:780, 1995.

96. Matick H, Anderson D, Brumlik J: Cerebral vasculitis associated with oral amphetamine overdose. *Arch Neurol* 40:253, 1983.

97. Giang DW: Central nervous system vasculitis secondary to infections, toxins, and neoplasms. *Semin Neurol* 14:313, 1994.

98. Moore PM: Diagnosis and management of isolated angiitis of the central nervous system. *Neurology* 39:167, 1989.

99. Moore PM, Cupps TR: Neurological complications of vasculitis. *Ann Neurol* 14:155, 1983.

100. Kumar R, Wijdicks EFM, Brown RD Jr, et al.: Isolated angiitis of the CNS presenting as subarachnoid haemorrhage. *J Neurol Neurosurg Psychiatry* 62:649, 1997.

101. Wijdicks EFM, Manno ED, Fulgham JR, et al.: Cerebral vasculitis mimicking posterior leukoencephalopathy. *J Neurol* 250:444, 2003.

102. Greenan TJ, Grossman RI, Goldberg HI: Cerebral vasculitis: MR imaging and angiographic correlation. *Radiology* 182:65, 1992.

103. Harris KG, Tran DD, Sickels WJ, et al.: Diagnosing intracranial vasculitis: the roles of MR and angiography. *AJNR Am J Neuroradiol* 15:317, 1994.

104. Brant-Zawadzki M, Anderson M, DeArmond SJ, et al.: Radiation-induced large intracranial vessel occlusive vasculopathy. *AJR Am J Roentgenol* 134:51, 1980.

105. Devinsky O: Radiation-induced cerebral vasculitis revisited. *Stroke* 19:784, 1988.

106. Alhalabi M, Moore PM: Serial angiography in isolated angiitis of the central nervous system. *Neurology* 44:1221, 1994.

107. Stone JH, Pomper MG, Roubenoff R, et al.: Sensitivities of noninvasive tests for central nervous system vasculitis: a comparison of lumbar puncture, computed tomography, and magnetic resonance imaging. *J Rheumatol* 21:1277, 1994.

108. Parisi JE, Moore PM: The role of biopsy in vasculitis of the central nervous system. *Semin Neurol* 14:341, 1994.

109. Vollmer TL, Guarnaccia J, Harrington W, et al.: Idiopathic granulomatous angiitis of the central nervous system. Diagnostic challenges. *Arch Neurol* 50:925, 1993.

110. Greaves M: Coagulation abnormalities and cerebral infarction. *J Neurol Neurosurg Psychiatry* 56:433, 1993.

111. Hart RG, Kanter MC: Hematologic disorders and ischemic stroke. A selective review. *Stroke* 21:1111, 1990.

112. Levine SR, Brey RL, Sawaya KL, et al.: Recurrent stroke and thrombo-occlusive events in the antiphospholipid syndrome. *Ann Neurol* 38:119, 1995.

113. Levine SR, Deegan MJ, Futrell N, et al.: Cerebrovascular and neurologic disease associated with antiphospholipid antibodies: 48 cases. *Neurology* 40:1181, 1990.

114. Cervera R, Piette JC, Font J, et al.: Antiphospholipid syndrome: clinical and immunologic manifestations and patterns of disease expression in a cohort of 1,000 patients. *Arthritis Rheum* 46:1019-1027, 2002.

115. Rand JH: The antiphospholipid syndrome. *Annu Rev Med* 54:409, 2003.

116. Lockshin MD: Antiphospholipid antibody syndrome. *JAMA* 268:1451, 1992.

117. Westney GE, Harris EN: Catastrophic antiphospholipid syndrome in the intensive care unit. *Crit Care Clin* 18:805, 2002.

118. Tanne D, D'Olhaberriague L, Schultz LR, et al.: Anticardiolipin antibodies and their associations with cerebrovascular risk factors. *Neurology* 52:1368, 1999.

119. Bousser M-G, Russell RR: Cerebral venous thrombosis. *Major Probl Neurol* 33:1, 1997.

120. Villringer A, Einhaupl KM: Dural sinus and cerebral venous thrombosis. *New Horiz* 5:332, 1997.

121. Jacobs K, Moulin T, Bogousslavsky J, et al.: The stroke syndrome of cortical vein thrombosis. *Neurology* 47:376, 1996.

122. Corvol JC, Oppenheim C, Manai R, et al.: Diffusion-weighted magnetic resonance imaging in a case of cerebral venous thrombosis. *Stroke* 29:2649, 1998.

123. Perkin GD: Cerebral venous thrombosis: developments in imaging and treatment. *J Neurol Neurosurg Psychiatry* 59:1, 1995.

124. Stolz E, Kaps M, Dorndorf W: Assessment of intracranial venous hemodynamics in normal individuals and patients with cerebral venous thrombosis. *Stroke* 30:70, 1999.

125. Wasay M, Bakshi R, Bobustuc G, et al.: Diffusion-weighted magnetic resonance imaging in superior sagittal sinus thrombosis. *J Neuroimaging* 12:267, 2002.

126. Lefebvre P, Lierneux B, Lenaerts L, et al.: Cerebral venous thrombosis and procoagulant factors—a case study. *Angiology* 49:563, 1998.

127. Ludemann P, Nabavi DG, Junker R, et al.: Factor V Leiden mutation is a risk factor for cerebral venous thrombosis: a case-control study of 55 patients. *Stroke* 29:2507, 1998.

128. Biousse V, Conard J, Brouzes C, et al.: Frequency of the 20210 G → A mutation in the 3′-untranslated region of the prothrombin gene in 35 cases of cerebral venous thrombosis. *Stroke* 29:1398, 1998.

129. Wingerchuk DM, Wijdicks EFM, Fulgham JR: Cerebral venous thrombosis complicated by hemorrhagic infarc-

tion: factors affecting the initiation and safety of anticoagulation. *Cerebrovasc Dis* 8:25, 1998.

130. de Bruijn SFTM, Stam J, for the Cerebral Venous Sinus Thrombosis Study Group: Randomized, placebo-controlled trial of anticoagulant treatment with low-molecular-weight heparin for cerebral sinus thrombosis. *Stroke* 30:484, 1999.

131. Frey JL, Muro GJ, McDougall CG, et al.: Cerebral venous thrombosis: combined intrathrombus rtPA and intravenous heparin. *Stroke* 30:489, 1999.

132. Breteau G, Mounier-Vehier F, Godefroy O, et al.: Cerebral venous thrombosis: 3-year clinical outcome in 55 consecutive patients. *J Neurol* 250:29, 2003.

Chapter 16
Acute Bacterial Infections of the Central Nervous System

Bacterial seeding of the brain may exert its destructive effect at an early stage in the clinical course. Delay in diagnosis due to difficulty to appreciate nonspecific symptoms or, equally common, failure to act timely when signs become apparent contributes to later morbidity.[1] Indeed, the vexing concern for any physician is to recognize a bacterial infection when obvious signs, such as fever, confusion, skin rash, and recent sinusitis or otitis, are absent. Without question, a medical debacle may evolve in the first hours after entry to the emergency department despite responding quickly and appropriately. Intracranial abscesses may be first unmasked only after a single seizure without fever. Purulent CSF is sometimes a physician's surprise in a patient with unexplained coma.

In adults, the most common causative organisms in community-acquired meningitis are *Streptococcus pneumoniae*, *Neisseria meningitidis*, *Listeria monocytogenes*, and *Haemophilus influenzae*.[2,3] From the onset, it is clear that the priorities in evaluation (computed tomography [CT] or cerebrospinal fluid [CSF]) of a presumed bacterial meningitis are complicated.[4] Also, management in bacterial meningitis caused by *S. pneumoniae* or *N. meningitidis* has become problematic with the emergence of organisms resistant to penicillin and cephalosporin. This chapter focuses on early aggressive management of common bacterial infections of the central nervous system. It emphasizes avoidance of pitfalls and provides guidelines to make simple and straightforward clinical decisions.

Acute Bacterial Meningitis

The pathophysiology of bacterial meningitis involves many pathways that may, at least in the most severe cases, lead to cerebral edema, brain tissue displacement, and, probably most important, cerebral infarction.[5] The consequences of meningeal inflammation are discussed in Box 16.1.

Clinical Presentation

In most adults, a healthy state is first interrupted by an upper respiratory tract infection or ear infection, and antibiotic therapy does not make any major progress. Thus, potential sources for acute bacterial meningitis, such as pneumonia, paranasal sinusitis, and middle ear infection, should be sought. These sources are more prevalent in patients with profound comorbidity, such as diabetes mellitus, prior transplantation, long-term dialysis, splenectomy, alcoholism, and certain malignancies such as Hodgkin's disease.

Characteristic symptoms and signs of acute bacterial meningitis are fever, headache, and reduced alertness. The degree of fever in bacterial meningitis may vary. Most patients have so-called hectic temperature, with an increase to 39°C or 40°C, but low-grade fever (or none at all) may be present in the elderly, immunosuppressed patients, or patients who have been taking oral antibiotics or antipyretic drugs, all of whom may have greatly reduced mechanisms to mount this febrile response.[2] Temperature is usually con-

Box 16.1. Pathogenesis of Bacterial Meningitis and Its Consequences

A common sequence in the development of bacterial meningitis is as follows: Nasopharyngeal colonization occurs and is dependent on fimbriae and specific surface cell receptors. Attachment may be facilitated by previous viral infection. It is followed by development of bacteremia. The polysaccharide capsule should counter the classic complement pathway or alternative complement pathway (common in patients with underlying sickle cell disease and splenectomy) and defy phagocytosis. Next is meningeal invasion and entrance into the CSF through the choroid plexus, again facilitated by receptors. The bactericidal activity in the subarachnoid space is poor because the complement activity needed to initiate phagocytosis is low. Then, an inflammatory response is mounted by components of the lysed bacterial cell mass (teichoic acid endotoxin), which induce production of inflammatory cytokines (tumor necrosis factor, interleukin-1, and macrophage inhibitory protein). Neutrophils invade, and blood–brain barrier permeability increases, finally causing vasogenic brain edema. The toxic oxygen metabolites cause cytotoxic edema, and CSF outflow resistance from protein-rich exudate in the subarachnoid space produces interstitial edema and hydrocephalus.

Cerebral infarcts from vasculitis, vasospasm of basal arteries, or thrombosis of the major venous sinuses may occur, possibly only in the most fulminant cases with virulent pathogens.[6-9] The urokinase plasminogen activator system may be involved in breaching of the CSF–blood-barrier (Fig. 16.1).[10]

stantly elevated, and marked temperature oscillations may therefore suggest a localized collection of pus (e.g., tonsillar, mastoid, or middle ear abscess).

More than 75% of patients with bacterial meningitis are confused, irritable, or stuporous. Most patients can be roused with a forcible command or painful stimulus. Elderly patients may simply have a blank expression and be motionless and withdrawn.[11,12]

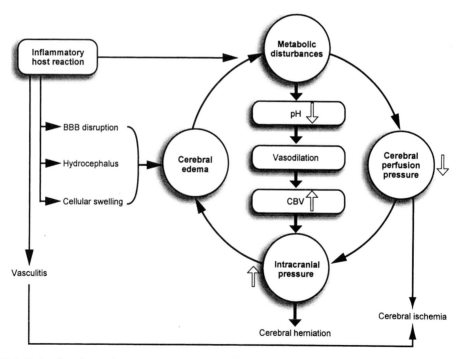

Figure 16.1 Pathophysiologic alterations causing a vicious cycle. BBB, blood–brain barrier; CBV, cerebral blood volume. (From Scheld et al., 2002,[5] with permission.)

Nuchal rigidity is common in bacterial meningitis. Flexion of the neck causes flexion in the hips and knees (Brudzinski's sign of meningismus, see Chapter 8). Cranial nerve involvement may include abducens nerve palsy as a false localizing sign of increased intracranial pressure, facial nerve palsy associated with mastoiditis, and, most worrisome, inflammation of the cochlear nerve leading to permanent hearing loss, reducing response to voice.

Seizures are more prevalent in children and young adults but may occur in up to 10% of adults or the elderly. Seizures, particularly focal, can be attributed to focal edema, early cortical venous thrombosis, and cerebral infarction from occlusion of penetrating branches encased by the basal purulent exudate.

Generalized myoclonus may occur and should immediately prompt measurement of the level of penicillin or cephalosporin. It is common in patients with coexistent renal disease, which reduces excretion and allows penicillin or cephalosporins to accumulate to toxic levels.[13]

Rapidly developing coma with pathologic motor responses is uncommon in adults, but when present, it signals a fulminant variant with diffuse cerebral edema or multiple cerebral infarcts from secondary inflammatory vasculitis.[14] Increased intracranial pressure leading to cerebral herniation syndromes occurs in approximately 10% of patients. Rarely, meningeal veins become necrotic or thrombosed, a condition leading to extensive hemorrhagic cortical infarction and bihemispheric swelling.

Meningococcal meningitis may progress to shock from adrenal hemorrhages. Petechiae, widespread purpuric rash with patches of necrotic skin (see Color Fig. 16.2 in separate color insert), conjunctival hemorrhage, and punctate lesions inside the mouth and on the lips are seen in conjunction with shock, profound hyponatremia and hyperkalemia (Addison's disease), and laboratory evidence of intravascular coagulation.

Tuberculous meningitis should be suspected in patients with human immunodeficiency virus (HIV) infection, malnutrition, drug abuse, homelessness, or any immunosuppressed state. Prodromal symptoms of coughing, weight loss, and night sweats followed by confusion and rapidly developing coma with cranial nerve deficits are frequent but nonspecific. Choroidal tubercles at ophthalmoscopy, hilar adenopathy on chest radiographs, and hydrocephalus on CT scan are additional indicators of tuberculous meningitis. In a recent series, 32 of 48 patients with adult tuberculous meningitis had an extrameningeal tuberculous location.[15] When younger patients are seen on admission, white cell counts of less than $10,000 \times 10^3$ per mL, age, and protracted history of illness are more common features seen with tuberculous meningitis than with bacterial meningitis.[16] Clear CSF with moderate number of lymphocytes and monocytes and a reduced ratio of cerebral fluid–blood glucose were important differentiating factors in a large study of tuberculous meningitis from Vietnam.[16]

Interpretation of Diagnostic Tests

Computed Tomography and Magnetic Resonance Imaging

CT scanning could precede CSF examination because images can be acquired very quickly with modern CT scanners. If CT scan cannot be rapidly obtained, empiric therapy should be administered first, followed by CT scan and CSF, in that order. The nonspecific presentation of fever, seizures, and neck stiffness may indicate a subdural empyema or an intracranial abscess with ventricular rupture rather than bacterial meningitis. When CT scanning is deferred, either of these conditions may theoretically worsen with lumbar puncture. If diffuse cerebral edema is present, herniation may occur with lumbar puncture despite removal of a small amount of CSF (e.g., 5 mL) or the use of a smaller needle (e.g., 22 gauge), although herniation from fulminant meningitis may occur irrespective of lumbar puncture. CT scan images are typically normal in bacterial meningitis.

Mild obstructive hydrocephalus (see Chapter 11), cerebral edema, and hypodensities from ischemic strokes have been reported in a small proportion of patients with acute bacterial meningitis.[3,17] However, CT scan findings are abnormal in 51% of patients with tuberculous meningitis. Ventricular dilatation, superficial meningeal enhancement, and hypodensity representing cerebral infarcts are common in tuberculous meningitis.

Magnetic resonance imaging (MRI), particularly fluid-attenuated inversion recovery (FLAIR) sequences, may reveal important findings in any type of bacterial meningitis because of its superb sensitivity; cerebral infarcts (Fig. 16.3) or the inflammatory exudate[18] (Fig. 16.4) may be detected. MRI may also document involvement of vestibular and cochlear structures in patients with hearing loss.[19]

Cerebrospinal Fluid

The CSF in acute bacterial meningitis is typically turbid or xanthochromic, with increased opening pressure (>200 mm H_2O) and polymorphonuclear pleocytosis (>1000 cells/mm^3). CSF leukocyte counts are increased less in meningitis associated with *S. pneumoniae* than in *N. meningitidis*, and could reflect a poor immunocompetent state.[20] Increased CSF protein (often >100 mg/dL) and decreased CSF glucose concentration (<40 mg/dL) are typical findings. CSF glucose should be compared with serum glucose, which may be increased as a stress response to the acute neurologic illness (normal ratio of CSF glucose to serum glucose is 0.6). Decreased CSF glucose concentration is typical of bacterial meningitis but may occur in fungal, tuberculous, or carcinomatous meningitis, in neurosarcoidosis, or, rarely, as a reflection of marked hypoglycemia. When CSF

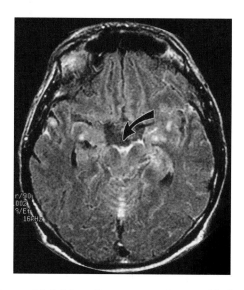

Figure 16.4 Magnetic resonance image with fluid-attenuated inversion recovery (FLAIR) sequences demonstrates purulent exudate (*arrow*) not visible on routine sequences or after gadolinium T_1 enhancement. (From Vernino et al.[18] By permission of the American Academy of Neurology.)

is bloody, the total white blood cell count is falsely increased, complicating interpretation. Red blood cells from a traumatic puncture increase the total cell count of 1 white blood cell per 700 red blood cells.

CSF lymphocytosis is most compatible with viral, fungal, and tuberculous meningitis. However, initial CSF lymphocytosis in bacterial meningitis was found in 6% of 428 patients and in 24% of patients with CSF leukocyte counts of fewer than 1000 cells/mm^3, irrespective of previous antibiotic use.[20] A predominant CSF lymphocytosis may occur early in the ictus, most often associated with *L. monocytogenes* meningitis in immunosuppressed patients. If glucose concentration is decreased, the presence of predominantly lymphocytes in the CSF formula should strongly point to the possibility of tuberculous or fungal meningitis.[20] At least three CSF samples are needed to obtain material for a smear; an enzyme-linked immunosorbent assay may visualize the tuberculous bacilli in 40% of smears. CSF cultures require up to 6 weeks for growth. However, fungal meningitis may not be detected with any of these tests, and meningeal biopsy may be needed. Other diagnostic tests are available to complement CSF cultures (Box 16.2).

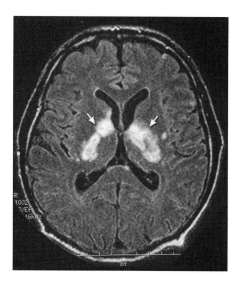

Figure 16.3 Magnetic resonance image with fluid-attenuated inversion recovery (FLAIR) sequences in patient with fulminant pneumococcal meningitis. Bilateral thalamic infarcts (*arrows*) from penetrating branch occlusions produce coma. (From Vernino et al.[18] By permission of the American Academy of Neurology.)

Box 16.2. Rapid Diagnostic Tests

Latex particle agglutination tests can rapidly detect bacterial antigens in purulent CSF. The specificity is close to 100%; the sensitivity depends on the organism (*H. influenzae*, 78%–86%; *S. pneumoniae*, 69%–100%; *N. meningitidis*, 33%–70%). Experience with polymerase chain reaction in acute bacterial infection is limited. The technique is useful in certain unusual causes of bacterial infections, but processing takes from 12 hours to 3 days. It has a sensitivity of 70%–80% in Lyme disease.

Gram stain has a positive yield in 60%–80% of patients, but the yield is much lower (40%–50%) with previous antibiotic use. Acid-fast stain may diagnose tuberculosis in 35%–80% of cases.[21]

First Priority in Management

Cephalosporins and vancomycin should be given intravenously at once, before any further diagnostic tests are ordered and, in fact, when the first purulent spinal fluid drops appear in the test tube. Recommended empirical therapy is shown in Figure 16.5. The addition of vancomycin is important to immediately preempt cephalosporin-resistant *S. pneumoniae*, which has become increasingly frequent.[22] Vancomycin administration should be closely monitored (aiming at a trough of 10 mg/mL and a peak serum level of 50 mg/mL) and

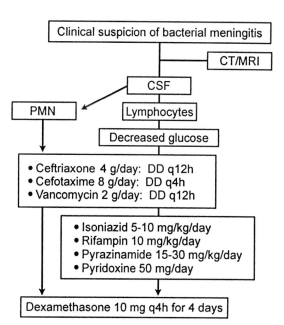

Figure 16.5 Empirical therapy for acute bacterial meningitis. CSF, cerebrospinal fluid; CT, computed tomography; DD, divided dose (intravenously); MRI, magnetic resonance imaging; PMN, polymorphonuclear cells.

continued for 14 days, if indicated. (Vestibular damage is uncommon from vancomycin and is much more likely from direct inflammation of the vestibular nerve due to meningitis.) Antibiotic therapy for specific organisms is summarized in Table 16.1.[23] A combination of three antituberculous drugs is additionally needed if tuberculous meningitis is likely on the basis of the initial CSF formula and clinical presentation.[24] Dexamethasone is reserved for fulminant variants (e.g., brain edema, impending brain herniation), including tuberculous meningitis;[25] and its use is proven in adult-onset bacterial meningitis[26] due to penicillin-susceptible streptococcus meningitis. In other conditions, dexamethasone may seriously reduce penetration of cephalosporins and, particularly, vancomycin (Box 16.3).[26] Nonetheless, dexamethasone, 10 mg every 6 hours for 4 days,[26] just before administration of antibiotics should be very seriously contemplated, if not considered standard. Rifampin, 600 mg/day, may increase the bioavailability of vancomycin and should be added if penicillin resistance becomes obvious.

Chemoprophylaxis is indicated in meningococcal meningitis and is administered to any person who had close contact with the patient. Recommendations for chemoprophylaxis, which should be discussed in the emergency department, are shown in Table 16.2.[30–33]

Predictors of Outcome

S. pneumoniae meningitis continues to cause sequelae such as hearing loss, seizures, personality change, and cognitive deficits.[34] In well-recovered patients with adult bacterial meningitis, neuropsychologic tests have noted reduced reaction speed and executive functioning but no memory deficits.[35] Drug-resistant strains of pneumococci

Table 16.1. Recommended Antimicrobial Therapy for Bacterial Meningitis

Organism	Antibiotic, Total Daily Dose (Dosing Interval)
Neisseria meningitidis	Penicillin G 20–24 million U/day IV q4h
	Or
	Ampicillin 12 g/day IV (q4h)
Streptococcus pneumoniae	Cefotaxime 8–12 g/day (q4h)
Gram-negative bacilli (except *Pseudomonas aeruginosa*)	Ceftriaxone 2–4 g/day IV (q12h)
	Or
	Cefotaxime 8–12 g/day IV (q4h)
Pseudomonas aeruginosa	Ceftazidime 6–12 g/day IV (q8h)
Haemophilus influenzae type b	Ceftriaxone 2–4 g/day (q12h)
	Or
	Cefotaxime 8–12 g/day q4h
Staphylococcus aureus	
Methicillin-sensitive	Oxacillin 9–12 g/day IV (q4h)
Methicillin-resistant	Vancomycin 2 g/day IV (q12h) or nafcillin 8–12 g/day IV (q4h)
Listeria monocytogenes	Ampicillin 12 g/day IV (q4h)
Enterobacteriaceae	Cefotaxime 8–12 g/day (q4h)
	Or
	Ceftriaxone 2–4 g/day (q12h)

Source: Modified from Roos et al.[23] By permission of the publisher.

cause significantly higher mortality than other pneumococcal bacteria. Coma at onset or focal seizures, focal neurologic deficits, and low CSF leukocyte counts increase the risk of poor outcome.[36] Acute complications such as brain edema and cerebral infarcts significantly increase the chance of a persistent vegetative state. Many predictors of poor outcome have been identified in tuberculous meningitis, including extremes of age, malnutrition, miliary disease, hydrocephalus, documented ischemic stroke, and low total CD4 cell count in a subset with HIV infection.[37]

Triage

- Urgent otolaryngologic evaluation.
- Admission to a neurologic intensive care unit is indicated to monitor the development of cerebral edema or, more commonly, hydrocephalus.
- If seizures have occurred, loading with fosphenytoin or phenytoin, 20 mg/kg intravenously.

Subdural Empyema and Epidural Abscess

Sinusitis,[38] recent sinus surgery, and, less commonly, otitis or traumatic brain injury are sources that may cause infection of the subdural space. Infection may spread directly, through erosion of the posterior wall of the frontal sinus or tegmen

tympani of the middle ear, or indirectly, through retrograde extension of thrombophlebitis.[39] This bacterial infection is uncommon in adults and often mistakenly diagnosed at first as bacterial meningitis.[40,41]

Epidural abscess is produced by sources similar to those in subdural empyema, but in this condition, the suppurative infection is localized between the dura and bone. Continuous infection is most common, and the abscess creates a mass effect, gradually lifting the dura from the overlying skull.

Clinical Presentation

Patients (often men in the second or third decade) with subdural empyema are very ill with fever, vomiting, excruciating headache, and, most commonly, localizing neurologic deficits, such as aphasia, apraxia, visuospatial neglect, hemiparesis, and focal seizures.[42] Most of these seizures arise in the premotor area of the frontal lobe (adversive seizures), with turning of the head and eyes, abduction of the contralateral arm, and flexion in the elbow with raised arm similar to the posture of a fencer. Other patients have speech arrest without impairment of consciousness or jacksonian seizures (the spread of the seizure reflects the cortical topography, beginning in the hand and moving to the face, the leg, and the foot).[43]

Clinical presentation is insidious and directly related to the mass effect, which may take weeks to

Box 16.3. Dexamethasone in Bacterial Meningitis

Dexamethasone reduces the production of cytokines and thus reduces the inflammatory response. It may reduce permeability of the blood–brain barrier and thus reduce cerebral edema. However, reduction of meningeal inflammation may reduce the penetration of antibiotics that require an impaired blood–brain barrier.

Dexamethasone reduces mortality, deafness, and neurologic deficits in children with bacterial meningitis caused by *H. influenzae*. It also reduces morbidity in tuberculous meningitis but only in the most severe cases. In fulminant bacterial meningitis, dexamethasone is arbitrarily recommended for 4 days. Preferably, dexamethasone should be administered 30 minutes or less prior to the first antibiotic dose. Antibiotic therapy causes bacteriolysis and release of endotoxin. Dexamethasone may preempt production of tumor necrosis factor initiated after release of endotoxin.[25,27–29] In adults, a dose of 10 mg q6h for 4 days reduces disability but not hearing loss.[26]

become prominent and critical. Papilledema may be observed in patients with a comparatively slow-growing abscess. This allows time for increased intracranial pressure to be transmitted to the optic nerve sheaths, with subsequent venous stasis and resultant disk swelling. Nuchal rigidity is present; and if localizing neurologic signs are absent and the classic association with recent pyogenic sinusitis or surgery is not appreciated, bacterial meningitis is often incorrectly diagnosed. Misdiagnosis may also be more prevalent when the epidural empyema overlies or collects between the hemispheres. Headache and fever may be the only symptoms in these patients. An uncommon but localizing symptom complex of facial pain (trigeminal nerve involvement), facial palsy, and abducens paresis can be observed if the petrous bone is involved in the process (Gradenigo's syndrome).

Interpretation of Diagnostic Tests

Computed Tomography and Magnetic Resonance Imaging
CT scanning or MRI demonstrates a fairly characteristic lesion (Fig. 16.6), usually supratentorially. Small collections may also be seen in the posterior fossa.[44] Noncontrast CT scanning shows a hypodensity over or between the hemispheres along the falx, but enhancement of the pus collection after contrast administration reveals the characteristic crescent shape of the mass. Imaging of the mastoid and paranasal sinuses to seek a potential source is imperative.[45,46]

MRI with gadolinium is superior to contrast CT because bone artifacts that may limit detection are absent.[41,47] MRI also clearly distinguishes between hydroma (similar T_1- and T_2-weighted signals to CSF) and pus (hyperintense to CSF on T_2-weighted image and hypointense to CSF on T_1).[48] MRI may also detect parenchymal involvement and development of cerebral venous thrombosis, but a separate magnetic resonance venogram may be needed.

In a patient with an epidural abscess, a lentiform mass overlying the cerebral convexity without hemispheric involvement is clearly evident on CT scans with contrast and is not uncommonly found after a prior craniotomy (Fig. 16.7).[49] MRI may further localize small locations and their extent.[50] Lack of gadolinium enhance-

Table 16.2. Chemoprophylaxis Options for Meningococcal Meningitis

Antibiotic	Dose
Rifampin (oral agent)	Adults: 600 mg q12h for 2 days
	Children >1 year: 10 mg/kg q12h for 2 days
	Children <1 year: 5 mg/kg q12h for 2 days
Ceftriaxone (intramuscular injection)	Adults: 250 mg
	Children: 125 mg
Ciprofloxacin (oral agent)	Single dose of 500 mg

See references 30–33.

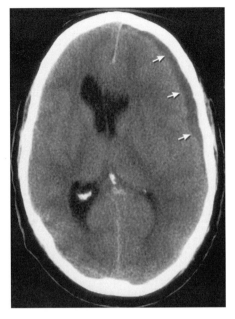

Figure 16.6 Computed tomographic scan showing subdural empyema with mass effect (*arrows*).

ment of the dura below the mass strongly favors epidural localization.[51]

Cerebrospinal Fluid

Lumbar puncture is contraindicated. One study suggested clinical deterioration after lumbar puncture.[52] When available (as mentioned earlier, often when bacterial meningitis was suspected), the findings include variable total cell counts (10–500/mm^3), increase in polymorphonucleated cells (fewer than 10 white blood cells may occur

in 10% of patients), increased protein (60%–80% of patients), normal glucose in CSF (at least 50% of cases), but often negative Gram stain and sterile culture (>90% of patients).[39,43] The CSF isolates are often *Streptococcus milleri* (otorhinogenic source), *Staphylococcus aureus*, or coagulase-negative staphylococcus (sinus, trauma, or surgery). When pneumonia is concomitantly present, *S. pneumoniae*, *Escherichia coli*, and *H. influenzae* are common infectious agents. Blood cultures are seldom diagnostic.

First Priority in Management

Surgical evacuation and immediate antibiotic coverage are therapeutic interventions in the first hours of presentation. Antibiotic therapy in the emergency department should start with a combination of a third-generation cephalosporin and metronidazole. However, anaerobic isolates are uncommon. Alternatively, a combination of piperacillin sodium and tazobactam sodium (Zosyn) can be considered (Table 16.3). Craniotomy rather than aspiration over multiple burr holes is preferred.[53–55] In a patient with an epidural abscess, grafting may be needed if the dura is destroyed or penetrated by the inflammation. Parenteral antibiotic therapy should continue for 2–6 weeks. Conservative management is seldom considered and perhaps an option only in the remote clinical situation of full alertness, tiny fluid collections (<1 cm in diameter), and rapid clinical improvement after intravenous antibiotics.[55] However, clinical deterioration may occur suddenly.

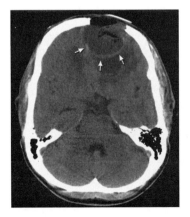
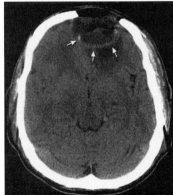
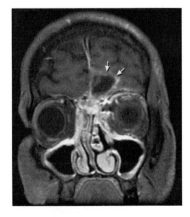

Figure 16.7 Computed tomographic scans and magnetic resonance image after frontal craniotomy show epidural pus collections (*arrows*).

Table 16.3. Empirical Antibiotic Therapy in Subdural Empyema and Epidural Abscess

Likely Source	Covers	Antimicrobial Therapy
Otitis media or mastoiditis	Streptococci Anaerobes Enterobacteria	Cefotaxime 8–12 g/day IV (q4h divided doses) Metronidazole 15 mg/kg loading, 7.5 mg/kg (q4h)
Sinusitis	Streptococci Anaerobes	*Or*
	Enterobacteria *Staphylococcus aureus* *Haemophilus* species	Piperacillin sodium and tazobactam sodium 3.375 g (q6h) IV

Predictors of Outcome

Subdural empyema is a potential calamity if not treated quickly.[56] Complacency leads to death in a matter of days, often from cerebral venous thrombosis as a result of cortical thrombophlebitis. Surgical drainage craniotomy rather than burr holes[52] and intravenous antibiotics are mandatory, resulting in the greatest chance of recovery with a minimal neurologic deficit. In a review of 102 patients with subdural empyema, treatment before the patients lapsed into stupor increased the chance of survival, reducing mortality to 10%.[57] Rhinogenic subdural empyema had the best prospects for good outcome.[52]

Triage

- Otolaryngologic evaluation.

- Start antibiotics and transport to the operating room.
- Consider mannitol, 1 g/kg, if CT scan shows a significant mass effect before transport.
- Intravenous loading with phosphenytoin or phenytoin, 20 mg/kg, if seizures have occurred.

Brain Abscess

In referral hospital emergency departments, the incidence of brain abscess may approximate 1 in 10,000 hospital admissions.[58] The causes are listed in Table 16.4. The paranasal sinuses, middle ear, and teeth remain the most common sources of entry. One should expect the cause in 30% of patients with a bacterial brain abscess to remain unresolved. Hematogenous source from endocardi-

Table 16.4. Brain Abscess: Predisposing Condition, Site of Abscess, and Microbiology

Predisposing Condition	Site of Abscess	Usual Microbial Isolates
Contiguous Focus or Primary Infection		
Otitis media or mastoiditis	Temporal lobe or cerebellum	Streptococci (anaerobic or aerobic), *Bacteroides fragilis*, Enterobacteriaceae
Frontoethmoidal sinusitis	Frontal lobe	Predominantly streptococci (anaerobic or aerobic), *Bacteroides* spp., Enterobacteriaceae, *Staphylococcus aureus*, *Haemophilus* spp.
Sphenoidal sinusitis	Frontal or temporal lobe	Same as frontoethmoidal sinusitis
Periodontal abscess	Frontal lobe	Mixed *Fusobacterium*, *Bacteroides*, and *Streptococcus* spp.
Penetrating head injury or postsurgical infection	Near the laceration	*S. aureus*, streptococci, Enterobacteriaceae, *Clostridium* spp.
Hematogenous Spread or Distant Site of Infection		
Congenital heart disease	Multiple sites	Streptococci (aerobic, anaerobic, or microaerophilic), *Haemophilus* spp.
Lung abscess, empyema, bronchiectasis	Multiple sites	*Fusobacterium* spp., *Actinomyces* spp., *Bacteroides* spp., *Streptococcus* spp., *Nocardia asteroides*
Bacterial endocarditis	Multiple sites	*Staphylococcus aureus*, *Streptococcus* spp.

tis, injected drugs, or tongue piercing should also be considered.[59,60]

Clinical Presentation

Brain abscess most often is manifested by dull headache and rarely by fever or papilledema.[61]

Neurologic signs depend on localization of the abscess and, as expected because of a lack of obvious symptoms, on localization in the frontal or occipital lobe. Clinical findings may become more

evident if edema surrounds the mass and certainly if rupture into the ventricular system occurs. Sudden worsening of headache and stupor may then be common clinical features. Level of consciousness depends on the timing of referral, and now significantly more patients seen in the emergency department are fully alert, with headache alone.[62] Seizures due to cerebral abscess are often generalized tonic-clonic seizures and have an estimated incidence of 40%.

Localization of an abscess in the cerebellum

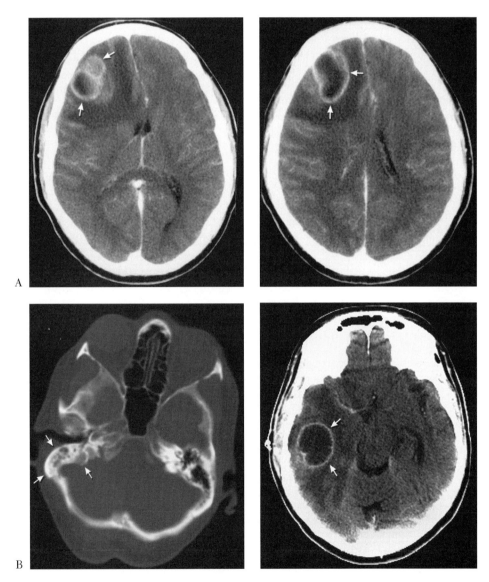

Figure 16.8 *A:* Computed tomographic scans showing abscess in the frontal lobe with perilesional edema (*arrows*). *B:* Temporal lobe abcess associated with oti-

tis media. Note absent air in mastoid and edema on magnetic resonance imaging (*arrows*).

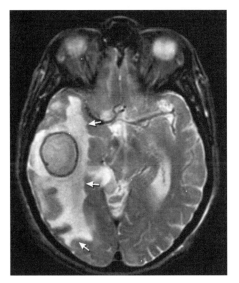 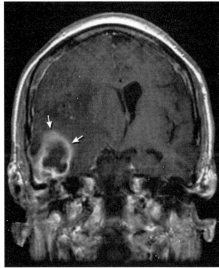

Figure 16.8 (*Continued*)

and brain stem is rare. The signs are ataxia, vomiting, appendicular dysmetria, and nystagmus.

Interpretation of Diagnostic Tests

CT scanning is diagnostic (Fig. 16.8).[63] A common misinterpretation of the abnormality in a noncontrast CT scan image, lacking the ring configuration, is a cerebral infarct. MRI may further define mass effect and demonstrate additional lesions. In T_1-weighted sequences, a hypodense center consisting of pus with a ring at the periphery is characteristic and may become evident only after contrast enhancement. T_2-weighted images show a hyperintense signal with edema, which should be separated from the actual lesion in assessment of its size.[64] MRI is also more sensitive in detecting newly developing lesions, particularly cerebritis, and it may demonstrate the proximity of the abscess to the ventricular system. Differentiation of brain abscess from cystic brain tumor remains difficult. In preliminary studies, results from magnetic resonance spectroscopy suggested that brain abscess could be distinguished on the basis of elevated acetate, succinate, and some amino acids.[65–67] Using diffusion-weighted imaging, hyperintensity was noted in abscess and hypodensity in necrotic brain tumors.[67]

Table 16.5. Suggested Empirical Therapy for Brain Abscess by Presumed Source

Putative Source	Antibiotic Therapy
Paranasal sinus	Cefotaxime 1–2 g IV (q4–8h, maximum dose 12 g/day)
	Metronidazole 500 mg IV (q6h)
Otogenic	Ceftazidime 1–2 g IV (q4–8h, maximum dose 12 g/day)
	Metronidazole 500 mg IV (q6h)
Spread from other sites	Nafcillin 2 g IV (q4–8h, maximum dose 12 g/day)
	Cefotaxime 1–2 g IV (q4–8h)
	Metronidazole 500 mg IV (q6h)
Penetrating trauma	Nafcillin 2 g IV (q4–8h, maximum dose 12 g/day)
	Cefotaxime 1–2 g IV (q4–8h)
Surgical procedure	Vancomycin 1 g IV (q12h)
	Ceftazidime 1–2 g IV (q4–8h)

First Priority in Management

Antibiotic therapy aimed at polymicrobial flora should be started immediately (Table 16.5). The decision to operate depends on several factors. Open craniotomy with debridement or stereotactic CT-guided aspiration is the first procedure in most cases. Early excision of an abscess should be considered if a thick, fibrotic capsule reduces the success of catheter drainage alone, predominantly in abscesses due to *Mycobacterium tuberculosis* and *Nocardia*. Impending rupture to the ventricular system is a reason for early surgical intervention.[68] However, surgery can be deferred if multiple abscesses are present, if the diameter of the abscess is less than 3 cm on CT scan images, or if *Toxoplasma* is considered. Corticosteroids (dexamethasone, 10 mg intravenously q6h) with multipronged antibiotic coverage should be considered if edema is profound and signs of early herniation are developing. The dose should be tapered over 3–7 days. Aggressive ventricular drainage with intraventricular administration of antibiotics is needed in patients with ventricular pus from rupture into the ventricular system. If the abscess is localized in the brain stem, stereotactic drainage is more cumbersome. Empirical therapy with antibiotics lasting up to 3 months may be preferred to surgical drainage with identification of the organism, but both approaches are successful.

Predictors of Outcome

Important factors predicting poor outcome in cerebral abscess are symptoms of short duration, decreased consciousness, rapidly progressive neurologic deficit, number and size of abscesses, and ventricular rupture.[69] Mortality is closely linked to initial presentation in coma, which increases the frequency to 50%–80% as opposed to a minimal risk of death in patients who are alert.

Triage

- To the operating room: patients with abscess and mass effect, close proximity to the ventricular system, or hydrocephalus.
- To the ward: patients with multiple small cerebral abscesses. Management is by intravenous administration of antibiotics with central venous catheter access.

REFERENCES

1. Aronin SI, Peduzzi P, Quagliarello VJ: Community-acquired bacterial meningitis: risk stratification for adverse clinical outcome and effect of antibiotic timing. *Ann Intern Med* 129:862, 1998.
2. Sigurdardottir B, Bjornsson OM, Jonsdottir KE, et al.: Acute bacterial meningitis in adults. A 20-year overview. *Arch Intern Med* 157:425, 1997.
3. Durand ML, Calderwood SB, Weber DJ, et al.: Acute bacterial meningitis in adults. A review of 493 episodes. *N Engl J Med* 328:21, 1993.
4. Saha S, Saint S, Tierney LM Jr: Clinical problem-solving. A balancing act. *N Engl J Med* 340:374, 1999.
5. Scheld WM, Koedel U, Nathan B, et al.: Pathophysiology of bacterial meningitis: mechanism(s) of neuronal injury. *J Infect Dis* 186(Suppl 2):S225, 2002.
6. Glimåker M, Kragsbjerg P, Forsgren M, et al.: Tumor necrosis factor-alpha (TNF alpha) in cerebrospinal fluid from patients with meningitis of different etiologies: high levels of TNF alpha indicate bacterial meningitis. *J Infect Dis* 167:882, 1993.
7. Pfister HW, Borasio GD, Dirnagl U, et al.: Cerebrovascular complications of bacterial meningitis in adults. *Neurology* 42:1497, 1992.
8. Quagliarello V, Scheld WM: Bacterial meningitis: pathogenesis, pathophysiology, and progress. *N Engl J Med* 327: 864, 1992.
9. Saez-Llorens X, Ramilo O, Mustafa MM, et al.: Molecular pathophysiology of bacterial meningitis: current concepts and therapeutic implications. *J Pediatr* 116:671, 1990.
10. Winkler F, Kastenbauer S, Koedel U, et al.: Role of the urokinase plasminogen activator system in patients with bacterial meningitis. *Neurology* 59:1350, 2002.
11. Behrman RE, Meyers BR, Mendelson MH, et al.: Central nervous system infections in the elderly. *Arch Intern Med* 149:1596, 1989.
12. Rasmussen HH, Sorensen HT, Moller-Petersen J, et al.: Bacterial meningitis in elderly patients: clinical picture and course. *Age Ageing* 21:216, 1992.
13. Herishanu YO, Zlotnik M, Mostoslavsky M, et al.: Cefuroxime-induced encephalopathy. *Neurology* 50:1873, 1998.
14. Igarashi M, Gilmartin RC, Gerald B, et al.: Cerebral arteritis and bacterial meningitis. *Arch Neurol* 41:531, 1984.
15. Verdon R, Chevret S, Laissy JP, et al.: Tuberculous meningitis in adults: review of 48 cases. *Clin Infect Dis* 22:982, 1996.
16. Thwaites GE, Chau TTH, Phu NH, et al.: Diagnosis of adult tuberculous meningitis by use of clinical and laboratory features. *Lancet* 360:1287, 2002.
17. Cabral DA, Flodmark O, Farrell K, et al.: Prospective study of computed tomography in acute bacterial meningitis. *J Pediatr* 111:201, 1987.
18. Vernino S, Wijdicks EFM, McGough PF: Coma in fulminant pneumococcal meningitis: new MRI observations. *Neurology* 51:1200, 1998.

19. Dichgans M, Jager L, Mayer T, et al.: Bacterial meningitis in adults: demonstration of inner ear involvement using high-resolution MRI. *Neurology* 52:1003, 1999.

20. Arevalo CE, Barnes PF, Duda M, et al.: Cerebrospinal fluid cell counts and chemistries in bacterial meningitis. *South Med J* 82:1122, 1989.

21. Maxson S, Lewno MJ, Schutze GE: Clinical usefulness of cerebrospinal fluid bacterial antigen studies. *J Pediatr* 125:235, 1994.

22. Jacobs MR: Drug-resistant *Streptococcus pneumoniae*: rational antibiotic choices. *Am J Med* 106:48S, 1999.

23. Roos KL, Tunkel AR, Scheld WM: Acute bacterial meningitis in children and adults. In WM Scheld, RJ Whitley, DT Durack (eds), *Infections of the Central Nervous System*, 2nd ed. Philadelphia: Lippincott-Raven, 1997, p. 335.

24. Gropper MR, Schulder M, Sharan AD, et al.: Central nervous system tuberculosis: medical management and surgical indications. *Surg Neurol* 44:378, 1995.

25. Girgis NI, Farid Z, Kilpatrick ME, et al.: Dexamethasone adjunctive treatment for tuberculous meningitis. *Pediatr Infect Dis J* 10:179, 1991.

26. de Gans J, van de Beek D: Dexamethasone in adults with bacterial meningitis. *N Engl J Med* 347:1549, 2002.

27. Lebel MH, Freij BJ, Syrogiannopoulos GA, et al.: Dexamethasone therapy for bacterial meningitis. Results of two double-blind, placebo-controlled trials. *N Engl J Med* 319:964, 1988.

28. Mustafa MM, Lebel MH, Ramilo O, et al.: Correlation of interleukin-1 beta and cachectin concentrations in cerebrospinal fluid and outcome from bacterial meningitis. *J Pediatr* 115:208, 1989.

29. Mustafa MM, Ramilo O, Olsen KD, et al.: Tumor necrosis factor in mediating experimental *Haemophilus influenzae* type B meningitis. *J Clin Invest* 84:1253, 1989.

30. Cuevas LE, Hart CA: Chemoprophylaxis of bacterial meningitis. *J Antimicrob Chemother* 31(Suppl B):79, 1993.

31. Feigin RD, McCracken GH Jr, Klein JO: Diagnosis and management of meningitis. *Pediatr Infect Dis J* 11:785, 1992.

32. Gaunt PN, Lambert BE: Single dose ciprofloxacin for the eradication of pharyngeal carriage of *Neisseria meningitidis*. *J Antimicrob Chemother* 21:489, 1988.

33. Schwartz B, Al-Tobaiqi A, Al-Ruwais A, et al.: Comparative efficacy of ceftriaxone and rifampicin in eradicating pharyngeal carriage of group A *Neisseria meningitidis*. *Lancet* 1:1239, 1988.

34. Wenger JD, Hightower AW, Facklam RR, et al.: Bacterial meningitis in the United States, 1986: report of a multistate surveillance study. *J Infect Dis* 162:1316, 1990.

35. van de Beek D, Schmand B, de Gans J, et al.: Cognitive impairment in adults with good recovery after bacterial meningitis. *J Infect Dis* 186:1047, 2002.

36. Kastenbauer S, Pfister H-W: Pneumococcal meningitis in adults. Spectrum of complications and prognostic factors in a series of 87 cases. *Brain* 126:1015, 2003.

37. Berenguer J, Moreno S, Laguna F, et al.: Tuberculous meningitis in patients infected with the human immunodeficiency virus. *N Engl J Med* 326:668, 1992.

38. Younis RT, Lazar RH, Anand VK: Intracranial complication of sinusitis: a 15-year review of 39 cases. *Ear Nose Throat J* 81:636, 2002.

39. Dill SR, Cobbs CG, McDonald CK: Subdural empyema: analysis of 32 cases and review. *Clin Infect Dis* 20:372, 1995.

40. Farkas AG, Marks JC: Subdural empyema: an important diagnosis not to miss. *BMJ* 293:118, 1986.

41. Greenlee JE: Subdural empyema. *Curr Treat Options Neurol* 5:13, 2003.

42. Bhandari YS, Sarkari NB: Subdural empyema. A review of 37 cases. *J Neurosurg* 32:35, 1970.

43. Brock DG, Bleck TP: Extra-axial suppurations of the central nervous system. *Semin Neurol* 12:263, 1992.

44. Morgan DW, Williams B: Posterior fossa subdural empyema. *Brain* 108:983, 1985.

45. Hoyt DJ, Fisher SR: Otolaryngologic management of patients with subdural empyema. *Laryngoscope* 101:20, 1991.

46. Kaufman DM, Litman N, Miller MH: Sinusitis: induced subdural empyema. *Neurology* 33:123, 1983.

47. Hodges J, Anslow P, Gillett G: Subdural empyema: continuing diagnostic problems in the CT scan era. *Q J Med* 59:387, 1986.

48. Sadhu VK, Handel SF, Pinto RS, et al.: Neuroradiologic diagnosis of subdural empyema and CT limitations. *AJNR Am J Neuroradiol* 1:39, 1980.

49. Gallagher RM, Gross CW, Phillips CD: Suppurative intracranial complications of sinusitis. *Laryngoscope* 108:1635, 1998.

50. Weingarten K, Zimmerman RD, Becker RD, et al.: Subdural and epidural empyemas: MR imaging. *AJR Am J Roentgenol* 152:615, 1989.

51. Tsuchiya K, Makita K, Furui S, et al.: Contrast-enhanced magnetic resonance imaging of sub- and epidural empyemas. *Neuroradiology* 34:494, 1992.

52. Nathoo N, Nadvi SS, Gouws E, et al.: Craniotomy improves outcomes for cranial subdural empyemas: computed tomography-era experience with 699 patients. *Neurosurgery* 49:872, 2001.

53. Bok AP, Peter JC: Subdural empyema: burr holes or craniotomy? A retrospective computerized tomography-era analysis of treatment in 90 cases. *J Neurosurg* 78:574, 1993.

54. Luken MG III, Whelan MA: Recent diagnostic experience with subdural empyema. *J Neurosurg* 52:764, 1980.

55. Mauser HW, Ravijst RA, Elderson A, et al.: Nonsurgical treatment of subdural empyema. Case report. *J Neurosurg* 63:128, 1985.

56. Nathoo N, Nadvi SS, Van Dellan JR, et al.: Intracranial subdural empyemas in the era of computed tomography: a review of 699 cases. *Neurosurgery* 44:529, 1999.

57. Mauser HW, Van Houwelingen HC, Tulleken CA: Factors affecting the outcome in subdural empyema. *J Neurol Neurosurg Psychiatry* 50:1136, 1987.

58. Yen PT, Chan ST, Huang TS: Brain abscess: with special

reference to otolaryngologic sources of infection. *Otolaryngol Head Neck Surg* 113:15, 1995.

59. Tunkel AR, Wispelwey B, Scheld WM. Brain abscess. In GL Mandell, RG Douglas Jr, JE Bennett (eds), *Principles and Practice of Infectious Diseases,* 5th ed. New York: Churchill Livingstone, 2000, p. 1016.

60. Martinello RA, Cooney EL: Cerebellar brain abscess associated with tongue piercing. *Clin Infect Dis* 36:e32, 2003.

61. Grigoriadis E, Gold WL: Pyogenic brain abscess caused by *Streptococcus pneumoniae*: case report and review. *Clin Infect Dis* 25:1108, 1997.

62. Yang SY, Zhao CS: Review of 140 patients with brain abscess. *Surg Neurol* 39:290, 1993.

63. Miller ES, Dias PS, Uttley D: CT scanning in the management of intracranial abscess: a review of 100 cases. *Br J Neurosurg* 2:439, 1988.

64. Smith RR, Caldemeyer KS: Neuroradiologic review of intracranial infection. *Curr Probl Diagn Radiol* 28:1, 1999.

65. Kim SH, Chang KH, Song IC, et al.: Brain abscess and brain tumor: discrimination with in vivo H-1 MR spectroscopy. *Radiology* 204:239, 1997.

66. Martinez-Perez I, Moreno A, Alonso J, et al.: Diagnosis of brain abscess by magnetic resonance spectroscopy. Report of two cases. *J Neurosurg* 86:708, 1997.

67. Lai PH, Ho JT, Chen WL, et al.: Brain abscess and necrotic brain tumor: discrimination with proton MR spectroscopy and diffusion-weighted imaging. *AJNR Am J Neuroradiol* 23:1369, 2002.

68. Zeidman SM, Geisler FH, Olivi A: Intraventricular rupture of a purulent brain abscess: case report. *Neurosurgery* 36:189, 1995.

69. Seydoux C, Francioli P: Bacterial brain abscesses: factors influencing mortality and sequelae. *Clin Infect Dis* 15:394, 1992.

Chapter 17
Acute Encephalitis

Unravelling the cause in patients with acute encephalitis is a burden with a dire need for specific management in many of them. There are a bewildering number of causes of acute encephalitis. Clinical findings that are often diagnostic of acute encephalitis are fever, agitation, localizing neurologic signs, and changes in personal behavior (Chapter 7). Progression to coma is expected in fulminant variants, and attending physicians may then feel pressured because little in the presentation discriminates among the possible triggering agents.

Viral infection remains the most common cause, but other infectious agents should be considered[1] (Table 17.1). In the United States, one new problem has emerged, West Nile encephalitis,[2] and one may happen in the future—anthrax meningoencephalitis.[3] Noninfectious causes should be considered in appropriate circumstances, and the diagnostic considerations of major importance are listed in Table 17.2. This chapter concentrates on patients with acute encephalitis with more defined management and diagnostic tests.

Herpes Simplex Encephalitis

Epidemiologic registries have demonstrated that herpes simplex encephalitis is uncommon (2 cases per 1 million population annually) and can be implicated in less than 10% of all reported encephalitides in middle-aged and elderly adults.[4] Untreated, it frequently leads to further deterioration of consciousness, brain death, and, in survivors, permanent morbidity. The primary concern is to treat early and preempt further progression. Prompt treatment with acyclovir has considerably improved the neurologic outcome; but even so, there may be ravaging consequences despite early treatment.

Clinical Presentation

The clinical diagnosis of herpes simplex encephalitis should be urgently considered in patients with abrupt onset of a triad of fever (up to 39°C–40°C), change in personality, and localizing neurologic findings (e.g., aphasia, hemiparesis, and apraxia).[5,6] Seizures, often focal and transient, are present in one-third of patients. As the disorder progresses, epilepsia partialis continua and temporal lobe seizures may reflect frontal or temporal lobe involvement. Auras of temporal lobe seizures may consist of hallucinations and dysgeusia. Progression to coma may take days but can be rapid, and even the interval between the development of febrile illness and the late stages of coma with extensor responses may be surprisingly short. Some patients may be healthy in the morning and fulfill the criteria for brain death at night. Unusual features are visual field defects, papilledema (only in moribund patients), and memory loss (more commonly apparent in late survivors). Autonomic dysfunction with profound instability in blood pressure, tachypnea, and sweating may occur (60% of biopsy-proven cases) and in exceptional cases

Table 17.1. Infectious Diseases That Can Masquerade as Viral Central Nervous System Infections

Bacteria
  Spirochetes
    Syphilis (secondary or meningovascular)
    Leptospirosis
    Borrelia burgdorferi infection (Lyme disease)
  Mycoplasma pneumoniae infection
  Cat-scratch fever
  Listeriosis
  Brucellosis (particularly due to *Brucella melitensis*)
  Tuberculosis
  Typhoid fever
  Parameningeal infections (epidural infection, petrositis)
  Partially treated bacterial meningitis
  Brain abscesses
  Whipple's disease
Fungi
  Cryptococcosis
  Coccidioidomycosis
  Histoplasmosis
  North American blastomycosis
  Candidiasis
Parasites
  Toxoplasmosis
  Cysticercosis
  Echinococcosis
  Trichinosis
  Trypanosomiasis
  Plasmodium falciparum infection
  Amebiasis (due to *Naegleria* and *Acanthamoeba*)

Source: Modified from Johnson RT: Acute encephalitis. *Clin Infect Dis* 23:219, 1996. By permission of the University of Chicago.

may further deteriorate into a sympathetic overdrive with catatonia and extensive rigidity (Chapter 5). For unclear reasons, herpes simplex encephalitis in immunocompromised patients seems to occur more often as a brain stem encephalitis with diplopia, dysarthria, and ataxia.[7,8]

Table 17.2. Noninfectious Diseases Mimicking Encephalitis

CNS vasculitis
Fulminant bacterial meningitis
ADEM
Thrombotic thrombocytopenic purpura
Fulminant hepatic failure, Reye's syndrome
Endocrine crisis (e.g., myxedema, Addison's disease)
Toxic encephalopathy (e.g., cyclosporine, tacrolimus, MTX, 5-FU, illicit drugs)

ADEM, allergic demyelinating encephalomyelitis; CNS, central nervous system; 5-FU, 5-fluorouracil; MTX, methotrexate.

An anterior operculum syndrome has been reported,[9] and failure to recognize its distinguishing features may potentially delay therapy. Involvement of the anterior operculum (the operculum is the cortex and white matter tissue overlying the insula) results in difficulty chewing, a tendency for the mouth to be half open, bifacial palsy, dysphagia, drooling, anarthria, and trismus. Automatic facial movements, such as yawning, are preserved.[9,10] Manic behavior (hallucinations, elevated mood, decreased need for sleep, increased sexual desire, flirtations) has been pointed out (patients feel "absolutely marvelous, relaxed and happy") but is highly uncommon.[11] Cerebellitis with profound swelling, a location more preferentially affected in children, has been reported in an adult.[12] These complex presentations should alert the neurologist to herpes simplex encephalitis, but the very untraditional presentation may not be linked to this encephalitis.

Interpretation of Diagnostic Tests

Time is needed to document the source and nature of any infection, whether for careful preparation of cerebrospinal fluid (CSF) for cultures, priming of a polymerase chain reaction (PCR), or awaiting the results of blood cultures. Certain laboratory tests are helpful in the emergency department and can be used in early assessment of prognosis.

Cerebrospinal Fluid
Pleocytosis with lymphocytes (50–2000/mm^3) and a fivefold increase in protein are common. CSF glucose may be decreased. CSF is normal only exceptionally, mostly in patients examined very early in the course of the illness. CSF PCR has a sensitivity of 98% and a specificity of 94% (Box 17.1, Table 17.3). Acyclovir may reduce PCR sensitivity, but herpes simplex DNA can still be detected in one-third of cases long after acyclovir treatment.[4]

Electroencephalography
In the electroencephalogram (EEG), typical but not-to-be-mistaken nonspecific abnormalities over the temporal regions are spike-and-slow-wave activity, delta waves, or triphasic waves evolving into unilateral periodic lateralized epileptiform discharges, which rapidly spread to both temporal hemispheres.[19] This pattern is seen

Box 17.1. Polymerase Chain Reaction Technology for Fulminant Encephalitis

PCR has revolutionized the diagnosis of herpes simplex, cytomegalovirus, and toxoplasmic encephalitides. Small quantities of viral DNA or RNA in the CSF can be selectively amplified. Target sequences of DNA are amplified by DNA polymerase, and with multiple repeating of cycles, large copies can be obtained. This amplified DNA is visualized on gel stained by ethidium bromide. PCR is the method of choice for diagnosis but not useful to monitor treatment efficacy. In addition, persistent viral load DNA does not correlate with outcome.[13] False-negative PCR may result from antiviral treatment or, more commonly, technical difficulty with primers.[14–16]

in 84% of typical cases of herpes simplex encephalitis but with a specificity of only 30%.[19]

Computed Tomography and Magnetic Resonance Imaging

Computed tomographic (CT) scanning is generally not useful in herpes simplex encephalitis, and the findings become abnormal only after days and predominantly in advanced cases evolving into coma. Abnormal CT scan findings in the temporal and insular regions (Fig. 17.1) develop in approximately 50% of patients, but the reported radiologic series are certainly skewed toward the more severe cases. Initial unilateral involvement may occur in almost 60% of cases.[20] Hypodensity and swelling in the temporal lobe may become prominent and hemorrhagic and be initially misinterpreted as a lobar hematoma or hemorrhagic infarct (Fig. 17.2). Unilateral swelling may suggest a glioma or an abscess (and sometimes it is).

Magnetic resonance imaging (MRI) is the definitive diagnostic test, with a high sensitivity and specificity for early T$_2$ changes in the temporal lobe and, to a lesser extent, in the frontobasal or cingulate gyrus of the frontal lobe, in the insular cortex, and across the splenium (Fig. 17.3). Increased signal solely present in the cerebellar hemispheres has been noted.[12] Fluid-attenuated

inversion recovery is more sensitive and may clearly show abnormal images not evident on routine T$_2$-weighted sequences.[21] MRI abnormalities may appear within 1 day of herpes simplex encephalitis. Conversely, normal MRI findings in a comatose patient virtually exclude herpes simplex encephalitis.

Single-Photon Emission Computed Tomography

With single-photon emission computed tomography (SPECT), in which technetium Tc 99m hexamethyl propyleneamine oxime is the radiopharmaceutical, unilateral hyperfusion is a common finding and, as expected, the tracer preferentially lodges in the temporal lobe and adjacent frontal lobe. This phenomenon of increased uptake is not

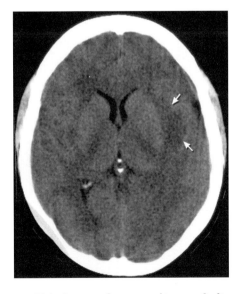

Figure 17.1 Computed tomographic scan findings of early herpes encephalitis with subinsular hypodensity (*arrows*).

Table 17.3. Sensitivity and Specificity of Polymerase Chain Reaction in Cerebrospinal Fluid

Agent	Sensitivity (%)	Specificity (%)
Herpes simplex[15]	98	94
Cytomegalovirus[17]	79	95
Toxoplasma[18]	42	100

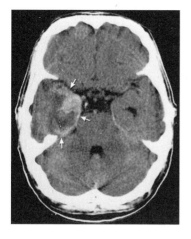
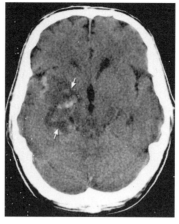
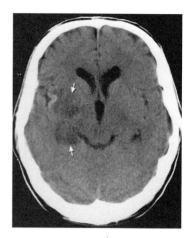

Figure 17.2 Computed tomographic scans showing unilateral swollen, hypodense, and partly hemorrhagic temporal lobe lesion from herpes simplex encephalitis (*arrows*).

specific for herpes simplex encephalitis and indicates only inflammation and early neuronal injury.

Approximately half of SPECT scans performed within days of symptoms yield normal results. It may become a preferred test in patients seen in the emergency department because data are rapidly acquired and, despite moderate sensitivity, it may be more helpful than EEG or MRI in the first days after presentation.

First Priority in Management

An immediate intravenous dose of acyclovir, 10 mg/kg, is needed, followed by maintenance with 10 mg/kg every 8 hours for 10 days. Intravenous loading with fosphenytoin, 18–20 mg/kg, is needed after presentation with seizures; but its use as prophylaxis is not established. Propofol is useful to control extreme agitation. With the introduction of PCR and MRI, earlier dilemmas about the need for brain biopsy have almost been resolved.[22,23] Biopsy should be considered if the PCR result is negative, if CSF pleocytosis is absent, and when, primarily to exclude a glioma, only unilateral temporal lobe swelling is present. Comatose patients with CT evidence of increased intracranial pressure (mass effect, obliteration of basal cisterns) should receive an intracranial pressure (ICP) monitor. In patients with a markedly swollen temporal lobe and shift and impending

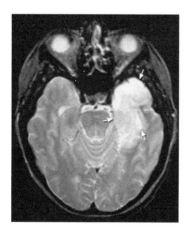
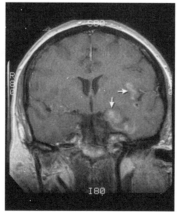
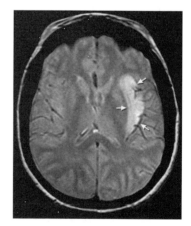

Figure 17.3 Magnetic resonance images with typical hyperintensities (T$_2$-weighted [*left*], T$_1$-weighted [*middle*], fluid attenuated inversion recovery [*right*]) in temporal, frontal lobe, and insular regions from herpes simplex encephalitis (*arrows*).

herniation despite conventional measures to reduce ICP, a craniotomy with dural grafting is indicated. Some of the necrotic tissue may need to be removed to decompress the supratentorial compartment.

Predictors of Outcome

Treatment with acyclovir within 5 days of onset of the first symptoms remains associated with a 25% incidence of fatal outcome. Fatal outcome is associated with brain edema but more commonly as a consequence of persistent vegetative state and terminal systemic infection. Good recovery with return to a similar productive life is possible in 50% of patients.[24] Mild forms of herpes simplex encephalitis have been reported in immunosuppressed patients with mostly involvement of the nondominant temporal lobe.[25] MRI abnormalities[26] and bilateral EEG abnormalities predict disability, with memory deficits[27] and inability to function at a normal intellectual level. A large study found a delay of more than 2 days between admission and that acyclovir was highly predictive of poor outcome. This, again, emphasizes that suspicion should be high and early treatment is needed while awaiting CSF/PCR results.[20]

SPECT may have some predictive value: a close association between focal hyperfusion on SPECT and poor outcome was emphasized in a large study of patients with acute encephalitis.[28]

Triage

- Supportive care, monitor and manage increased ICP in the neurologic intensive care unit.
- Consider video EEG monitoring in the intensive care unit if the patient has had seizures and impaired consciousness.

Arthropod-Borne Viral Encephalitis

Arthropod-borne (ARBO) viral encephalitides are widespread geographically and commonly endemic; sporadic cases are seasonal during the summer months, and cluster cases may signal an outbreak. Fatality depends on the type of virus and amplifying host. The virus is transmitted through ticks and mosquitoes after replication in wild animals. The most common viruses are *bunyavirus* (La Crosse, California), *alphavirus* (eastern and western equine), and *flavivirus* (St. Louis, West Nile).[29,30]

Clinical Presentation

Differences in presentation are apparent. La Crosse (California) encephalitis is most commonly reported to the Centers for Disease Control and predominates in children younger than 15 years. The hosts for the mosquito are chipmunks and squirrels, and the mosquito breeds in rainwater-filled tires and birdhouses. In California encephalitis, seizures are common (50%) and seizure disorder develops later in many patients. Within 2 weeks after prodromal fever, the patient may experience malaise, very severe headaches, confusion, drowsiness, and coma, in roughly that order.

The equine encephalitides (western and eastern) differ substantially in mortality.[31] The mosquito breeds in freshwater swamps, and birds (sparrows, ducks, and pheasants) are the hosts. It is prevalent along the Atlantic and Gulf coasts, but eastern encephalitis is infrequent. Evolution to coma from massive cerebral edema is rapid, usually within 1 week, but unusual.[31,32] The virus causes an acute encephalitis in horses, and it can be isolated from brain tissue specimens.[32] Western equine encephalitis peaks in August and September, and outbreaks have been reported from the midwestern United States. Improved vector control has reduced the incidence of both types of encephalitis.

St. Louis encephalitis occurs commonly in the United States. Its manifestations appear to be milder in children than in adults. The susceptible populations are persons living in public housing projects and, possibly, patients infected with human immunodeficiency virus (HIV).

In the tropics, Venezuelan equine encephalitis is most common, particularly in Central and South America, and is very comparable to western equine encephalitis in prevalence, clinical presentation, morbidity, and mortality. Japanese encephalitis is endemic in Southeast Asia and India. Vaccination of children has markedly decreased its prevalence in Japan, but vaccination for travelers to endemic areas is recommended. Most cases occur in China, India, and Thailand.[33] Japanese encephalitis peaks during the rainy season. It may occur during only brief stays, such as a vacation,[34] although the risk of exposure increases with a longer stay.

The clinical features of Japanese encephalitis are nonspecific, but seizures are very common,[35] with elements of diffuse involvement of both hemispheres; spinal cord involvement (often leading to the incorrect diagnosis of fulminant multiple sclerosis) has been noted.[33,36]

Flaviviruses are transmitted by tick bites. Encephalitis develops in only 1 of 10 infected persons, usually after a flu-like illness. Tick-borne encephalitis has become a serious health problem in forested areas of Europe and Russia.[37–40]

West Nile encephalitis swept the western and midwestern United States in the summer of 2002, and in 2003 moved to western states such as Colorado. The outbreaks are severe, and the ravages in survivors are not yet entirely known. The flavivirus is amplified in mosquitoes in the characteristic spring to fall season and is spread through birds. The virus is commonly found in all continents, with prior outbreaks in Africa, Romania, Russia, and Israel. The risk of developing encephalitis is estimated to be 1 in 150 infected persons and increases with age and prior poor immunologic state. Parkinsonism is a common feature. Fatalities have been common. The combination of neck stiffness, pleocytosis in the CSF, hyponatremia (30%), and clinical or electrophysiologic signs of asymmetric flaccid paralysis should suggest the diagnosis. Polio-like syndromes (marked asymmetry and pure motor involvement, Fig. 17.4) involving facial, cervical, and limb muscles have been described, with early indications of poor outcome.[2,41–43]

Interpretation of Diagnostic Tests

Diagnosis of arthropod-borne viral encephalitis is often delayed, and no specific neuroimaging finding has been reported that would link it to a certain types of encephalitis.

Computed Tomography and Magnetic Resonance Imaging

CT scans are normal or may show diffuse cerebral edema (see Chapter 9). Abnormal MRI findings have been described in a large series of patients with a predilection for basal ganglionic and thalamic lesions in all types of arbovirus en-

cephalitis. The midbrain and cortex may be involved in some. In one study, MRI findings were abnormal in 11 comatose patients, but other arboviruses can produce coma without MRI abnormalities in the earlier diagnostic phase.[31] MRI abnormalities, however, can be present soon after the onset of neurologic symptoms, if any. Diffuse cerebral edema appears after several days of coma. Similar MRI findings have been reported in Japanese encephalitis[44–46] and European tick-borne encephalitis. The sensitivity of MRI in these types of encephalitis is not known.

Cerebrospinal Fluid and Serology

As expected, pleocytosis with lymphocytosis is found along with increased protein. A CSF profile mimicking bacterial meningitis has been described in eastern equine encephalitis. The diagnosis of arbovirus encephalitis is based on determination of immunoglobulin M (IgM) antibodies by an enzyme-linked immunosorbent assay, which has a high sensitivity, but needs confirmation with a plaque reduction neutralization test. Isolation of the virus from blood or CSF is unrewarding. One study documented positive findings in 10% of tested specimens of CSF.[47] PCR detection of virus-derived DNA is available but not very sensitive (±50%) and thus the diagnosis is based on detectable IgM in the CSF or a fourfold increase in IgM in serum measured in the convalescent phase of the illness.

First Priority in Management

No specific antiviral therapy is available, but acyclovir (10 mg/kg intravenously every 3 hours) should be administered until PCR results are confirmed negative. Supportive therapy consists of antiepileptic drugs, mechanical ventilation, and prevention of medical complications in the more severe cases. Corticosteroids are not effective.[48] Reduction of increased intracranial pressure is not a typical feature of management in many ARBO encephalitides.

Predictors of Outcome

Mortality in La Crosse and California encephalitides is fortunately low, but neurologic sequelae with hemiparesis or aphasia are possible in 15% of patients. Eastern equine encephalitis may cause

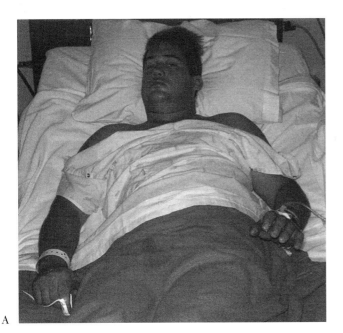

A

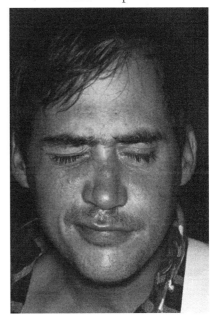

B

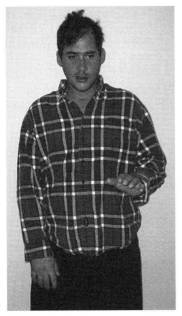

C

Figure 17.4 *A:* Patient with confirmed West Nile encephalitis. Marked pleocytosis and asymmetric pure motor weakness of arms ("man in the barrel"), able to lift only left hand. Follow-up photographs 1 month later show asymmetric eyelid closing when asked to forcefully close eyelids (*B*) and only partial lifting of left arm when instructed (*C*). Right arm remained flaccid and paralyzed.[41]

numerous deaths, and up to 70% of patients have severe neurologic disability. In western equine encephalitis, in contrast, full recovery occurs, although elderly patients may die. The death rate in St. Louis encephalitis is approximately one in four for elderly patients. Neuropsychologic sequelae seem more common than overt localizing neurologic signs in tick-borne encephalitis. Fatality is high in West Nile encephalitis,[41,42] but it appears that several patients awaken from coma without residual symptoms.[42]

Triage

- Neurologic or medical intensive care unit for supportive care.

Cytomegalovirus and Varicella-Zoster Virus Encephalitis

Cytomegalovirus (CMV) is an opportunistic infectious agent. In a review of 676 patients, 85%

with CMV encephalitis were infected with the acquired immunodeficiency syndrome (AIDS) virus.[17,49] CMV ventriculoencephalitis is the hall-mark of the infection and the cause of death.

The patterns of varicella-zoster virus (VZV) encephalitis have been classified by Amlie-Lefond et al.[13] and Kleinschmidt-DeMasters et al.[50] into three major categories: (1) large- or medium-vessel vasculopathy involving large vessels at the base of the brain or convexity, which may affect large territories and cause hemorrhagic infarc-tions (arteritis and the virus inside the artery have been well documented); (2) small-vessel vascu-lopathy producing demyelinating ischemic lesions with a more subacute clinical course; and (3) ven-triculitis. VZV encephalitis has been associated with hematologic–oncologic malignant disease, sarcoidosis, rheumatoid arthritis, tuberculosis, transplantation, and AIDS.

Clinical Presentation

Confusion and lethargy in a patient with a history of CMV retinitis or pneumonitis should suggest the diagnosis. The clinical features include con-fusion (60% of patients), coma (45%), cranial nerve palsy (40%), and seizures (25%).[49] Ventric-ulitis and hydrocephalus may be the cause of re-duced consciousness. Hyponatremia from CMV adrenalitis is common and an important labora-tory indicator in patients with AIDS and rapidly developing encephalitis.

VZV encephalitis should be the first considera-tion in immunosuppressed (e.g., HIV-infected) pa-tients with recent shingles.[51] In most reported cases, however, a rash developed days to months before the onset but was not always remembered by the patients. In several reports, VZV encephali-tis actually occurred without a skin eruption.

Progressive multifocal neurologic deficits oc-cur, often leading to visual field defects, aphasia, apraxia, hemiparesis, and more specific neu-rocognitive syndromes, such as Gerstmann's syn-drome (acalculia, finger agnosia, right–left con-fusion, and agraphia) and Anton's syndrome (cor-tical blindness). Progressive mental impairment with frontal release signs and spastic paraparesis has been observed in patients with a type of small-vessel vasculopathy causing widespread white mat-ter demyelination without cortical involvement.

Interpretation of Diagnostic Tests

Computed Tomography and Magnetic Resonance Imaging

MRI in CMV encephalitis may show nonspecific brain atrophy and enlarged ventricles with typical ependymal signal enhancement.[49] Brain stem and cerebellar abnormalities after gadolinium have been reported in isolated cases.

In patients with VZV encephalitis, both neu-roimaging studies show multiple T_1-weighted hy-pointensity and T_2-weighted hyperintensity in-volving the white and gray matter. Subcortical enhancing, coalescing lesions followed by gray matter involvement are characteristic.[52] Involve-ment of multiple territories is compatible with several large intracranial vasculitides representing infarction (Fig. 17.5).

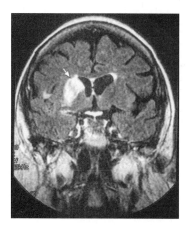 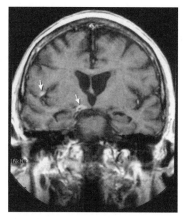 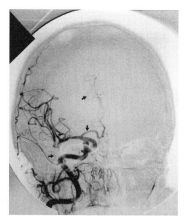

Figure 17.5 Varicella-zoster virus encephalitis with multiple infarcts (*white arrows*) and vasculitis (*black arrows*) on carotid angiogram.

Cerebrospinal Fluid

The CSF formula is normal in many instances, complicating detection. PCR of CMV has significantly increased the ability to make the diagnosis (sensitivity, 79%; specificity, 95%).

In VZV encephalitis, a marked variation in inflammatory response is known, from only a few to several hundred cells, with accompanying increase in protein. Glucose concentration is normal. PCR has become available for VZV encephalitis, but the diagnostic validity is not yet known.[53]

First Priority in Management

Ganciclovir is the preferred agent (10 mg/kg), with maintenance of 5 mg/kg once a day for 14 days. Patients previously receiving a maintenance dose of ganciclovir need the addition of foscarnet, 180 mg/kg. The efficacy of cidofovir is not clear in these infections, although successful in retinitis.[54]

Predictors of Outcome

The outcome in CMV-associated encephalitis is poor because of underlying HIV infection and, commonly, concomitant opportunistic infection. The outcome in VZV encephalitis is entirely determined by associated vasculitis; without it, full recovery is possible.

Triage

- Neurologic intensive care unit.
- Consider ventriculostomy in patients with hydrocephalus.

Encephalitis from Rickettsiae

Rickettsial diseases are transmitted through ticks, mites, lice, and fleas. The stings are often not remembered because they are painless and may not be followed by a rash at the injection site. The most important and potentially fatal disorder is Rocky Mountain spotted fever, which causes a generalized vasculitis and meningoencephalitis. It emerges in late spring and summer, predominantly in the southeast region of the United States[55] (regardless of its name, which suggests the west).

Other rickettsial infections that may involve the central nervous system are encephalitides from the typhus group. The typhus group includes Q fever, epidemic typhus, murine typhus, and scrub typhus. The epidemic can be worldwide and produce similar neurologic manifestations, with typical maculopapular rash and multifocal central nervous system manifestations.[55]

Clinical Presentation

Rocky Mountain spotted fever is evident in patients with fever who have a marked purpuric rash involving the palms and soles. The flexor surfaces of the hands and feet are involved first before the rash spreads over the body. The purpuric lesions are a consequence of rickettsiae invading small blood vessels and causing occlusion and necrosis. This rash (see Color Fig. 17.6 in separate color insert) may be absent early in the disease.[56]

Neurologic manifestations are protean, but severe headache, profound neck stiffness, and clouding of consciousness are common, with progression to stupor in more than one-fourth of affected patients.[57,58]

Q fever occurs as a result of exposure to farm animals, rabbits, or deer and may result in fever, pneumonia, myocarditis, endocarditis, and meningoencephalitis. The involvement of the central nervous system is less common in Q fever but may mimic herpes simplex encephalitis.[59] Neurologic involvement from the responsible agent, Coxiella burnetii, is uncommon but can be dramatic. Severe headache and myalgias are common.[60] Neurologic manifestations that may precede stupor are cranial nerve involvement and cerebellar signs.[59] Acute confusion evolving into acute manic behavior has been reported as well. Epidemic, murine, and scrub types, which occur widely in Southeast Asia, the Pacific Islands, India, and Nepal, are not further considered here.

Interpretation of Diagnostic Tests

Computed Tomography and Magnetic Resonance Imaging

The findings in Rocky Mountain spotted fever are multiple small subcortical infarcts (often in the basal ganglia), development of cerebral edema with loss of gray–white matter differentiation, and sulci effacement.[5] A survivor in one report had multiple punctate areas of increased intensity throughout the white matter in the distribution of the perivascular (Virchow-Robin) spaces, possibly representing a perivascular inflammatory response.[61,62] Meningeal enhancement after gadolinium is typical.

Cerebrospinal Fluid and Serum

Increased protein occurred in only one-third of patients, with only mild pleocytosis (<50 mm^3) in most cases. PCR detection in blood samples from infected patients has been successful, even in those obtained on the day of onset.[63]

Predictors of Outcome

These types of encephalitides are typically diagnosed at autopsy because patients deteriorate rapidly from brain edema.

No early clinical predictors are known other than brain edema, which may be difficult to control. Increased ICP (>40 mm Hg) despite aggressive mannitol therapy predicts poor outcome.

First Priority in Early Management

Early treatment of rickettsial or tick-borne encephalitis with oral tetracycline is needed (25–50 mg/kg daily in two or four divided doses). A relapse can be treated with chloramphenicol, but tetracycline remains the agent for first-line therapy.[64]

Triage

- Neurologic intensive care unit for monitoring of ICP.
- Cardiac consultation in Q fever for possible myocarditis.

Encephalitis from Anthrax

Exemplary of the potential of effective bioweaponry, anthrax may cause a fatal meningoencephalitis. The clinical presentation emerging from a cutaneous infection is dramatic and involves multiorgan failure. (An important review by Lanska is available.[3]) It may also cause a gastrointestinal symptom when spores are ingested from uncooked meat.

Clinical Presentation

Cutaneous or gastrointestinal symptoms are common and found in association with fever. Seizures appear in 40% of reported cases, followed by marked decline in consciousness. Pleural effusions, widened mediastinum, and soft tissue edema are additional clues.

Interpretation of Diagnostic Tests

Computed Tomography and Magnetic Resonance Imaging

Due to its nonspecific appearance, multiple diagnostic tests are needed to point in this direction. Focal hemorrhages, subarachnoid hemorrhages, diffuse edema, and meningeal enhancement have been noted; but the experience is limited.[65,66] Contrast-enhanced CT scan may document, next to parenchymal hematoma, noticeable enhancement after contrast administration.[66] The combination of subarachnoid hemorrhage, lobar hematoma with pulmonary infiltrates, and cutaneous lesions could suggest the diagnosis.

Cerebrospinal Fluid and Serum

Blood and tissue cultures may document the gram-positive spore-forming *Bacillus anthracis*. The CSF is pink or bloody, with pleocytosis varying from a few increased polymorphonuclear leukocytes to several thousand. A high yield of positive rods has been claimed on gram staining.

First Priority in Early Management

Management includes treatment of the rapid evolution of multiorgan failure, hypotension, and therapy-resistant shock, with a high probability of death. Ciprofloxacin and doxycycline are the preferred drugs. Rifampin with vancomycin has been suggested as adjuvant therapy.

Triage

- To medical intensive care unit for management of multiorgan failure

Toxoplasmic Encephalitis

Normal host immunity contains an infection with *Toxoplasma gondii*. Therefore, toxoplasmic encephalitis is a leading cause of acute encephalitis in patients with AIDS or in immunosuppressed patients.[67] HIV encephalitis has a more protracted course. *Toxoplasma* infestation can be a defining illness in previously HIV-positive patients. It is much less common in transplant recipients, patients with Hodgkin's disease, or patients with systemic lupus erythematosus.[68] Its incidence may be lower in patients with AIDS receiving trimethoprim-sulfamethoxazole prophylaxis for *Pneumocystis carinii*.

Clinical Presentation

Toxoplasma infection may result in a single mass effect, multiple abscesses, or multiple hemorrhages in abscesses mimicking coagulopathy-associated hemorrhages. The total parasite burden to the brain determines the clinical manifestations, but many of these abscesses do not produce clinical signs other than headache and lethargy. Progression may be in days or protracted over months. Decreasing alertness, onset of seizures, and persisting headache should alert one to the diagnosis.[69] *Toxoplasma* has a predilection for the basal ganglia and cerebellum, but hemichorea, hemiballismus, and ataxia are uncommon manifestations.

Interpretation of Diagnostic Tests

The diagnosis is confirmed by CSF PCR, MRI of the brain, or biopsy of the brain in selected cases.

Computed Tomography and Magnetic Resonance Imaging

CT scanning underestimates the number of abscesses, even when contrast material is administered in double doses; therefore, its use is limited to initial screening.[70] Acute hydrocephalus without defined abscesses may point to the diagnosis in the proper clinical situation. Multiple intracerebral hemorrhages in patients with AIDS often indicate *Toxoplasma* (or *Aspergillus*) rather than a coagulopathy.[71,72]

MRI of toxoplasmic encephalitis, which displays multiple abscesses, is nonspecific because very similar signal abnormalities and ring enhancement can be seen with lymphoma, tuberculous abscesses, nocardiosis, cryptococcosis, and, less commonly, syphilitic gummas.

Hyperintensity on T_2-weighted images is common, but after treatment, it evolves into T_2-weighted isointensity comparable with that of necrotizing abscesses (Fig. 17.7).[73] Marked perilesional edema is typical.

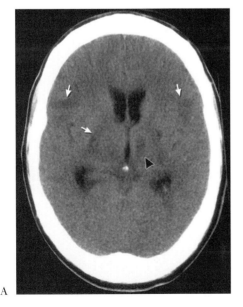
A

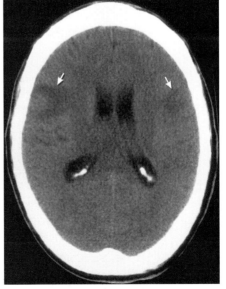
B

Figure 17.7 Toxoplasmic encephalitis with multiple abscesses (*arrows and arrowhead*). The abscesses are poorly defined by computed tomographic scan (*A,B*) and more evident by magnetic resonance imaging fluid-attenuated inversion recovery (*C*) and postcontrast T_1-weighted scan (*D*).

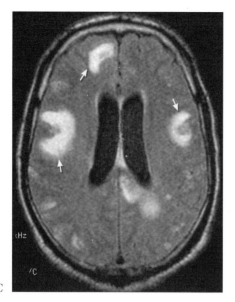
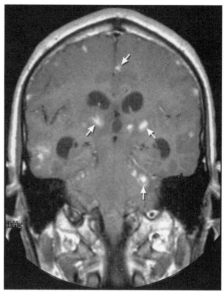

C   D

Figure 17.7 (*Continued*)

Cerebrospinal Fluid

An inflammatory profile is present in the CSF, with increased protein concentration and, rarely, marked mononuclear pleocytosis (fewer than 100 cells). The sensitivity of PCR for *Toxoplasma* is 42%, but the specificity is 100%.[18,74] The comparatively low sensitivity is determined by intraparenchymal localization of *Toxoplasma*, so it is more likely that CSF does not contain *Toxoplasma* DNA. Its diagnostic value, therefore, is limited, but PCR technology has reduced the number of brain biopsies for confirmation.

Single-Photon Emission Computed Tomography

SPECT of the brain with thallium-201 may differentiate lymphoma from toxoplasmic encephalitis. The high mitotic activity of the lymphoma increases uptake, causing a "hot" region. Its accuracy in predicting lymphoma is questionable despite impressive predictive value in a first series of patients.[75-77]

Serum Serology

Low or absent antitoxoplasmic antibody titers (IgG) are common in immunosuppressed patients, and IgM titers are negative. Variation is great, from 1:8 to titers exceeding 1:1024. A significant increase in serum titer over time has no significance because it may occur in immunocompromised patients without active *Toxoplasma* infection.

First Priority in Management

The standard therapeutic agents for toxoplasmic encephalitis are pyrimethamine, 50–100 mg, and sulfadiazine, 4–8 g, daily, combined with folinic acid, 10 mg/day, to reduce bone marrow depression.[78]

Adverse reactions are a rash and anemia, leukopenia, or thrombocytopenia, occurring in 20% of patients. Any allergic reaction should result in replacement of sulfadiazine by clindamycin (600–900 mg every 8 hours).[79] When *Toxoplasma* is the culprit, within 3 weeks radiologic improvement (defined as less edema and isointense signals rather than hyperintense signals on MRI) or complete resolution should be expected in 70% of patients.

Predictors of Outcome

Fatal outcome occurs in patients with multiple hemorrhagic abscesses. The response to therapy determines outcome.[78,80] Often, underlying central nervous system lymphoma (together with toxoplasmic encephalitis) reduces prospects of full recovery.

Triage

- Most patients can be initially managed on wards rather than in an intensive care unit.

- Surgical drainage of a large abscess should be considered if a mass effect is present.
- Biopsy should be strongly considered when PCR is negative, primarily to exclude lymphoma. Immunofluorescence techniques can confirm *Toxoplasma* in brain tissue with the use of monoclonal antibodies in the tissue samples.[81]

Fungal Encephalitis

Viral meningoencephalitis is the most common cause in patients with progressive headache, nuchal rigidity, confusion, and lymphocytic predominance, but a fungal cause should always be considered.[81] One should be especially alert if an acute presentation is followed by an insidious course, particularly in endemic regions. Prompt diagnosis and therapy with amphotericin B result in survival and reduced morbidity.

Clinical Presentation

The lung is the port of entry of the fungus and generally the primary site of infection. Evidence of infection in organ systems outside the central nervous system, such as skin, bone, and prostate, is commonly needed to implicate fungal infection. Typical clinical features are headaches, myalgia, fever, intermittent nausea, and photophobia. Cognition may rapidly become impaired, and patients may have marked abulia and lethargy due to irreversible, devastating brain damage. The presentation often is nonspecific and atypical, making the diagnosis very difficult.

Coccidioides immitis is endemic to the southwestern United States and the central valley of California. Dissemination is usually seen only in immunosuppressed patients but occurs in 1% of infected patients. Central nervous system involvement is typically severe and fatal if untreated.

Other fungal causes must be considered in the differential diagnosis. Organisms include *Cryptococcus neoformans*, *Blastomyces dermatitidis*, *Histoplasma capsulatum*, *Aspergillus* species, and a number of uncommon pathogens, all with possibly similar presentations and CSF formulae. Meningitis is the most common manifestation of infection by *C. neoformans* and is generally found in immunocompromised patients. It is

ubiquitous and protean in its presentation, ranging from indolent changes in cognitive function to florid meningoencephalitis.[82,83] *H. capsulatum* is found in the Ohio and Mississippi river valleys, and most persons in endemic areas have positive skin tests for previous infection. Active disease is rare and, again, seen most commonly in immunocompromised hosts. *Aspergillus* is a common fungal pathogen with a predilection for the brain parenchyma over the meninges. Abscess formation is common, as is central nervous system vasculitis.

Case reports of blastomycotic meningitis are noteworthy for the frequent misdiagnosis of tuberculous meningitis (see Chapter 16).[84,85] The similar clinical characteristics and the nodular appearance of meningeal enhancement on MRI in both diseases make distinction between the two difficult. Not infrequently, patients have been treated with antituberculous agents before the accurate diagnosis of blastomycotic meningitis. This can further confuse the diagnosis, because rifampin has some therapeutic benefit in treating blastomycosis and incomplete treatment with that drug may lead to reactivation of disease.

Interpretation of Diagnostic Tests

Magnetic Resonance Imaging
Prominent enhancement of the meninges can be found. A nodular appearance may suggest a fungal cause. Scattered hyperintensities in the basal ganglia may represent extension of infection along penetrating arteries (Fig. 17.8).[86]

Cerebrospinal Fluid
Typical findings are lymphocytic pleocytosis, borderline decreased glucose concentration, and mildly increased protein level. CSF serology for *C. neoformans*, *C. immitis*, *H. capsulatum*, and *B. dermatitidis* should be done; but the results may be negative.

Brain Biopsy
Brain biopsy should be considered early, but the poor sensitivity of microscopy in identifying the organism in biopsied specimens is often remarkable. Culture of CSF and brain tissue obtained at operation remains the prime diagnostic test.

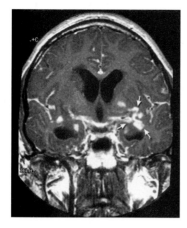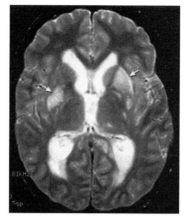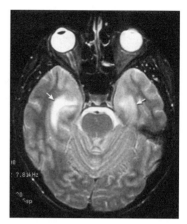

Figure 17.8 Magnetic resonance images showing diffuse nodular enhancement of basal meninges, with abnormal T_2 signal in the basal ganglia bilaterally and bitemporal lesions representing encephalitis (*arrows*). The fungus isolated from brain biopsy culture was *Blastomyces*. (From Friedman et al.[86])

First Priority in Management

Ketoconazole or, more recently, itraconazole is the first-line agent for pulmonary blastomycosis.[87] Amphotericin B is usually reserved for more serious clinical situations or refractory disease, but many experts believe that it is the drug of choice in patients with meningeal involvement. Most authorities recommend a total dose of amphotericin B of 2–3 g. One should also consider intrathecal (using the Ommaya reservoir) amphotericin B (test dose of 0.01–0.1 mg for 3 days followed by 0.5 mg 3 times a week). Hydrocephalus may become considerable, and ventriculostomy is needed. This provides the opportunity to culture CSF, but brain biopsy may be needed to unveil the fungus.[88]

Predictors of Outcome

These disorders are rare, but morbidity is substantial. Amphotericin therapy may be successful in arresting progression of neurologic manifestations. Despite early initiation of empirical treatment with amphotericin, death has been reported.

Triage

• Brain biopsy to confirm the diagnosis, and surgery may be indicated if a single abscess has formed.
• Ventriculostomy may be needed to relieve hydrocephalus.
• To the ward for intravenous amphotericin B therapy.

Paraneoplastic Limbic Encephalitis

The rare disorder paraneoplastic limbic encephalitis should be considered when infectious agents seem highly unlikely. A history of depression, agitation, paranoia, and feelings of depersonalization and memory loss may be obtained.[89] The pathologic substrate can be extensive, with neuronal loss, perivascular monocytic infiltrates, and microglial nodules, predominantly in the limbic and insular cortices but also located in the brain stem, spinal cord, and dorsal root ganglia.[90] It is uncommon to find a neoplasm during life, but the condition can be the first manifestation or appear in a patient with a previous diagnosis of small cell (oat cell) carcinoma, Hodgkin's disease, or testicular seminoma.[91–94]

Clinical Presentation

Rapid onset of mood changes, usually sadness, detachment, and loss of recent memory, is the characteristic presentation, but more fulminant forms are manifested by agitation, hallucinations, and bizarre behavior preceding a decrease in alertness. (The diagnosis is often suggested when the psychiatric symptoms progress despite psychotropic drugs.) Lack of topographic orientation has been noted.[95] Coma is uncommon and, if present, mostly from secondary causes, such as infections, sepsis, and acute metabolic derangements.

Neurologic examination clearly demonstrates only poor recall, clinical signs of major depression, and, if the patient is specifically asked, behavioral abnormalities and hallucinations. Subtle brain stem or cerebellar signs and symptoms may be evident in some patients.

Interpretation of Diagnostic Tests

Full evaluation for a possible malignancy workup is therefore needed and should include CT scan of the chest and lymph node biopsy in patients with lymphadenopathy because of the common association with Hodgkin's disease and lung cancer. However, diagnostic evaluation may be extended to exclude gastrointestinal, kidney, and gynecologic malignant diseases and thus should include mammogram, pelvic examination, testicular ultrasonography, serum cancer markers, and antineuronal nuclear antibodies.[92,93,96–98]

Electroencephalography
The EEG may be normal early in the course but will show progressive nonspecific slowing of the background rhythm with temporal slow waves and spike foci. Epileptiform activity is uncommon.

Computed Tomography and Magnetic Resonance Imaging
Normal findings are common and often suggest the diagnosis in the proper situation. However, T_2-weighted hyperintensity changes in the medial temporal lobes may appear with contrast enhancement in the temporal lobes, amygdala, and hippocampus (Fig. 17.9).[94] MR abnormalities may improve with successful treatment of underlying cancer.[99]

Cerebrospinal Fluid and Serum
CSF is under normal opening pressures, but an increased protein and mononuclear pleocytosis varied from 30 to 150 total nucleated cells in more than 50% of the reported cases. Normal CSF or only mildly increased protein is less common.

Anti-HU (term derived from a patient's initials) denotes an autoantibody in patients with cancer, predominantly small cell lung cancer (Chapter 2). It is found mostly in patients with subacute sensory neuropathy leading to severe ataxia but can be found in paraneoplastic limbic encephalitis.[96] Anti-HU is a polyclonal IgG antibody reacting with neuron nuclei in vitro. The HU antigen has been cloned, and a cell-mediated response toward one of the HU antigens (HUD) has been documented.[97] The specificity and sensitivity for the anti-HU test are not exactly known, but low titers can be found in patients with cancer and no neurologic involvement. Antibodies to voltage-gated potassium channels were detected and seem to correlate with clinical manifestation.[100]

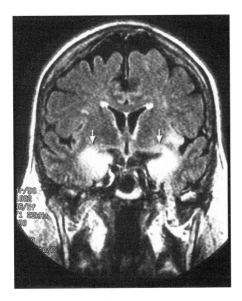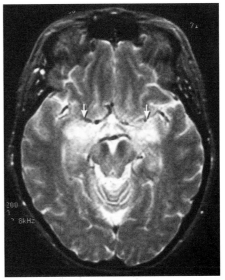

Figure 17.9 Magnetic resonance images of limbic paraneoplastic encephalitis, showing symmetric T_2 signal in mesial temporal lobe (*arrows*).

Brain Biopsy

Stereotactic brain biopsy may show perivascular infiltrates with predominantly B cells, and microglia-like cells may be observed surrounding neurons.[101]

Predictors of Outcome

The clinical course is progressive, but fluctuations may occur. The interval from initial psychiatric signs to death due to infections varies greatly, from 1 month to 2 years. Treatment of underlying cancer has resulted in substantial improvement in only some patients. Plasma exchange resulted in improvement in a patient with potassium channel antibodies.[100]

Triage

- Supportive measures and hospital admission for full medical evaluation and a search for the underlying cancer are needed.
- Management of respiratory complications from aspiration or sepsis and brain biopsy to exclude other treatable disorders may justify brief intensive care unit admission.

REFERENCES

1. Johnson RT: Acute encephalitis. Clin Infect Dis 23:219, 1996.
2. Campbell GL, Marfin AA, Lanciotti RS, et al.: West Nile virus. Lancet Infect Dis 2:519, 2002.
3. Lanska DJ: Anthrax meningoencephalitis. Neurology 59:327, 2002.
4. Koskiniemi M, Piiparinen H, Mannonen L, et al.: Herpes encephalitis is a disease of middle aged and elderly people: polymerase chain reaction for detection of herpes simplex virus in the CSF of 516 patients with encephalitis. J Neurol Neurosurg Psychiatry 60:174, 1996.
5. Bonawitz C, Castillo M, Mukherji SK: Comparison of CT and MR features with clinical outcome in patients with Rocky Mountain spotted fever. AJNR Am J Neuroradiol 18:459, 1997.
6. Sköldenberg B: Herpes simplex encephalitis. Scand J Infect Dis Suppl 100:8, 1996.
7. Chretien F, Belec L, Hilton DA, et al.: Herpes simplex virus type 1 encephalitis in acquired immunodeficiency syndrome. Neuropathol Appl Neurobiol 22:394, 1996.
8. Hamilton RL, Achim C, Grafe MR, et al.: Herpes simplex virus brainstem encephalitis in an AIDS patient. Clin Neuropathol 14:45, 1995.
9. McGrath NM, Anderson NE, Hope JK, et al.: Anterior opercular syndrome, caused by herpes simplex encephalitis. Neurology 49:494, 1997.
10. van der Poel JC, Haenggeli CA, Overweg-Plandsoen WC: Operculum syndrome: unusual feature of herpes simplex encephalitis. Pediatr Neurol 12:246, 1995.
11. Fisher CM: Hypomanic symptoms caused by herpes simplex encephalitis. Neurology 47:1374, 1996.
12. Ciardi M, Giacchetti G, Fedele CG, et al.: Acute cerebellitis caused by herpes simplex virus type 1. Clin Infect Dis 36:50, 2003.
13. Amlie-Lefond C, Kleinschmidt-DeMasters BK, Mahalingam R, et al.: The vasculopathy of varicella-zoster virus encephalitis. Ann Neurol 37:784, 1995.
14. Jeffery KJ, Read SJ, Peto TE, et al.: Diagnosis of viral infections of the central nervous system: clinical interpretation of PCR results. Lancet 349:313, 1997.
15. Lakeman FD, Whitley RJ: Diagnosis of herpes simplex encephalitis: application of polymerase chain reaction to cerebrospinal fluid from brain-biopsied patients and correlation with disease. J Infect Dis 171:857, 1995.
16. Wildemann B, Ehrhart K, Storch-Hagenlocher B, et al.: Quantitation of herpes simplex virus type 1 DNA in cells of cerebrospinal fluid of patients with herpes simplex virus encephalitis. Neurology 48:1341, 1997.
17. Arribas JR, Storch GA, Clifford DB, et al.: Cytomegalovirus encephalitis. Ann Intern Med 125:577, 1996.
18. Novati R, Castagna A, Morsica G, et al.: Polymerase chain reaction for Toxoplasma gondii DNA in the cerebrospinal fluid of AIDS patients with focal brain lesions. AIDS 8:1691, 1994.
19. Smith JB, Westmoreland BF, Reagan TJ, et al.: A distinctive clinical EEG profile in herpes simplex encephalitis. Mayo Clin Proc 50:469, 1975.
20. Raschilas F, Wolff M, Delatour F, et al.: Outcome of and prognostic factors for herpes simplex encephalitis in adult patients: results of a multicenter study. Clin Infect Dis 35:254, 2002.
21. White ML, Edwards-Brown MK: Fluid attenuated inversion recovery (FLAIR) MRI of herpes encephalitis. J Comput Assist Tomogr 19:501, 1995.
22. Revello MG, Manservigi R: Molecular diagnosis of herpes simplex encephalitis. Intervirology 39: 185, 1996.
23. Tebas P, Nease RF, Storch GA: Use of the polymerase chain reaction in the diagnosis of herpes simplex encephalitis: a decision analysis model. Am J Med 105:287, 1998.
24. Preiser W, Weber B, Klos G, et al.: Unusual course of herpes simplex virus encephalitis after acyclovir therapy. Infection 24:384, 1996.
25. Kennedy PGE, Chaudhuri A: Herpes simplex encephalitis. J Neurol Neurosurg Psychiatry 73:237, 2002.
26. Takanashi J, Sugita K, Ishii M, et al.: Longitudinal MR imaging and proton MR spectroscopy in herpes simplex encephalitis. J Neurol Sci 149:99, 1997.
27. Hokkanen L, Salonen O, Launes J: Amnesia in acute herpetic and nonherpetic encephalitis. Arch Neurol 53:972, 1996.

28. Launes J, Siren J, Valanne L, et al.: Unilateral hyperfusion in brain-perfusion SPECT predicts poor prognosis in acute encephalitis. *Neurology* 48:1347, 1997.

29. Lowry PW: Arbovirus encephalitis in the United States and Asia. *J Lab Clin Med* 129:405, 1997.

30. Mancao MY, Law IM, Roberson-Trammell K: California encephalitis in Alabama. *South Med J* 89:992, 1996.

31. Deresiewicz RL, Thaler SJ, Hsu L, et al.: Clinical and neuroradiographic manifestations of eastern equine encephalitis. *N Engl J Med* 336:1867, 1997.

32. Komar N, Spielman A: Emergence of eastern encephalitis in Massachusetts. *Ann NY Acad Sci* 740:157, 1994.

33. Igarashi A: Epidemiology and control of Japanese encephalitis. *World Health Stat Q* 45:299, 1992.

34. Wittesjö B, Eitrem R, Niklasson B, et al.: Japanese encephalitis after a 10-day holiday in Bali. *Lancet* 345:856, 1995.

35. Misra UK, Kalita J: Seizures in Japanese encephalitis. *J Neurol Sci* 190:57-60, 2001.

36. Jelinek T, Nothdurft HD: Japanese encephalitis vaccine in travelers. Is wider use prudent? *Drug Saf* 16:153, 1997.

37. Haglund M, Forsgren M, Lindh G, et al.: A 10-year follow-up study of tick-borne encephalitis in the Stockholm area and a review of the literature: need for a vaccination strategy. *Scand J Infect Dis* 28:217, 1996.

38. Prokopowicz D, Bobrowska E, Bobrowski M, et al.: Prevalence of antibodies against tick-borne encephalitis among residents of north-eastern Poland. *Scand J Infect Dis* 27:15, 1995.

39. Roggendorf M: Epidemiology of tick-borne encephalitis virus in Germany. *Infection* 24:465, 1996.

40. Treib J, Haass A, Mueller-Lantzsch N, et al.: Tick-borne encephalitis in the Saarland and the Rhineland-Palatinate. *Infection* 24:242, 1996.

41. Flaherty ML, Wijdicks EFM, Stevens JC, et al.: Clinical and electrophysiologic patterns of flaccid paralysis due to West Nile virus. Mayo Clin Proc 78:1245, 2003.

42. Sejvar JJ, Haddad MB, Tierney BC, et al.: Neurologic manifestations and outcome of West Nile virus infection. JAMA 290:511, 2003; Erratum in: JAMA 290:1318, 2003.

43. Li J, Loeb JA, Shy ME, et al. Asymmetric flaccid paralysis: A neuromuscular presentation of West Nile virus infection. *Ann Neurol* 53:703, 2003.

44. Kumar S, Misra UK, Kalita J, et al.: MRI in Japanese encephalitis. *Neuroradiology* 39:180, 1997.

45. Misra UK, Kalita J, Jain SK, et al.: Radiological and neurophysiological changes in Japanese encephalitis. *J Neurol Neurosurg Psychiatry* 57:1484, 1994.

46. Shoji H, Murakami T, Murai I, et al.: A follow-up study by CT and MRI in 3 cases of Japanese encephalitis. *Neuroradiology* 32:215, 1990.

47. Huang C, Chatterjee NK, Grady LJ.: Diagnosis of viral infections of the central nervous system. *N Engl J Med* 340:483, 1999.

48. Hoke CH Jr, Vaughn DW, Nisalak A, et al.: Effect of high-dose dexamethasone on the outcome of acute encephalitis due to Japanese encephalitis virus. *J Infect Dis* 165:631, 1992.

49. Pierelli F, Tilia G, Damiani A, et al.: Brainstem CMV encephalitis in AIDS: clinical case and MRI features. *Neurology* 48:529, 1997.

50. Kleinschmidt-DeMasters BK, Amlie-Lefond C, Gilden DH: The patterns of varicella zoster virus encephalitis. *Hum Pathol* 27:927, 1996.

51. Case records of the Massachusetts General Hospital. Weekly clinicopathological exercises. Case 36-1996. A 37-year-old man with AIDS neurologic deterioration and multiple hemorrhagic cerebral lesions. *N Engl J Med* 335:1587, 1996.

52. Weaver S, Rosenblum MK, DeAngelis LM: Herpes varicella zoster encephalitis in immunocompromised patients. *Neurology* 52:193, 1999.

53. Bergstrom T: Polymerase chain reaction for diagnosis of varicella zoster virus central nervous system infections without skin manifestations. *Scand J Infect Dis Suppl* 100:41, 1996.

54. Maschke M, Kastrup O, Diener HC: CNS manifestations of cytomegalovirus infections: diagnosis and treatment. *CNS Drugs* 16:303, 2002.

55. Marrie TJ, Raoult D: Rickettsial infections of the central nervous system. *Semin Neurol* 12:213, 1992.

56. Horney LF, Walker DH: Meningoencephalitis as a major manifestation of Rocky Mountain spotted fever. *South Med J* 81:915, 1988.

57. Katz DA, Dworzack DL, Horowitz EA, et al.: Encephalitis associated with Rocky Mountain spotted fever. *Arch Pathol Lab Med* 109:771, 1985.

58. Kirk JL, Fine DP, Sexton DJ, et al.: Rocky Mountain spotted fever. A clinical review based on 48 confirmed cases, 1943-1986. *Medicine* (Baltimore) 69:35, 1990.

59. Sempere AP, Elizaga J, Duarte J, et al.: Q fever mimicking herpetic encephalitis. *Neurology* 43:2713, 1993.

60. Silpapojakul K, Ukkachoke C, Krisanapan S, et al.: Rickettsial meningitis and encephalitis. *Arch Intern Med* 151:1753, 1991.

61. Baganz MD, Dross PE, Reinhardt JA: Rocky Mountain spotted fever encephalitis: MR findings. *AJNR Am J Neuroradiol* 16(Suppl 4):919, 1995.

62. Lorenzl S, Pfister HW, Padovan C, et al.: MRI abnormalities in tick-borne encephalitis. *Lancet* 347:698, 1996.

63. Tzianabos T, Anderson BE, McDade JE: Detection of *Rickettsia rickettsii* DNA in clinical specimens by using polymerase chain reaction technology. *J Clin Microbiol* 27:2866, 1989.

64. Shaked Y: Rickettsial infection of the central nervous system: the role of prompt antimicrobial therapy. *Q J Med* 79:301, 1991.

65. Domínguez E, Bustos C, Garcia M, et al.: Anthrax meningoencephalitis: radiologic findings. *AJR Am J Roentgenol* 169:317, 1997.

66. Kim HJ, Jun WB, Lee SH, et al.: CT and MR findings of anthrax meningoencephalitis: report of two cases and review of the literature, *AJNR Am J Neuroradiol* 22:1303, 2001.

67. Peacock JE Jr, Folds J, Orringer E, et al.: *Toxoplasma gondii* and the compromised host. Antibody response in

the absence of clinical manifestations of disease. *Arch Intern Med* 143:1235, 1983.

68. Deleze M, Mintz G, del Carmen Mejia M: *Toxoplasma gondii* encephalitis in systemic lupus erythematosus. A neglected cause of treatable nervous system infection. *J Rheumatol* 12:994, 1985.

69. Porter SB, Sande MA: Toxoplasmosis of the central nervous system in the acquired immunodeficiency syndrome. *N Engl J Med* 327:1643, 1992.

70. Knobel H, Guelar A, Graus F, et al.: Toxoplasmic encephalitis with normal CT scan and pathologic MRI. *Am J Med* 99:220, 1995.

71. Casado-Naranjo I, Lopez-Trigo J, Ferrandiz A, et al.: Hemorrhagic abscess in a patient with the acquired immunodeficiency syndrome. *Neuroradiology* 31:289, 1989.

72. Wijdicks EFM, Borleffs JC, Hoepelman AI, et al.: Fatal disseminated hemorrhagic toxoplasmic encephalitis as the initial manifestation of AIDS. *Ann Neurol* 29:683, 1991.

73. Brightbill TC, Post MJ, Hensley GT, et al.: MR of toxoplasma encephalitis: signal characteristics on T2-weighted images and pathologic correlation. *J Comput Assist Tomogr* 20:417, 1996.

74. Roberts TC, Storch GA: Multiplex PCR for diagnosis of AIDS-related central nervous system lymphoma and toxoplasmosis. *J Clin Microbiol* 35:268, 1997.

75. Campbell BG, Hurley J, Zimmerman RD: False-negative single-photon emission CT in AIDS lymphoma: lack of effect of steroids. *AJNR Am J Neuroradiol* 17:1000, 1996.

76. O'Malley JP, Ziessman HA, Kumar PN, et al.: Diagnosis of intracranial lymphoma in patients with AIDS: value of [201]TI single-photon emission computed tomography. *AJR Am J Roentgenol* 163:417, 1994.

77. Ruiz A, Ganz WI, Post MJ, et al.: Use of thallium-201 brain SPECT to differentiate cerebral lymphoma from toxoplasma encephalitis in AIDS patients. *AJNR Am J Neuroradiol* 15:1885, 1994.

78. Fung HB, Kirschenbaum HL: Treatment regimens for patients with toxoplasmic encephalitis. *Clin Ther* 18:1037, 1996.

79. Dannemann BR, Israelski DM, Remington JS: Treatment of toxoplasmic encephalitis with intravenous clindamycin. *Arch Intern Med* 148:2477, 1988.

80. Green JA, Spruance SL, Cheson BD: Favorable outcome of central nervous system toxoplasmosis occurring in a patient with untreated Hodgkin's disease. *Cancer* 45:808, 1980.

81. Treseler CB, Sugar AM: Fungal meningitis. *Infect Dis Clin North Am* 4:789, 1990.

82. Minamoto GY, Rosenberg AS: Fungal infections in patients with acquired immunodeficiency syndrome. *Med Clin North Am* 81:381, 1997.

83. Lyons RW, Andriole VT: Fungal infections of the CNS. *Neurol Clin* 4:159, 1986.

84. Gonyea EF: The spectrum of primary blastomycotic meningitis: a review of central nervous system blastomycosis. *Ann Neurol* 3:26, 1978.

85. Harley WB, Lomis M, Haas DW: Marked polymorphonuclear pleocytosis due to blastomycotic meningitis: case report and review. *Clin Infect Dis* 18:816, 1994.

86. Friedman J, Wijdicks EFM, Fulgham J, et al.: Meningoencephalitis due to blastomycosis dermatitis: a case report and literature review. *Mayo Clin Proc* 75:403, 2000.

87. Sarosi GA, Davies SF: Therapy for fungal infections. *Mayo Clin Proc* 69:1111, 1994.

88. Ward BA, Parent AD, Raila F: Indications for the surgical management of central nervous system blastomycosis. *Surg Neurol* 43:379, 1995.

89. Newman NJ, Bell IR, McKee AC: Paraneoplastic limbic encephalitis: neuropsychiatric presentation. *Biol Psychiatry* 27:529, 1990.

90. Camara EG, Chelune GJ: Paraneoplastic limbic encephalopathy. *Brain Behav Immun* 1:349, 1987.

91. Corsellis JA, Goldberg GJ, Norton AR: "Limbic encephalitis" and its association with carcinoma. *Brain* 91:481, 1968.

92. Deodhare S, O'Connor P, Ghazarian D, et al.: Paraneoplastic limbic encephalitis in Hodgkin's disease. *Can J Neurol Sci* 23:138, 1996.

93. Wingerchuk DM, Noseworthy JH, Kimmel DW: Paraneoplastic encephalomyelitis and seminoma: importance of testicular ultrasonography. *Neurology* 51:1504, 1998.

94. Kodama T, Numaguchi Y, Gellad FE, et al.: Magnetic resonance imaging of limbic encephalitis. *Neuroradiology* 33:520, 1991.

95. Hirayama K, Taguchi Y, Sato M, et al.: Limbic encephalitis presenting with topographical disorientation and amnesia. *J Neurol Neurosurg Psychiatry* 74:110, 2003.

96. Greenlee JE, Lipton HL: Anticerebellar antibodies in serum and cerebrospinal fluid of a patient with oat cell carcinoma of the lung and paraneoplastic cerebellar degeneration. *Ann Neurol* 19:82, 1986.

97. Benyahia B, Liblau R, Merle-Beral H, et al.: Cell-mediated autoimmunity in paraneoplastic neurological syndromes with anti-Hu antibodies. *Ann Neurol* 45:162, 1999.

98. Almera C, Soussi N, Molko N, et al.: Paraneoplastic limbic encephalitis, a complication of the testicular cancer. *Urology* 58:105, 2001.

99. Messori A, Lanza C, Serio A, et al.: Resolution of limbic encephalitis with detection and treatment of lung cancer: clinical–radiological correlation. *Eur J Radiol* 45:78, 2003.

100. Buckley C, Oger J, Clover L: Potassium channel antibodies in two patients with reversible limbic encephalitis. *Ann Neurol* 50:73, 2001.

101. Jean WC, Dalmau J, Ho A, et al.: Analysis of the IgG subclass distribution and inflammatory infiltrates in patients with anti-Hu-associated paraneoplastic encephalomyelitis. *Neurology* 44:140, 1994.

Chapter 18
Acute White Matter Diseases

Devastating white matter disorders are fulminant multiple sclerosis (MS), transverse myelitis, and disseminated encephalomyelitis. Even in academic institutions, they are sporadically seen. They are included in this book because it is important to diagnose and manage these disorders quickly.

Acute demyelination of the neuraxis may turn out catastrophic, and treatment in the acute phase remains problematic. Generally, rapid cures remain few and far between. However, aggressive immunosuppression or plasma exchange may shorten the relapse and, in certain disorders, resolve some or virtually all of its manifestations.

A related disorder, often with an acute onset, is acute leukoencephalopathy, occurring in a diverse group of patients. In this entity, demyelination or edema is part of a more global involvement of white matter structures. Toxicity from immunosuppressive and chemotherapeutic agents is commonly implicated or a hypertensive crisis may touch off white matter edema or demyelination. These disorders may resolve quickly after elimination of the trigger alone.

Acute Disseminated Encephalomyelitis

Acute disseminated encephalomyelitis (ADEM) is a dramatic monophasic illness resulting from an autoimmune response activated by a viral infection or vaccination. ADEM occurs more often in children and young adults, and most infections are mundane viral respiratory episodes. ADEM may also follow any well-defined illness (e.g., rubeola, varicella, mycoplasmal pneumonia,[1,2] infectious mononucleosis, and hepatitis C[3]) or may occur without an identifiable antecedent event.

Even in the most severe fatal cases, use of polymerase chain reaction analysis to recover a virus (e.g., enterovirus, adenovirus, herpesvirus, and respiratory syncytial virus) from the brain during autopsy has not been successful (no virus has been isolated from the cerebrospinal fluid [CSF]). More recently, human herpesvirus 6 has been associated with ADEM.[4] Neurologic manifestation occurs after a delay of 1–3 weeks but progresses rapidly to a maximum within days. Widespread involvement of the central nervous system may affect many eloquent areas of the brain and cord. White matter destruction involving the optic tract, brain stem, and spinal cord that resembles acute transverse myelitis is a classic finding if the disorder progresses. Pathologic features of ADEM include multifocal patchy perivenous demyelination.

Clinical Presentation

Patients or their consulted family members recall a flu-like illness with a variable combination of fever, aching joints, swollen lymph nodes, and fatigue. Some of these constitutional symptoms may still be present at onset.

Initially, headaches with transient focal neurologic signs may be prominent and fluctuating.

Neurologic findings further reflect acute myelin destruction and may consist of any degree of impairment of consciousness, with several prompts needed to alert patients to their surroundings. In others, ophthalmoplegia, cerebellar ataxia, and speech abnormality may evolve to muteness. Fever, loss of consciousness, and meningism, if present, are more common in patients with a single event.[5]

Spinal cord involvement may be the first presenting symptom or may quickly merge into a more diffuse or multifocal neurologic symptom complex. Progressive quadriparesis may result in early inability to walk, but level of consciousness should also become involved at this time.

Progression is within days, but a clinical course with up to 2 months of gradual, protracted change has been documented. ADEM can be mistaken for central nervous system lymphoma, vasculitis, viral encephalitis, and manifestations of flaring up rheumatologic disorders, some of which have yet to be diagnosed (Table 18.1).

Interpretation of Diagnostic Tests

Computed Tomography and Magnetic Resonance Imaging

Computed tomographic (CT) and magnetic resonance imaging (MRI) findings are fairly typical but may be rather subtle in earlier stages. The typical appearance in ADEM is multiple discrete lesions in the cerebral white matter and rarely in periventricular areas, a location much more typical of fulminant MS. The lesions predominate in occipital-parietal white matter (Fig. 18.1A,B) but may involve the basal ganglia, thalamus, and brain stem.[6,7] A single bout confined to the brain stem has been recorded.[8] Symmetrical cerebellar white

Table 18.1. Disorders Mimicking Acute Disseminated Encephalomyelitis

Acute viral encephalitis (arboviruses)
Herpes simplex encephalitis
Central nervous system vasculitis
Intravascular lymphoma
Progressive multifocal leukoencephalopathy
Neurosarcoidosis
Systemic lupus erythematosus
Sjögren's disease

matter and basal ganglia involvement may differentiate it from MS.[9,10] All of these abnormalities may hardly be detected by CT, and only some decreased attenuation in the white matter of the centrum semiovale is seen, even at the stage of prominent neurologic manifestations. MRI remains a crucial determinant for its diagnosis. Gadolinium enhancement is a reflection of the blood–brain barrier breakdown in the earlier stages of demyelination. Enhancement may appear in some lesions on MRI and not in others, suggesting different stages in demyelination.[11,12] Enhancement may be marginal because of corticosteroid treatment, which reduces the blood–brain barrier permeability.[13] If enhancement is found, abnormal signal intensity is more commonly found in the optic nerves (as opposed to unilateral optic neuritis in MS). Generally, these MRI features cannot be easily differentiated from those of MS nor has a more distinct histologic feature been identified in brain tissue specimens.

Hemorrhagic changes (Fig. 18.1C,D) suggest an acute hemorrhagic leukoencephalitis (Weston Hurst disease); and this disorder, noted after similar triggering circumstances, may primarily be an aggressive variant of ADEM. Not infrequently, it presents with massive brain edema.[14,15] Hyperintense lesions on T_2-weighted images, with ring-like solid enhancing lesions and perifocal edema, have been reported as well. Cortical involvement is compatible with the diagnosis, albeit less extensively distributed.

Cerebrospinal Fluid
CSF may show moderate pleocytosis (up to 200 cells/mm^3). In ADEM, the CSF contains lymphocytes; in Weston Hurst disease, polymorphonuclear leukocytes are prominent.[14] The pleocytosis is usually out of proportion to what is expected during a flare-up of MS. Oligoclonal bands can be found in up to 50% of cases[5] and may disappear after treatment (oligoclonal bands commonly persist in MS).

First Priority in Management

High-dose methylprednisolone (1000 mg intravenously daily) remains the first therapy of choice. Excellent recovery has also been observed with plasma exchange, and failure to improve rapidly

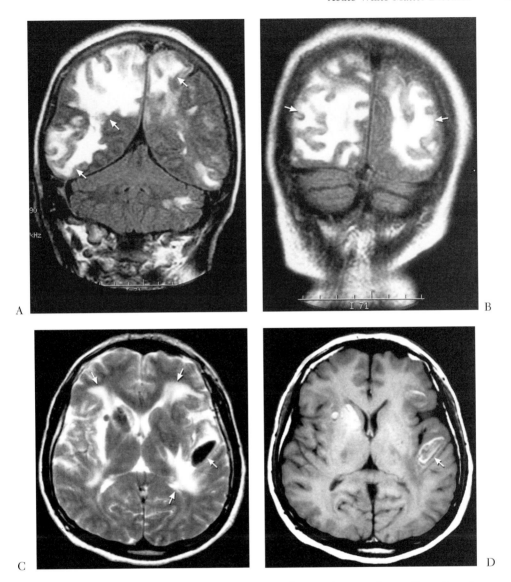

Figure 18.1 *A,B:* Magnetic resonance imaging with coronal views of acute disseminated encephalomyelitis. *C,D:* Hemorrhagic leukoencephalitis (Weston Hurst).

(arbitrarily defined as 1–2 days) with corticosteroids should prompt its use. The exact number of plasma exchanges is unknown, although exchanges for up to 10 days (or until improvement) have been proposed.[16–18] Alternatively, intravenous immunoglobulin, 0.4 g/kg for 5 days, can be used,[19,20] again, typically in patients worsening while receiving methylprednisolone.[21,22]

Predictors of Outcome

Improved arousal can be rather rapid and is followed by improvement in diplopia, bulbar dysfunction, and, more gradually, ambulation. Residual symptoms may remain but are in a minority disabling. MRI findings should closely parallel clinical improvement. Full recovery after Weston

Hurst disease has been described in several cases. One study suggested that one of three patients with ADEM develops MS within 3 years; this included patients with well-established triggers such as infection or vaccination.[5] This report also emphasized that the diagnosis of ADEM as a monophasic demyelinating disorder becomes likely only if the patient has remained asymptomatic for at least 1 year.[5]

Triage

- A brief period of observation in the intensive care unit and support with mechanical ventilation may be needed, but many patients are soon able to protect their airway and ventilate normally.
- Brain biopsy should be deferred until the effect of immunosuppressive therapy or plasma exchange has been evaluated.

Fulminant Multiple Sclerosis

Patients with clinically definitive or laboratory-supported MS may have very severe exacerbations. Progression into a devastating condition or death rarely is the first presentation. The designation *fulminant* in this condition is usually defined by symptoms and signs emerging in days rather than weeks and presupposes involvement of multiple areas in the cerebral white matter and often the brain stem. Demyelination, which leads to loss of ambulation from weakness or ataxia, may involve the bulbar function and respiratory control. A brain biopsy, usually performed to characterize the source of a new mass, shows fairly typical neuropathologic features of marked inflammatory perivascular infiltrates, extensive myelin breakdown that spares the nerve cell bodies and axis cylinders, and diffuse macrophage infiltration.

Clinical Presentation

Earlier descriptions of this fulminant variant emphasized an accelerated development of ataxia, hemiparesis, or paraparesis; blindness or progressive ophthalmoplegia; and notable bulbar involvement leading to dysphagia and aspiration. Brain stem involvement is a common feature in acute fulminant MS. Quadriparalysis and involvement of the lower cranial nerves with sparing of only the oculomotor nerves closely resemble a locked-in syndrome and often are linked to a fatal outcome.[23,24]

The most dramatic variant, one with high mortality, is the Marburg variant.[25,26] Within days, progressive ophthalmoplegia, dysarthria, dysphagia, and blindness may develop and the patient becomes comatose. An uncal brain herniation pattern appears when a large inflammatory demyelinating tumefactive lesion shifts brain tissue.

Mechanical ventilation is often needed in patients whose condition deteriorates to coma and in patients with bulbar signs. Neurogenic pulmonary edema as a result of sympathetic disinhibition may accompany the fulminant form.[27] In most patients, marked bulbar failure and inability to swallow secretions lead to aspiration pneumonitis, and upper cervical or spinal cord involvement impairs pulmonary mechanics.[28]

Interpretation of Diagnostic Tests

The diagnostic criteria of MS, including laboratory abnormalities, have been expertly outlined. A modification of the Poser criteria is shown in Box 18.1.[29]

Computed Tomography and Magnetic Resonance Imaging

MRI assists in the diagnosis, but findings are nonspecific. MRI suggests demyelination when lesions are hypointense or isointense on T_1-weighted images, occasionally display hyperintense edges, and are small, irregular, or confluent. White matter lesions are invariably located in the pons, medulla, additional hemispheric areas involving the junctions of gray and white matter, and corpus callosum. Larger confluent areas in periventricular white matter can be seen as well.[30,31] Ovoid lesions at right angles to the ventricular surface are characteristic (Fig. 18.2). Unilateral mass effect with developing edema may occur. Mass effect may be the most prominent CT scan manifestation (Fig. 18.3). Ringlike structures may appear, corresponding to layers of macrophages, which generate free radicals to produce this paramagnetic effect.[32] However, magnetic resonance spectroscopy studies have found that these rings

Box 18.1. Diagnostic Criteria for Multiple Sclerosis

Category	Subcategory	No. of Clinical Attacks	No. of Clinically Evident Lesions	Paraclinical Evidence°	CSF Oligoclonal Bands
CDMS	A1	2	2	N/A	N/A
	A2	2	1	and 1 (or more)	N/A
	A3	1	1	2[†]	N/A
LSDMS	B1	2	1	or 1 (or more)	+
	B2	1	2	—	+
	B3	1	1	and 1 (or more)	+

CDMS, clinically definite multiple sclerosis; CSF, cerebrospinal fluid; LSDMS, laboratory-supported definite multiple sclerosis; N/A, not applicable; +, present.

°Implies magnetic resonance imaging, evoked potentials, or CSF.

[†]A diagnosis of CDMS A3 requires paraclinical evidence for dissemination in time as well as space.

Source: Paty DW, Noseworthy JH, Ebers GC: Diagnosis of multiple sclerosis. In DW Paty, GC Ebers (eds), *Multiple Sclerosis. Contemporary Neurology Series.* Philadelphia: FA Davis, 1998, p. 48. By permission of Oxford University Press.

more than likely represent central edema in the core of the ring plaque.[33]

Evoked Potentials

Evoked potential studies may detect asymptomatic lesions.[34,35] Pattern reversal visual evoked potential is sensitive for lesions in the optic nerve and chiasm, and findings are abnormal in 40%–60% of patients with early MS.[31] The sensitivity in median nerve somatosensory evoked potentials is similar. Brain stem auditory evoked potentials are less sensitive and positive in only 20%–25% of patients with MS.[34]

Evoked potentials probably are most useful for providing supportive laboratory evidence of MS when additional diagnostic tests are abnormal.[35]

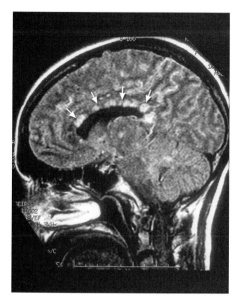
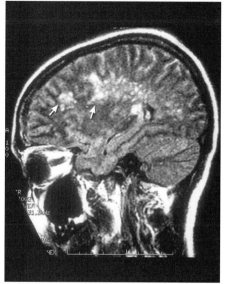

Figure 18.2 Fulminant multiple sclerosis with multiple periventricular white matter lesions and characteristic scattered lesions in the corpus callosum and brain stem.

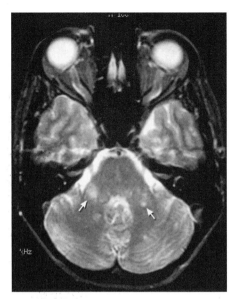
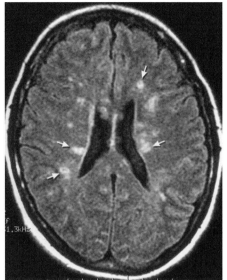

Figure 18.2 (*Continued*)

Cerebrospinal Fluid

Cell count can vary from 10 to 50 lymphocytes/mm³, with a mixture of monocytes, plasma cells, and macrophages. Total protein is mildly increased, and immunoglobulin G (IgG) is increased in 70% of clinically definite MS. Two or more oligoclonal bands in the gamma field may be detected in only 40% of patients with first presentation of MS. Intrathecal immunoglobulin in the CSF is a result of increased plasma cell synthesis and leakage from the brain through a defective blood–brain barrier. Oligoclonal bands in the CSF (at least two different and distinct bands) but not in the serum are typical for MS but can occur in 8% of patients with other neurologic diseases that may superficially mimic MS (viral meningoen-

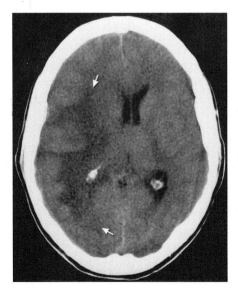
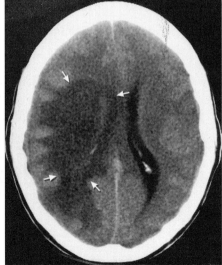

Figure 18.3 Marked mass effect and edema common in the Marburg variant of multiple sclerosis.

cephalitis, neurosyphilis, sarcoidosis, and fungal meningitis). The sensitivity of oligoclonal bands in CSF for MS is more than 90%.[36]

First Priority in Management

Intravenous administration of methylprednisolone, 1 g per day for 3–5 days, is followed by 60 mg of prednisone.[37] The number of contrast-enhancing lesions is significantly reduced.[38] Tapering of oral prednisone should be completed in 14 days. Overall prognosis is not affected by corticosteroids. Azathioprine, methotrexate, cyclophosphamide, and cyclosporine have no demonstrated benefit in acute progressive MS.

High doses of corticosteroids may not be sufficient to counter the fulminant attack, and evidence in patients with fulminant MS suggests that plasma exchange may be useful.[39,40] Improvement begins within several days, reversing quadriplegia and dependence on a mechanical ventilator. Plasmapheresis has shown no effect in long-term outcome of progressive MS, but it may be beneficial in fulminant exacerbations by removing soluble factors involved in the process of demyelination. The number of plasma exchanges is unknown, but up to six exchanges every other day may be needed.[39,40]

Two forms of recombinant interferon-beta should be considered. These agents decrease clinical relapses by 30%, halve the number of severe relapses, and lengthen time to first relapse. They are administered subcutaneously (interferon-beta-1b, 8 million units every other day) or intramuscularly (interferon-beta-1a, 6 million units weekly). The effects of a new agent, glatiramer acetate (20 mg subcutaneously daily), are similar.[41] An evidence-based report on therapy in MS has been made available by the American Academy of Neurology, and some of the pertinent conclusions are summarized in Table 18.2. There is insufficient proof of effect and concern of more harm using sulfasalazine, mitoxantrone, cyclophosphamide, and cladribine.[42]

Predictors of Outcome

Fulminant MS is associated with a high probability of permanent disability and with a somewhat shortened life span, strongly dependent on the degree of disability. Unfavorable prognostic factors are age over 40, male gender, and extensive MRI abnormalities (increased T_2 lesion load and number of active enhancing lesions). The relapse rate varies after a first major attack but decreases over time. After the first attack, approximately 25% of patients have a relapse within 1 year and 50% within 3 years. The extent of disability 5 years after the diagnosis strongly determines the future clinical course.[29] Recovery may be protracted, lasting 3–4 weeks; and intercurrent infections may contribute to early mortality.

Triage

- Early aspiration pneumonia, fever, or major oropharyngeal involvement justifies admission to an intensive care unit.
- Placement of an intracranial pressure device is warranted in the Marburg variant of MS, to monitor clinical progression and treat increased intracranial pressure.

Table 18.2. Therapy in Multiple Sclerosis (MS)

Drug/Procedure	Specific Effect	Effectiveness
Glucosteroids	Shorten acute attack	Established
	Reduce attack rate of relapsing-remitting MS	Possible
Interferon-β	Reduces attack rate in MS or isolated syndromes at high risk of developing MS	Probable
Intravenous immunoglobulin	Reduces attack rate in relapsing-remitting MS	Possible
Glatiramer acetate	Reduces attack rate in relapsing-remitting MS	Possible
Methotrexate	Alters disease in progressive MS	Possible
Azathioprine	Reduces relapse rate	Possible
Cyclosporine	Some benefit in progressive MS	Possible
Plasma exchange	Severe acute episodes in previously nondisabled patients	Possible

Data from Goodin et al.[42]

- Neurosurgical consultation for craniotomy or biopsy may be needed to pathologically confirm the diagnosis.

Acute Transverse Myelitis

Acute transverse myelitis is an uncommon, potentially devastating disorder associated with many illnesses (Table 18.3). Diagnostic criteria for idiopathic transverse myelitis have been published.[43] It is not a likely consideration if there had been prior radiation to the spine within the last 10 years, evidence of connective tissue disease, or a variety of infectious agents.[43] A vigorously mounted immune response is attributed to its pathogenesis. Demyelination and inflammation involve the spinal cord at any level, but often the effects are limited to a few segments. However, patients presenting with acute paraparesis and a distinct sensory level more commonly have extramedullary cord compression or another cause of myelitis. Chapter 12 presents the overall evaluation of acute spinal cord compression.

Clinical Presentation

Rapid ascending sensory deficit and difficulty walking within days are hallmarks of the disorder.[44] Fever and nuchal rigidity may occur in 27% and 13% of patients, respectively.[45] Paresthesias may be widespread, but usually a sensory level below which sensation is abnormal is pointed out by the patient.

Table 18.3. Causes of Acute Transverse Myelitis

Echovirus
Varicella
Herpes zoster
Herpes simplex (HSV1, HSV2)
Influenza
Epstein-Barr virus
Cytomegalovirus
Mycoplasma
Parasite infection (e.g., schistosomiasis)
Vaccination
Multiple sclerosis
Lupus erythematosus
Sjögren's syndrome
Syphilis
Lyme disease

Motor weakness may vary substantially, with a maximum deficit usually within 1–2 days, although subacute progression up to 2 months is known. However, maximal motor deficit may be reached within several hours.

The neurologic findings are typical of a functional cord transection at one segment, with loss of motor and sensory function and areflexia. All spinal cord levels can become involved. Partial variants have been described, with incomplete involvement, patchy and dissociated sensory symptoms, and sparing of the bladder.

Interpretation of Diagnostic Tests

Magnetic Resonance Imaging
MRI is preferred, to exclude causes that are potentially reversible. The rarity of the disorder implies that other causes of paraplegia are more frequent in clinical practice. MRI should be performed at once and, if necessary, patients should be referred to a tertiary center.

MRI findings are swelling of the cord, increased T_2-weighted signal, and often abnormal enhancement throughout the cord.[46–50]

More extensive involvement may be found on MRI than is clinically evident and vice versa (Fig. 18.4). A swollen cord is difficult to differentiate from an intramedullary neoplasm or dural arteriovenous malformation causing venous hypertension (see Chapter 12), but follow-up MRI, usually within weeks, should demonstrate complete resolution or substantial improvement. MRI of the brain and visual evoked potentials are useful to demonstrate other demyelinating lesions that increase the probability of MS or Devic's disease, with acute transverse myelitis as the first defining lesion.

Cerebrospinal Fluid
CSF examination may show pleocytosis of up to 10,000 cells (both lymphocytes and polymorphonuclear leukocytes), but CSF cell count can be almost normal. CSF protein is commonly increased (in more than three-fourths of patients) and may reach values as high as 500 mg/dL.

Miscellaneous
Vasculitis (e.g., systemic lupus erythematosus) and a vascular malformation are important con-

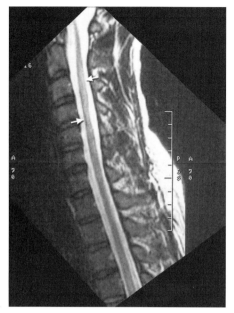
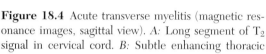
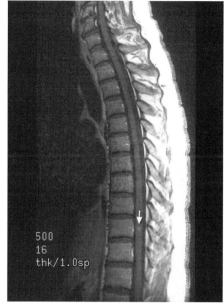

A   B

Figure 18.4 Acute transverse myelitis (magnetic resonance images, sagittal view). *A:* Long segment of T$_2$ signal in cervical cord. *B:* Subtle enhancing thoracic cord abnormality. Both patients had complete cord lesions on examination.

siderations, and spinal angiography should be performed if involvement is at a high or middle thoracic level. This localization in a spinal watershed zone may suggest a vascular rather than an autoimmune mechanism.

Viral serology may be useful because well-known viruses may cause acute transverse myelitis.[51]

First Priority in Management

Treatment with corticosteroids is controversial. No measurable effect has been reported, and with marked variability in recovery time, improvement cannot be attributed to this treatment without a formal clinical trial. Most physicians, however, prefer a brief course with methylprednisolone (1000 mg/day).

It is unknown whether specific antibiotic or antiviral therapy improves outcome. Experience with plasmapheresis and intravenous immunoglobulin is lacking. It is important to place an indwelling catheter in patients with minimal bladder reflex activity. Dysautonomia may occur alone from a distended bladder when the lesion is above the sympathetic outflow (T6), and any stimulus may produce severe hypertension. Prophylaxis for deep venous thrombosis (heparin subcutaneously or intermittent compression devices) should begin early.

Predictors of Outcome

One-third of patients with acute transverse myelitis do not recover ambulation or bladder or bowel control. Partial recovery with a considerable handicap and good recovery each account for one-third of patients.[52] Transverse myelitis has a much better prognosis if there is no progression to a complete cord syndrome and sensation remains preserved. MRI findings are not predictive of outcome. No correlation has been found with extent of the initial deficit, neurologic deficit and prognosis, and MRI findings[53] (Fig. 18.4).

Triage

- MRI of the spine on an urgent basis.
- Neurology ward or rehabilitation unit.

Acute Leukoencephalopathy

Selective white matter damage has become more apparent with the introduction of immunosuppressive agents and chemotherapeutic agents. These lipophilic substances preferentially target myelin because of its high lipid content. MRI predominance in the bilateral parieto-occipital hemispheric regions justifies the term *posterior leukoencephalopathy*.[54–58] The term *posterior reversible encephalopathy syndrome* (PRES) has been suggested, connotating a relationship with hypertension. This section describes acute leukoencephalopathy in adults. Causes are presented in Table 18.4. Chronic, protracted leukoencephalopathies consist of a very wide array of disorders, including aminoacidopathy, organic acid disorders, and lysosomal storage disease.

Clinical Presentation

Decrease in level of consciousness and marked cognitive decline, but also behavioral changes alone, may be presenting symptoms. Headache is prominent. Seizures are prevalent, mostly generalized tonic-clonic but focal onset has been noted. The disorder may progress rapidly to cortical blindness, marked ataxia, and speech or language abnormalities. Akinetic mutism may occur if the disorder is not recognized in the earlier stages of presentation. Akinetic mutism (summarized by Cairns et al.[59] as "motionless, mindless wakefulness") can be explained by extensive involvement of the thalamofrontal fibers and isolation of the anterior cingulate cortex.

Immunosuppressive agents (cyclosporine and tacrolimus) in transplantation recipients have

Table 18.4. Acute Leukoencephalopathy in Adults

Immunosuppressive agents (cyclosporine, tacrolimus)
Hypertensive crises
Eclampsia, HELLP syndrome
Chemotherapeutic agents (methotrexate, 5-fluorouracil, levamisole, intra-arterial nimustine [ACNU])
Fulminant multiple sclerosis
Postradiation period
Human immunodeficiency virus encephalopathy
Erythropoietin
Interferon-α
Heroin inhalation
Progressive multifocal leukoencephalopathy

ACNU, 1-(4-amino-2-methyl-5-pyrimidinyl)-methyl-(2-chloroethyl)-3-nitrosourea); HELLP, hemolysis, elevated liver enzymes, and low platelet count.

been used in many well-documented cases of acute leukoencephalopathy. Breakdown of the blood–brain barrier or facilitated transport is required for these immunosuppressive drugs to enter the brain. Cyclosporine or tacrolimus may have a direct damaging effect on the vasculature, leading to microvascular damage and access to the brain.

Tremors, vivid visual hallucinations, and behavioral changes with paranoid behavior and wide mood swings are common and associated with rambling, nonsensible speech.[60] Commonly, the speech disorder is characterized by stuttering when words are spoken rapidly or even at a normal pace but normal output when the patient is instructed to speak slowly. Speech may be distorted, with similarity to a foreign accent, and a single, generalized tonic-clonic seizure may be the only clue to toxicity. Less common presentations are blindness, cerebellar syndrome, orofacial dyskinesias, and mutism.[60] Presentation is similar in tacrolimus and cyclosporine neurotoxicity: less severe signs and symptoms regress rapidly after discontinuation but may recur after a different immunosuppressive agent is substituted. With the oral microemulsion of cyclosporine (Neoral), neurotoxicity is less severe, mostly tremor and headache only.[61] There are no reports of neurotoxicity with sirolimus (the term suggests a pharmacologic similarity with tacrolimus, but although receptor linkage is similar, the two agents differ in structure).

Another well-identified leukoencephalopathy has been associated with chemotherapeutic agents, predominantly 5-fluorouracil and levamisole. The estimated incidence of this toxic leukoencephalopathy is 2%.[62]

The lesions are more confluent and multifocal when tissue is examined. Perivascular lymphocytic inflammation is found next to demyelination. A more delayed manifestation, often with seizures, has been reported with chemotherapeutic agents. In these patients, a history of insidious decline in intellectual function is obtained together with clinical evidence of a progressive disorder characterized by spasticity and bulbar palsy. Its clinical presentation can be nothing more specific than depression and withdrawal, sometimes mistaken for a psychological response to the diagnosis of cancer. Ataxia, impaired thinking, slurring of speech, and memory impairment follow, and profound stupor or coma may ensue. The predominant trigger of neurotoxicity is 5-fluorouracil,[62–64] but toxicity with levamisole alone has been reported.[65]

Methotrexate is used intravenously, intrathecally, and orally.[66] All of these modes of administration may be associated with toxic damage to the white matter.[67,68] Methotrexate barely crosses the blood–brain barrier because it is an ionized and lipid-insoluble compound, but prior radiation-induced damage to the integrity of the blood–brain barrier may facilitate its transport. Intra-arterially administered nimustine (ACNU) has produced leukoencephalopathy in the treatment of glioma.[69] However, combined use of radiation and chemotherapy may complicate finding a precise cause-and-effect relationship. It may occur without prior radiation.[70] The mechanism is unclear, but reversible cerebral vasospasm has been documented.[71]

In the management of leukemia, three recognized chemotherapy-associated leukoencephalopathy syndromes have been described: (1) an acute syndrome within 24 hours after intrathecal administration of methotrexate, cranial irradiation, or use of cytarabine, resulting in an acute confusional state and seizures resolving in 2–3 days; (2) subacute leukoencephalopathy 1–2 weeks after intravenous administration of methotrexate, with focal motor neurologic signs, behavioral changes, and seizures; and (3) insidious leukoencephalopathy progressing over months, with personality changes, marked intellectual decline, and spasticity.[72]

Leukoencephalopathy may occur after heroin abuse, particularly after inhalation of heroin vapor ("chasing the dragon").[73,74] Progression from cerebellar symptoms to extrapyramidal involvement to spasticity to akinetic mutism is due to involvement of both cerebral hemispheres, the cerebellar peduncles, and the midbrain.

Anecdotal reports of acute leukoencephalopathy with erythropoietin,[75] amphotericin,[76] and interferon[57] have appeared. Hypertensive encephalopathy and eclampsia may cause headache, seizures, cortical blindness, and papilledema and may produce reversible posterior leukoencephalopathy syndrome.[77,78]

It remains important to exclude multifocal leukoencephalopathy associated with human immunodeficiency virus (HIV) and progressive multifocal leukoencephalopathy associated with JC virus by examination of CSF, polymerase chain reaction, or brain biopsy.[79–82] In addition, we noted that posterior leukoencephalopathy can be the first manifestation of CNS vasculitis, with progression in other vascular territories when untreated.[83] Finally a link with hypercalcemia has been suggested.[84]

Interpretation of Diagnostic Tests

Computed Tomography and Magnetic Resonance Imaging

CT scanning is not nearly as diagnostic as MRI in leukoencephalopathy, and a CT scan may be surprisingly normal. A comatose patient with any of the toxins or triggers mentioned above should therefore undergo MRI.

Routine MRI sequences, gadolinium enhancement, and, if available, diffusion-weighted imaging may further delineate the white matter lesion. Restricted diffusion on diffusion-weighted MRI may support cytotoxic edema, which indicates ischemia and is associated with reduced ADC values (see Chapter 9).[85]

The extensive lesions are nonspecific, but some MRI characteristics may point to a certain cause. These are sparing of the U fibers (cytomegalovirus and HIV encephalopathy); capping of the lateral ventricles, centrum semiovale, and corpus callosum (MS); additional gray matter involvement (central nervous system vasculitis, organic acidurias, postanoxic–ischemic encephalopathies, including carbon monoxide and cyanide); enhancement with gadolinium (ADEM, MS, Alexander's disease, Schilder's diffuse sclerosis); and sparing of the basal ganglia (lysosomal disorders, including sphingolipidosis). Several examples of acute leukoencephalopathies are shown in Figures 18.5–18.7. Most patients with mild forms of cyclosporine or tacrolimus neurotoxicity do not have MRI abnormalities,[86,87] which are typically seen in the most severe instances,[88–90] often in patients with seizures at presentation. Progressive multifocal leukoencephalopathy may mimic these disorders. Little or no mass effect or gadolinium enhancement is noted. The lesions are in focal areas of the gray–white junction (Fig. 18.8).

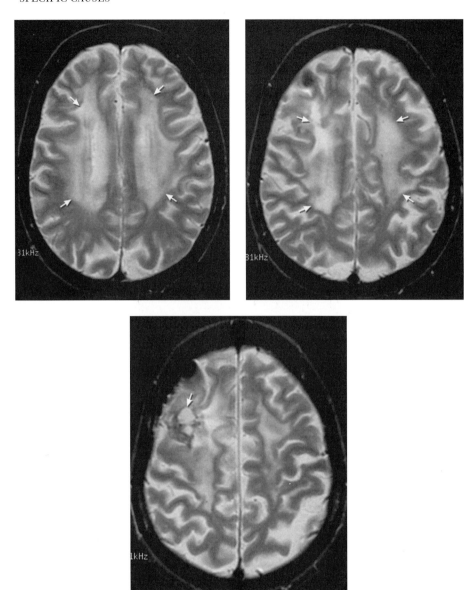

Figure 18.5 Magnetic resonance images demonstrate radiation leukoencephalopathy (radiation for glioma).

Cerebrospinal Fluid and Serum

CSF examination is useful to obtain material for detecting the JC virus, and the test has 100% specificity in immunosuppressed patients after transplantation. Oligoclonal bands and IgG index are not diagnostic and can be seen in many demyelinating disorders.

The correlation of cyclosporine and tacrolimus

with blood or plasma levels is unreliable, and in some patients progression may occur despite declining blood levels. In only 30%–40% of reported cases, trough plasma levels are increased or show a significant upward trend. Plasma levels of these immunosuppressive agents are more likely to be increased when leukoencephalopathy is demonstrated on MRI, but correlation remains poor.

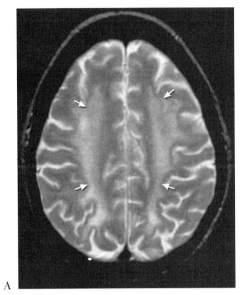
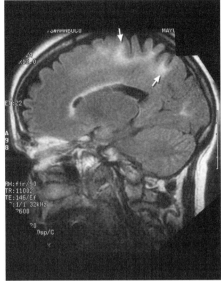

A   B

Figure 18.6 Methotrexate leukoencephalopathy on axial T$_2$-weighted (*A*) and sagittal fluid-attenuated inversion recovery (*B*) magnetic resonance imaging

(similar findings possible with 5-fluorouracil and levamisole).

First Priority in Management

Discontinuation of therapy with the causative drug may resolve most of the symptoms within 2 days. Cyclosporine or tacrolimus can be replaced by mycophenolate mofetil (CellCept) or

sirolimus. Methylprednisolone (1 g for 3–5 days) has been administered intravenously in inflammatory leukoencephalopathies associated with chemotherapeutic agents, with a successful result but no proof of its effect.[65] Suspicion of progressive multifocal leukoencephalopathy should be

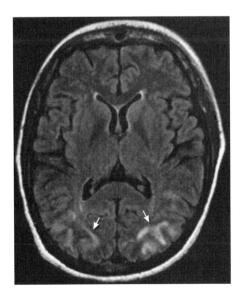
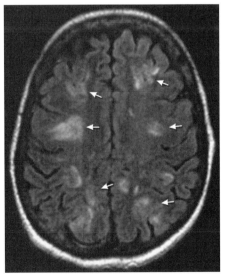

Figure 18.7 Cyclosporine-associated leukoencephalopathy, with multiple areas of involvement but normal diffusion-weighted imaging, suggesting edema.

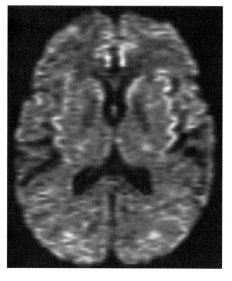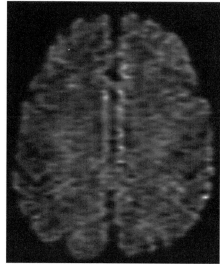

Figure 18.7 (*Continued*)

high in patients who have acquired immunodeficiency syndrome (AIDS) and in transplantation recipients. Treatment with cytarabine (2 mg/kg) should await biopsy determination, but it may retard progression only for several months.

Predictors of Outcome

The prognosis for complete recovery in drug-associated leukoencephalitis is excellent, and both clinical resolution and MRI resolution are expected after cessation of the immunosuppressive and chemotherapeutic agents. Incomplete recovery has been noted, however, particularly in comatose patients.[62] The median survival with progressive multifocal leukoencephalopathy in HIV infection is 10 weeks, but survival appears prolonged when leukoencephalopathy emerges in patients receiving highly active antiretroviral therapy, increasing to 46 weeks.[91]

Triage

- Most patients can be treated with supportive care on the ward.
- Status epilepticus or focal partial status epilepticus is very uncommon, but a prolonged series of seizures may justify 24-hour observation with video and electroencephalographic monitoring in an intensive care unit.

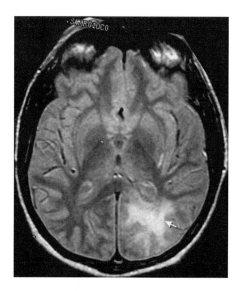

Figure 18.8 Focal posterior leukoencephalopathy due to biopsy-proven progressive multifocal leukoencephalopathy.

REFERENCES

1. Kornips HM, Verhagen WI, Prick MJ: Acute disseminated encephalomyelitis probably related to a *Mycoplasma pneumoniae* infection. *Clin Neurol Neurosurg* 95:59, 1993.
2. Mills RW, Schoolfield L: Acute transverse myelitis associated with *Mycoplasma pneumoniae* infection: a case report and review of the literature. *Pediatr Infect Dis J* 11:228, 1992.

3. Sacconi S, Salviati L, Merelli E: Acute disseminated encephalomyelitis associated with hepatitis C virus infection. *Arch Neurol* 58:1679, 2001.

4. Carrigan DR, Harrington D, Knox KK: Subacute leukoencephalitis caused by CNS infection with human herpesvirus-6 manifesting as acute multiple sclerosis. *Neurology* 47:145, 1996.

5. Schwarz S, Mohr A, Knauth M, et al.: Acute disseminated encephalomyelitis: a follow-up study of 40 adult patients. *Neurology* 56:1313, 2001.

6. Atlas SW, Grossman RI, Goldberg HI, et al.: MR diagnosis of acute disseminated encephalomyelitis. *J Comput Assist Tomogr* 10:798, 1986.

7. Mader I, Stock KW, Ettlin T, et al.: Acute disseminated encephalomyelitis: MR and CT features. *AJNR Am J Neuroradiol* 17:104, 1996.

8. Tateishi K, Takeda K, Mannen T: Acute disseminated encephalomyelitis confined to brainstem. *J Neuroimaging* 12:67, 2002.

9. Kesselring J, Miller DH, Robb SA, et al.: Acute disseminated encephalomyelitis. MRI findings and the distinction from multiple sclerosis. *Brain* 113:291, 1990.

10. Orrell RW: Grand Rounds—Hammersmith Hospitals. Distinguishing acute disseminated encephalomyelitis from multiple sclerosis. *BMJ* 313:802, 1996.

11. Caldemeyer KS, Harris TM, Smith RR, et al.: Gadolinium enhancement in acute disseminated encephalomyelitis. *J Comput Assist Tomogr* 15:673, 1991.

12. Caldemeyer KS, Smith RR, Harris TM, et al.: MRI in acute disseminated encephalomyelitis. *Neuroradiology* 36:216, 1994.

13. Burnham JA, Wright RR, Dreisbach J, et al.: The effect of high-dose steroids on MRI gadolinium enhancement in acute demyelinating lesions. *Neurology* 41:1349, 1991.

14. Case records of the Massachusetts General Hospital (case 1-1999). *N Engl J Med* 340:127, 1999.

15. Kuperan S, Ostrow P, Landi MK, et al.: Acute hemorrhagic leukoencephalitis vs ADEM: FLAIR MRI and neuropathology findings. *Neurology* 60:721, 2003.

16. Markus R, Brew BJ, Turner J, et al.: Successful outcome with aggressive treatment of acute haemorrhagic leukoencephalitis. *J Neurol Neurosurg Psychiatry* 63:551, 1997.

17. Kanter DS, Horensky D, Sperling RA, et al.: Plasmapheresis in fulminant acute disseminated encephalomyelitis. *Neurology* 45:824, 1995.

18. Stricker RB, Miller RG, Kiprov DD: Role of plasmapheresis in acute disseminated (postinfectious) encephalomyelitis. *J Clin Apheresis* 7:173, 1992.

19. Hahn JS, Siegler DJ, Enzmann D: Intravenous gammaglobulin therapy in recurrent acute disseminated encephalomyelitis. *Neurology* 46:1173, 1996.

20. Kleiman M, Brunquell P: Acute disseminated encephalomyelitis: response to intravenous immunoglobulin. *J Child Neurol* 10:481, 1995.

21. Sahlas DJ, Miller SP, Guerin M, et al.: Treatment of acute disseminated encephalomyelitis with intravenous immunoglobulin. *Neurology* 54:1370, 2000.

22. Marchioni E, Marninou-Aktipi K, Uggetti C, et al.: Effectiveness of intravenous immunoglobulin treatment in adult patients with steroid-resistant monophasic or recurrent acute disseminated encephalomyelitis. *J Neurol* 249:100, 2002.

23. Blunt SB, Boulton J, Wise R, et al.: Locked-in syndrome in fulminant demyelinating disease. *J Neurol Neurosurg Psychiatry* 57:504, 1994.

24. Forti A, Ambrosetto G, Amore M, et al.: Locked-in syndrome in multiple sclerosis with sparing of the ventral portion of the pons. *Ann Neurol* 12:393, 1982.

25. Johnson MD, Lavin P, Whetsell WO Jr: Fulminant monophasic multiple sclerosis, Marburg's type. *J Neurol Neurosurg Psychiatry* 53:918, 1990.

26. Khoshyomn S, Braff SP, Penar PL: Tumefactive multiple sclerosis plaque. *J Neurol Neurosurg Psychiatry* 73:85, 2002.

27. Melin J, Usenius JP, Fogelholm R: Left ventricular failure and pulmonary edema in acute multiple sclerosis. *Acta Neurol Scand* 93:315, 1996.

28. Pittock SJ, Weinshenker BG, Wijdicks EFM: Mechanical ventilation and tracheostomy in multiple sclerosis (abstract). *Ann Neurol* 54:S63, 2003.

29. Paty DW, Noseworthy JH, Ebers GC: Diagnosis of multiple sclerosis. In DW Paty, GC Ebers (eds), *Multiple Sclerosis. Contemporary Neurology Series*. Philadelphia: FA Davis, 1998, p. 48.

30. Niebler G, Harris T, Davis T, et al.: Fulminant multiple sclerosis. *AJNR Am J Neuroradiol* 13:1547, 1992.

31. Paty DW, Oger JJ, Kastrukoff LF, et al.: MRI in the diagnosis of MS: a prospective study with comparison of clinical evaluation, evoked potentials, oligoclonal banding, and CT. *Neurology* 38:180, 1988.

32. Powell T, Sussman JG, Davies-Jones GA: MR imaging in acute multiple sclerosis: ringlike appearance in plaques suggesting the presence of paramagnetic free radicals. *AJNR Am J Neuroradiol* 13:1544, 1992.

33. Landtblom A-M, Sjöqvist L, Söderfeldt B, et al.: Proton MR spectroscopy and MR imaging in acute and chronic multiple sclerosis—ringlike appearances in acute plaques. *Acta Radiol* 37:278, 1996.

34. Chiappa KH: *Evoked Potentials in Clinical Medicine*, 3rd ed. Philadelphia: Lippincott-Raven, 1997.

35. Nuwer MR: Evoked potentials in multiple sclerosis. In CS Raine, HF McFarland, WW Tourtellotte (eds), *Multiple Sclerosis: Clinical and Pathogenetic Basis*. London: Chapman & Hall, 1997:43.

36. Ebers GC, Paty DW: CSF electrophoresis in one thousand patients. *Can J Neurol Sci* 7:275, 1980.

37. Miller DH, Thompson AJ, Morrissey SP, et al.: High dose steroids in acute relapses of multiple sclerosis: MRI evidence for a possible mechanism of therapeutic effect. *J Neurol Neurosurg Psychiatry* 55:450, 1992.

38. Rao AB, Richert N, Howard T, et al.: Methylprednisolone effect on brain volume and enhancing lesions in MS before and during IFNβ-1b. *Neurology* 59:688, 2002.

39. Rodriguez M, Karnes WE, Bartleson JD, et al.: Plasmapheresis in acute episodes of fulminant CNS inflammatory demyelination. *Neurology* 43:1100, 1993.

40. Weinshenker BG: Natural history of multiple sclerosis. *Ann Neurol* 36(Suppl):S6, 1994.

41. Rudick RA, Cohen JA, Weinstock-Guttman B, et al.: Management of multiple sclerosis. *N Engl J Med* 337:1604, 1997.

42. Goodin DS, Frohman EM, Garmany GP Jr, et al.: Disease modifying therapies in multiple sclerosis: report of the Therapeutics and Technology Assessment Subcommittee of the American Academy of Neurology and MS Council for Clinical Practice Guidelines. *Neurology* 58:169, 2002.

43. Transverse Myelitis Consortium Working Group: Proposed diagnostic criteria and nosology of acute transverse myelitis. *Neurology* 59:499, 2002.

44. Kelley CE, Mathews J, Noskin GA: Acute transverse myelitis in the emergency department: a case report and review of the literature. *J Emerg Med* 9:417, 1991.

45. Berman M, Feldman S, Alter M, et al.: Acute transverse myelitis: incidence and etiologic considerations. *Neurology* 31:966, 1981.

46. Barakos JA, Mark AS, Dillon WP, et al.: MR imaging of acute transverse myelitis and AIDS myelopathy. *J Comput Assist Tomogr* 14:45, 1990.

47. Fukazawa T, Hamada T, Tashiro K, et al.: Acute transverse myelopathy in multiple sclerosis. *J Neurol Sci* 100:217, 1990.

48. Fukazawa T, Miyasaka K, Tashiro K, et al.: MRI findings of multiple sclerosis with acute transverse myelopathy. *J Neurol Sci* 110:27, 1992.

49. Sanders KA, Khandji AG, Mohr JP: Gadolinium-MRI in acute transverse myelopathy. *Neurology* 40:1614, 1990.

50. Tartaglino LM, Heiman-Patterson T, Friedman DP, et al.: MR imaging in a case of postvaccination myelitis. *AJNR Am J Neuroradiol* 16:581, 1995.

51. Baig SM, Khan MA: Cytomegalovirus-associated transverse myelitis in a non-immunocompromised patient. *J Neurol Sci* 134:210, 1995.

52. Ford B, Tampieri D, Francis G: Long-term follow-up of acute partial transverse myelopathy. *Neurology* 42:250, 1992.

53. Austin SG, Zee CS, Waters C: The role of magnetic resonance imaging in acute transverse myelitis. *Can J Neurol Sci* 19:508, 1992.

54. Arnoldus EP, Van Laar T: A reversible posterior leukoencephalopathy syndrome. *N Engl J Med* 334:1745, 1996.

55. Donnan GA: Posterior leukoencephalopathy syndrome. *Lancet* 347:988, 1996.

56. Eaton JM: A reversible posterior leukoencephalopathy syndrome. *N Engl J Med* 334:1744, 1996.

57. Hinchey J, Chaves C, Appignani B, et al.: A reversible posterior leukoencephalopathy syndrome. *N Engl J Med* 334:494, 1996.

58. Williams EJ, Oatridge A, Holdcroft A, et al.: Posterior leukoencephalopathy syndrome. *Lancet* 347:1556, 1996.

59. Cairns H, Oldfield RC, Pennybacker JB, et al.: Akinetic mutism with an epidermoid cyst of the third ventricle (with a report on associated disturbance of brain potentials). *Brain* 64:273, 1941

60. Wijdicks EF: Neurotoxicity of immunosuppressive drugs. *Liver Transpl* 7:937-942, 2001.

61. Wijdicks EFM, Dahlke LJ, Wiesner RH: Oral cyclosporine decreases severity of neurotoxicity in liver transplant recipients. *Neurology* 52:1708, 1999.

62. Figueredo AT, Fawcet SE, Molloy DW, et al.: Disabling encephalopathy during 5-fluorouracil and levamisole adjuvant therapy for resected colorectal cancer: a report of two cases. *Cancer Invest* 13:608, 1995.

63. Critchley P, Abbott R, Madden FJ: Multifocal inflammatory leukoencephalopathy developing in a patient receiving 5-fluorouracil and levamisole. *Clin Oncol (R Coll Radiol)* 6:406, 1994.

64. Hook CC, Kimmel DW, Kvols LK, et al.: Multifocal inflammatory leukoencephalopathy with 5-fluorouracil and levamisole. *Ann Neurol* 31:262, 1992.

65. Kimmel DW, Wijdicks EFM, Rodriguez M: Multifocal inflammatory leukoencephalopathy associated with levamisole therapy. *Neurology* 45:374, 1995.

66. Worthley SG, McNeil JD: Leukoencephalopathy in a patient taking low dose oral methotrexate therapy for rheumatoid arthritis. *J Rheumatol* 22:335, 1995.

67. Chamberlain MC, Kormanik PA, Barba D: Complications associated with intraventricular chemotherapy in patients with leptomeningeal metastases. *J Neurosurg* 87:694, 1997.

68. Lemann W, Wiley RG, Posner JB: Leukoencephalopathy complicating intraventricular catheters: clinical, radiographic and pathologic study of 10 cases. *J Neurooncol* 6:67, 1988.

69. Tsuboi K, Yoshii Y, Hyodo A, et al.: Leukoencephalopathy associated with intra-arterial ACNU in patients with gliomas. *J Neurooncol* 23:223, 1995.

70. Gowan GM, Herrington JD, Simonetta AB: Methotrexate-induced toxic leukoencephalopathy. *Pharmacotherapy* 22:1183-1187, 2002.

71. Henderson RD, Rajah T, Nicol AJ, et al.: Posterior leukoencephalopathy following intrathecal chemotherapy with MRA-documented vasospasm. *Neurology* 60:326-328, 2003.

72. Gay CT, Bodensteiner JB, Nitschke R, et al.: Reversible treatment-related leukoencephalopathy. *J Child Neurol* 4:208, 1989.

73. Tan TP, Algra PR, Valk J, et al.: Toxic leukoencephalopathy after inhalation of poisoned heroin: MR findings. *AJNR Am J Neuroradiol* 15:175, 1994.

74. Wolters EC, van Wijngaarden GK, Stam FC, et al.: Leucoencephalopathy after inhaling "heroin" pyrolysate. *Lancet* 2:1233, 1982.

75. Delanty N, Vaughan C, Frucht S, et al.: Erythropoietin-associated hypertensive posterior leukoencephalopathy. *Neurology* 49:686, 1997.

76. Walker RW, Rosenblum MK: Amphotericin B-associated leukoencephalopathy. *Neurology* 42:2005, 1992.

77. Dahmus MA, Barton JR, Sibai BM: Cerebral imaging in eclampsia: magnetic resonance imaging versus computed tomography. *Am J Obstet Gynecol* 167:935, 1992.

78. Primavera A, Audenino D, Mavilio N, et al.: Reversible posterior leukoencephalopathy syndrome in systemic lupus and vasculitis. *Ann Rheum Dis* 60:534, 2001.

79. Anders KH, Becker PS, Holden JK, et al.: Multifocal necrotizing leukoencephalopathy with pontine predilection in immunosuppressed patients: a clinicopathologic review of 16 cases. *Hum Pathol* 24:897, 1993.

80. Gray F, Chimelli L, Mohr M, et al.: Fulminating multiple sclerosis-like leukoencephalopathy revealing human immunodeficiency virus infection. *Neurology* 41:105, 1991.

81. Poon TP, Tchertkoff V, Win H: Fine needle aspiration biopsy of progressive multifocal leukoencephalopathy in a patient with AIDS. A case report. *Acta Cytol* 41:1815, 1997.

82. Zunt JR, Tu RK, Anderson DM, et al.: Progressive multifocal leukoencephalopathy presenting as human immunodeficiency virus type 1 (HIV)–associated dementia. *Neurology* 49:263, 1997.

83. Wijdicks EFM, Manno EM, Fulgham JR, et al.: Cerebral angiitis mimicking posterior leukoencephalopathy. *J Neurol* 250:444, 2003.

84. Kastrup O, Maschke M, Wanke I, et al.: Posterior reversible encephalopathy syndrome due to severe hypercalcemia. *J Neurol* 249:1563, 2002.

85. Schaefer PW, Buonanno FS, Gonzalez RG, et al.: Diffusion-weighted imaging discriminates between cytotoxic and vasogenic edema in a patient with eclampsia. *Stroke* 28:1082, 1997.

86. Wijdicks EFM, Wiesner RH, Dahlke LJ, et al.: FK506-induced neurotoxicity in liver transplantation. *Ann Neurol* 35:498, 1994.

87. Wijdicks EFM, Wiesner RH, Krom RA: Neurotoxicity in liver transplant recipients with cyclosporine immunosuppression. *Neurology* 45:1962, 1995.

88. Thyagarajan GK, Cobanoglu A, Johnston W: FK506-induced fulminant leukoencephalopathy after single-lung transplantation. *Ann Thorac Surg* 64:1461, 1997.

89. Jarosz JM, Howlett DC, Cox TC, et al.: Cyclosporine-related reversible posterior leukoencephalopathy: MRI. *Neuroradiology* 39:711, 1997.

90. Lanzino G, Cloft H, Hemstreet MK, et al.: Reversible posterior leukoencephalopathy following organ transplantation. Description of two cases. *Clin Neurol Neurosurg* 99:222, 1997.

91. Clifford DB, Yiannoutsos C, Glicksman M, et al.: HAART improves prognosis in HIV-associated progressive multifocal leukoencephalopathy. *Neurology* 52:623, 1999.

Chapter 19
Traumatic Brain and
Spine Injury

The management of accidental traumatic brain and spine injuries commonly involves patients who have had motor vehicle accidents or have fallen— some from significant heights. On arrival in the emergency department, the medical complexities in these highly unstable patients and in those with nonpenetrating trauma to the central nervous system may be a predicament for most neurologists. The life-threatening potential of injuries to vital organs encompasses most of the activity in the emergency department. On closer examination, it appears in some instances that neurologists and neurosurgeons may have only a peripheral role and be consulted only after many hours or even days of stabilization of vital organ functions. (As the adage goes, many patients are "too sick to operate."[1]) Quite frankly, the priority to manage chest and abdominal trauma in multitraumatized patients may undermine the management of head and spine trauma. Also, intoxication often leads to trauma (e.g., bar brawls, intravenous drug use), and its drugging effect on the brain may confound clinical assessment. Some of these patients are found on the street or in the recesses of buildings, often in deplorable clinical condition. This chapter discusses how to determine the severity of the initial injury, accomplish medical management of traumatic brain edema and contusions, and assess the need for acute neurosurgical intervention.

Traumatic Brain Injury

The severity of injury is graded on the basis of the Glasgow coma score (see Chapter 8, Table 8.4, Fig.

8.5) and the presentation computed tomography (CT) scan. Head injury can be classified into several characteristic categories, and each may have different triage options (Table 19.1). Coexisting categories are common in catastrophic trauma.

Clinical Presentation

Traumatic brain injury frequently impairs level of alertness, but the mechanism is diverse. Coma may occur from bihemispheric contusions, extracerebral hematoma causing a mass effect on the opposite hemisphere or thalamus and, rarely, an isolated brain stem lesion.

The Glasgow coma score reliably measures the degree of traumatic coma. Eye opening and motor responses remain the most important leads and often closely correspond with other changes in the brain stem reflexes, such as pupillary and oculocephalic responses. In addition, the Glasgow coma score predicts outcome after traumatic brain injury irrespective of the underlying structural lesion. Assessment is most reliable after cardiopulmonary resuscitation and at least 6 hours after injury.[2] Coma is closely linked to a Glasgow coma sum score of 8 or less (e.g., ability to open eyes only to pain, E_2; incomprehensible sounds, V_2; and arm withdrawal to pain, M_4).

Pupillary light response and pupil size further localize and measure degree of impact. Unilaterally enlarged pupil is often due to an evolving intracranial mass lesion and may become oval when intracranial pressure (ICP) is increased. The fixed pupil of an extracranial hematoma is on the same side; but occasionally a falsely localizing con-

Table 19.1. Classification of Traumatic
Brain Injury

Closed
  Parenchymal
    Hemorrhagic contusion
    Contrecoup contusion
    Shear lesion
    Malignant brain edema
    Diffuse axonal injury
  Extracerebral
    Epidural
    Subdural
Penetrating
  Parenchymal
    Intracerebral hematoma
  Extracerebral
    Subdural hematoma
Skull fracture
  Vault
    Linear or stellate
    Depressed
    Open or closed
  Basilar
    With spinal fluid leak
    With facial nerve palsy
    With carotid artery trauma

tralateral pupil is seen, an observation not adequately explained. Mydriasis of one pupil after head injury indicates a swollen temporal lobe causing traction of the third nerve or direct compression. However, when a patient with a fixed pupil is seen early after trauma, the most frequent cause is an ipsilateral epidural or large subdural hematoma.

Fixed pupils of midposition size (diameter 5–6 mm) may indicate a mesencephalic stage of herniation and may be the first indication of brain death in the emergency department. Brain death in head injury is a result of massive cerebral edema, multiple hemorrhagic contusions, or a rapidly evolving epidural hematoma causing an irreversible shift of the brain stem. It is often observed in subtentorial epidural hematomas, which are not accommodated for in the small compartment of the posterior fossa.

In the midst of multiple trauma to limbs, abdomen, or chest, facial trauma may receive less attention; and neurologists are often the first to point out the injuries when the cranial nerves are examined. Causes of hypotension (e.g., abdominal/thoracic bleeding source) should be aggressively sought. Scalp avulsions may cause significant blood loss and shock and should be repaired immediately. However, hypotension in adults is almost never a direct result of central nervous system trauma. In a few instances, hypotension may result from major external scalp bleeding, spinal shock, and brain death; and in children it may occur with a large epidural hematoma.[3] Orbital swelling can be profound and may prevent full examination of fundi and eye movements. If the swelling is associated with ecchymosis of the eyelids (so-called raccoon or panda bear eyes) *(see Color Fig. 19.1 in separate color insert)*, it may indicate a fracture of the orbital roof or, more commonly, a Le Fort III (nasal-orbital-ethmoid midface) or zygomatic fracture. The orbital roof fracture may extend through the ethmoid or cribriform–ethmoid junction and result in a cerebrospinal fluid (CSF) fistula. Petrous bone fractures may result in facial paralysis from direct injury to the facial nerve, ecchymosis over the mastoid (Battle's sign), and a CSF leak from the external canal. The Battle and raccoon eye signs, however, take several hours to develop, and specificity for basal skull fracture is low. Abrasions of the chin are clues to possible retroflexion trauma of the spine and should prompt precautionary measures, such as a collar, until a cervical spine radiograph or CT scan has excluded a fracture or dislocation.

Seizures are associated with traumatic brain injury in only up to 10% of patients and are more common in patients with a cortical contusion or traumatic intracerebral hematoma, depressed skull fracture, and dural tear.

Dysautonomia may coexist, but if so, it indicates catastrophic diffuse axonal brain trauma.[4] Patients clench both fists, burying the thumbs into the palms; grind teeth; lock the jaw; and bite the endotracheal tube. Other manifestations are profuse sweating (Fig. 19.2) and tachycardia.

Many algorithms and trauma scores have been devised and may be helpful in triage; however, it is more important to weigh factors that would justify rapid transportation to a neurotrauma center or neurologic–neurosurgical intensive care unit (Table 19.2).

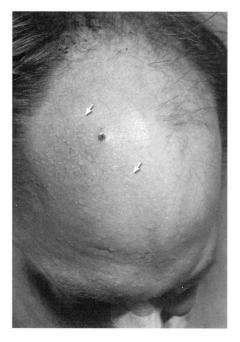

Figure 19.2 Profuse sweating (*arrows*) from dysautonomia in a patient with axonal brain injury.

Interpretation of Diagnostic Tests

Computed Tomography and Magnetic Resonance Imaging

CT scan imaging is imperative in any patient with facial lacerations or hematoma, reduced level of consciousness, significant impact to the cranium (particularly from a fall or fist fight), and certainly any evidence of focal neurologic signs or pupillary inequality during transport.[5] CT scan of the brain should be part of a complete evaluation in a patient with multitrauma and not be deferred to a later time. Magnetic resonance imaging (MRI) is

Table 19.2. Severity Indicators of Traumatic Brain Injury

Inability to remember trauma
Fall, fist fight, car collision
Age >60 years
Tachypnea
Hypotension
Scalp or face injury
Penetrating injury
Pupils fixed to light
Abnormal findings on computed tomographic scan

Table 19.3. Coma in Traumatic Brain Injury but "Normal" Findings on Computed Tomographic Scanning

Drug or alcohol overdose
Postanoxic insult to both hemispheres from asphyxia (vomiting, aspiration, foreign body)
Postictal state after seizures or nonconvulsive status epilepticus
Vertebral artery dissection with basilar artery occlusion (rare)

considered when CT scans do not fully explain the clinical presentation, but it is not readily available and is probably unsafe in mechanically ventilated patients with unstable multiple traumatic lesions to vital organs. Major dissimilarities between CT scan findings after trauma and the patient's state of impaired consciousness should point to confounding factors, including additional insults to the brain, some of which are reversible (Table 19.3).

Several CT scan patterns can be recognized, and they are illustrated in the figures of this chapter. The severity of head injury in comatose patients can be further classified. Absence of visualization of the basal cisterns, midline shift, and a mass lesion are strong predictors of increased ICP. Mass effect with absence of a third ventricle and trapping of the temporal horn correlates strongly with increased ICP.

Most parenchymal injuries are a direct effect of a blow to the brain. These contusions are created when brain tissue becomes impacted against the bony protuberances of the base of the skull. They are further subdivided into fracture contusions, contrecoup contusions, and shear lesions.

Contusions are common in the frontal and temporal lobes (Fig. 19.3) and can be seen in association with a fracture of the anterior fossa. This abnormality may be accompanied by an epidural or subdural hematoma, which may be responsible for the clinical symptoms. In patients with acute subdural hematoma, follow-up CT scans show lacerated brain tissue at the same site or this becomes apparent during craniotomy and removal of the extradural hematoma.

Contrecoup contusions (Fig. 19.4A,B) are often two or more lesions diametrically opposite to one another. Shear lesions (Fig. 19.5) are punctate lesions from disruption of small penetrating arter-

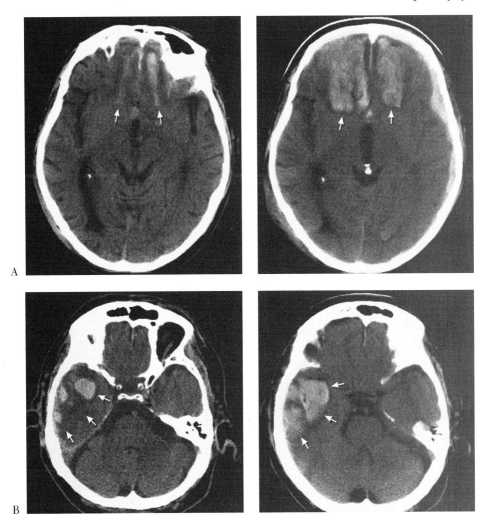

Figure 19.3 *A:* Frontal lobe contusions *(arrows). B:* Temporal lobe burst hematoma *(arrows).*

ies due to rotational forces at impact. The localization of shear lesions varies, but often they are identified at the gray–white matter junction. Basal ganglia (predominantly putamen) may be involved.

Hemorrhagic contusions may not be evident on initial CT scanning, are unmasked only after repeat studies, and are not always associated with clearly documented clinical deterioration (Fig. 19.6). Mass effect from cortical contusions is seldom severe initially but may increase from pericontusional swelling.

Another rather frequent CT scan image is diffuse axonal injury.[6] The pathologic damage is caused by acceleration–deceleration forces,[7] and

the overwhelming evidence of axonal destruction may be noted only microscopically at autopsy.[8] CT scan findings may appear initially normal, but often subtle changes are present, such as intraventricular blood (small amounts from corpus callosum tearing), punctate shear lesions, or sulci effacement. Later CT scans may show (ex vacuo) enlargement of the ventricles from reduction of the white matter tissue.

Corpus callosum lesions may be demonstrated on MRI but seldom are found by CT scanning. Corpus callosum lesions are in the splenium and posterior body because relative fixation from the posterior falx results in a tensile force rather than release with rotation. Brain stem lesions have

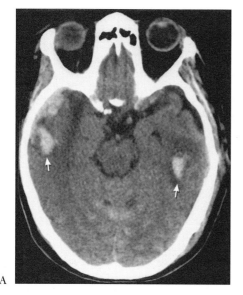
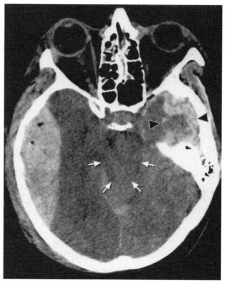

Figure 19.4 *A:* Contrecoup contusions (*arrows*). *B:* Epidural hematoma with contrecoup temporal lobe contusion (*arrowheads*) and basal cistern effacement (*arrows*).

been noted, often with multiple hemispheric lesions. A focal hemorrhage is most commonly seen in the dorsolateral aspect of the brain stem from a blow to the edge of the tentorium or in the interpeduncular cistern. Diffuse cerebral swelling (Fig. 19.7) occasionally is seen early after impact and indicates severe axonal damage. Typically, the differentiating features of the white matter and gray matter disappear and the basal cisterns are obliterated, resulting in a "featureless grayout of the brain." This malignant edema is often fatal and may occur after an asymptomatic interval and "trivial" impact (fall off a horse or bicycle).

A subdural hematoma typically is recognized as

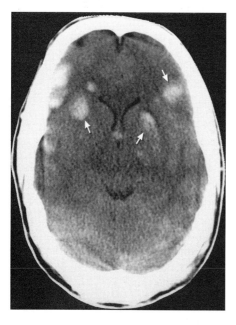
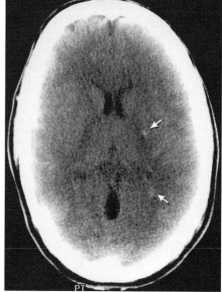

Figure 19.5 Shear lesions (*arrows*), including basal ganglia.

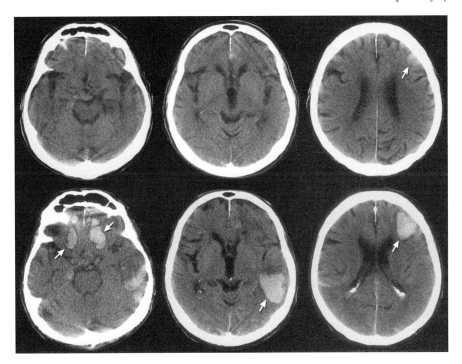

Figure 19.6 Delayed abnormalities on computed tomographic scans. *Top row*, Contusion (*arrow*) is barely seen. *Bottom row*, Multiple lobar contusions (*arrows*) develop later.

a hyperdense lesion with a characteristic crescentic (curving with the skull) collection.[9] Acute subdural hematomas are hyperdense, but when marked anemia (hemoglobin <8 g/dL) is present, they may approach the density of brain tissue.

When hyperdensity is seen within an isodense collection, rebleeding is likely. A fluid–blood interface may suggest rebleeding (Fig. 19.8). Usually, a subdural hematoma isodense to the gray matter is evident 3 weeks after onset. A change to a hy-

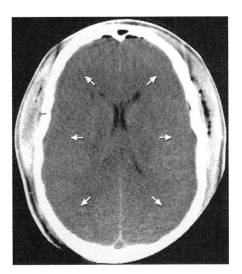
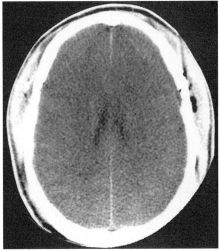

Figure 19.7 Axonal injury to the brain and diffuse swelling (*arrows*), with so-called featureless grayout.

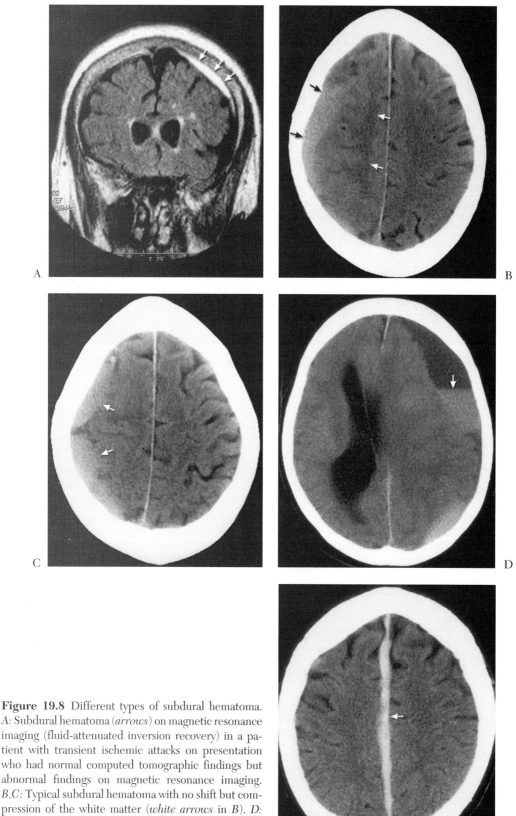

Figure 19.8 Different types of subdural hematoma.
A: Subdural hematoma (*arrows*) on magnetic resonance
imaging (fluid-attenuated inversion recovery) in a patient with transient ischemic attacks on presentation
who had normal computed tomographic findings but
abnormal findings on magnetic resonance imaging.
B,C: Typical subdural hematoma with no shift but compression of the white matter (*white arrows* in *B*). *D:*
Rebleeding subdural hematoma with fluid interface
(*arrow*) between recent and older collections of blood.
E: Falx subdural hematoma (*arrow*).

podense collection follows, but estimation of the age of the hematoma on CT images is difficult. In elderly patients, isodense subdural hematomas may only be recognized by loss of sulci and small ventricles (false CT-age mismatch). Small layers of subdural hematoma may go undetected on CT scans because they can hardly be distinguished from bone; MRI visualizes them (Fig. 19.8A).

Subdural hematoma can be seen as an inter-hemispheric collection along the falx, and this collection tends to enlarge (Fig. 19.8E).

Epidural hematomas (Fig. 19.9) are associated with fracture in more than 95% of cases. The hematoma, which is due to a tear in a meningeal artery, strips the dura away from the inner table of the skull, producing a biconvex, or lens-shaped,

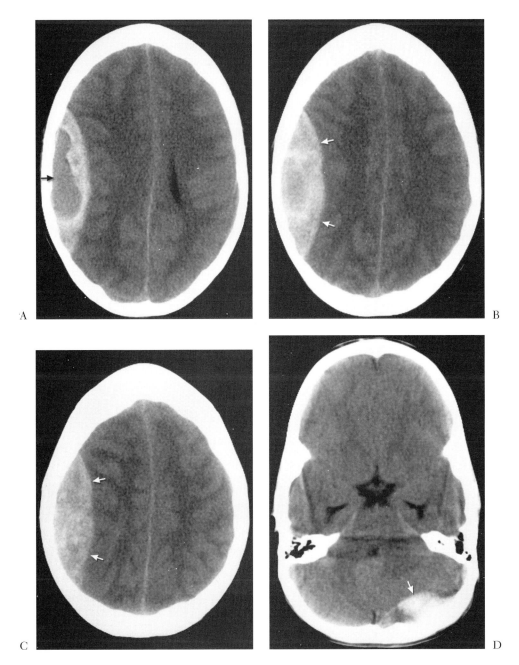

Figure 19.9: A–C: Supratentorial epidural hematoma (*arrows*, see hyperlucent areas). D: Subtentorial epidural hematoma.

configuration. Anterior–posterior extension is usually limited by the skull sutures. Its mass effect is significant in both the supratentorial and the infratentorial spaces and may rapidly lead to brain herniation syndromes. An ominous CT scan feature is a hyperlucent area, which should be recognized on CT images (Fig. 19.9A). It indicates active bleeding because a completed epidural hematoma is uniformly dense. An epidural hematoma in the posterior fossa is caused by a torn dural sinus (Fig. 19.9D); it may become large enough to cause full effacement of the brain stem cisterns. Vertex epidural hematomas, which are very rare, are caused by rupture of the superior sagittal sinus. Unlike the rapid evolution of arterial epidural hematomas, involvement of the dural sinus may not become clinically noticeable for several hours.[10]

Traumatic subarachnoid collections in sulci and fissures should not involve any of the suprasellar cisterns.[11] Occasionally, some sediment is seen in the ambient cistern (see Chapter 13). Blood from traumatic subarachnoid hemorrhage may have collected in the sylvian fissure alone. The distinction between a ruptured middle cerebral artery aneurysm, with blood deposited in the sylvian fissure, that causes the patient to fall and subarachnoid hemorrhage from trauma alone is impossible if no clear history of a thunderclap headache is volunteered by the patient. Cerebral angiography is always needed. Traumatic intraventricular hemorrhages are commonly associated with other contusional lesions, which may become apparent on follow-up CT scan.[12–14] Coma and traumatic intraventricular hemorrhage are associated with poor outcome, but isolated intraventricular blood in an alert patient is associated with good outcome and more often seen with use of warfarin. The source of bleeding is typically the choroid plexus. Primary intraventricular hemorrhage may be associated with a fall and additional traumatic lesion, further obfuscating the etiology. Thus, in young patients with frank intraventricular hemorrhage, a cerebral angiogram is warranted.

Bone Window Computed Tomography
Bone windows on CT scans are important to show linear fractures in the skull and are equivalent to routine skull radiographs. In many instances, they indicate the site of the blow and are next to the contused area of the brain. In one study, skull frac-

ture was present in 77% of patients with contusion, 87% with an extradural hematoma, 72% with a subdural hematoma, and 66% with an intracerebral hematoma.[15] The degree of depression of skull fracture can be easily visualized. Linear fractures are more commonly associated with epidural or subdural hematomas than are depressed skull fractures (Fig. 19.10).[15] Of specific note is the presence of blood in the sphenoid, which is typical of a foramen lacerum fracture and may indicate damage to the carotid artery (Fig. 19.10).

Serum
Next to a routine laboratory survey, obtaining a serum (and urinary) toxicologic screen is of value. Blood alcohol level is imperative not only for medicolegal reasons but also for judging its influence on level of consciousness. Increased serum osmolality may also indicate alcohol intoxication (a more detailed discussion is in Chapter 8). Laboratory support of disseminated intravascular coagulation needs to be sought and includes prolonged prothrombin time, thrombocytopenia (<60,000 platelets), increase in fibrin degradation products, red cell fragments in smears, and increased D-dimer. Early appearance of disseminated intravascular coagulation indicates massive destruction of brain tissue, releasing thrombogenic substances such as thromboplastin into vascular space.

Miscellaneous
Routine X-ray imaging in a head-injured patient should include the cervical spine with lateral and odontoid views and, when relevant, plain films of the abdomen and pelvis. Diagnostic peritoneal lavage or CT scan of the abdomen or chest is indicated in patients with fluctuating blood pressure after adequate fluid replacement.

First Priority in Management

The main principle of management of traumatic head injury is immediate treatment of increased ICP, which may involve removal of an extracranial hematoma or contusion with mass effect.[16,17]

Immediate stabilization is summarized in Table 19.4. Rapid triage to CT scanning is essential because it determines the cause of impaired con-

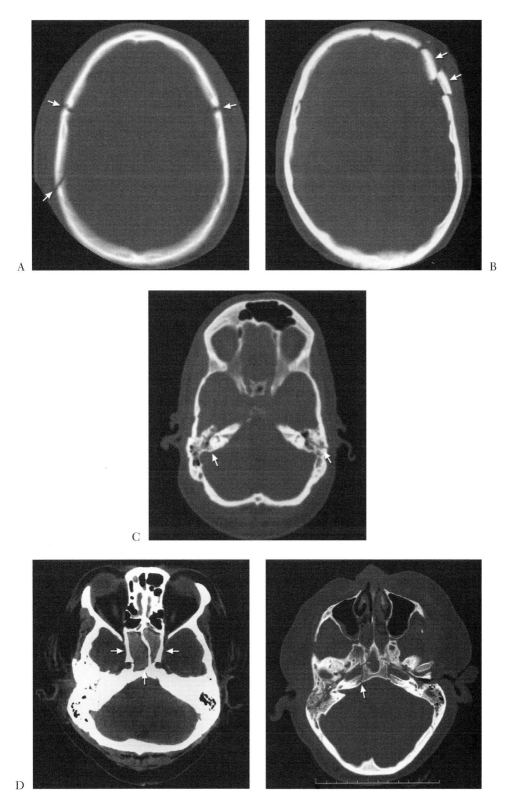

Figure 19.10 Major skull fractures. *A:* Nondepressed. *B:* Depressed. *C:* Petrous. *D:* Blood in the sphenoid sinus is typical of a fracture of the foramen lacerum.

Table 19.4. Immediate Priorities in
Head Injury

Secure airway
Remove foreign body
Endotracheal intubation
Immobilize spine
Inspect for scalp laceration and depressed fracture
Peritoneal lavage with hypotension
Secure venous access with two catheters
Normal saline resuscitation in hypotension
Obtain cervical spine X-ray
Chest radiography
Computed tomographic scan of brain
Computed tomographic scan of abdomen (if appropriate)

sciousness in most instances. Scalp lacerations should be temporarily repaired in the emergency department unless they are contaminated. It is important to secure the airway, provide fluids with two large-bore catheters, and exclude abdominal trauma with peritoneal lavage if blood pressure remains marginal despite fluid loading with hypertonic saline or dextran.[18,19] Some experts argue for a flat body position to maximize cerebral perfusion pressure (CPP). Early fluid resuscitation in an attempt to improve organ and brain perfusion may seem beneficial but could also worsen bleeding due to increase in blood flow. Others have argued that fluid administration may reduce blood viscosity, dilute clotting factors, or interfere with hemostasis (particularly, use of starch). Administration of poorly warmed fluids may also contribute to a coagulopathy. A reasonable consensus is to use aliquots of 250 ml normal saline in traumatized patients.[20]

The focus of management involves not only reduction of ICP but also maintenance of interrelated CPP (Box 19.1). It is prudent to hyperventilate the patient (frequency of more than 20 breaths per minute or squeezing the anesthesia [Ambu] bag every 3 seconds) and to give a single loading dose of mannitol (20%), 1 g/kg over 10 minutes, but only if blood pressure has remained stable throughout. Mannitol in multiple doses may have the opposite effect by accumulating within the brain and thus reversing the osmotic gradient between edematous brain and plasma.[22] However, en route to the operating room, mannitol in a dose of 1.4 g/kg was significantly better than lower doses

when infused in patients with contusional expanding temporal lobe hematoma.[23]

A restless patient may require intubation and sedation with propofol (infusion of 0.5 mg/kg hourly)[24] or, less attractive, morphine (infusion of 1 mg hourly) if the endotracheal tube and mechanical ventilator are not tolerated. Because propofol also reduces increased ICP, it is a useful drug in agitated patients with early brain swelling.[24] There is no rationale for use of corticosteroids or barbiturates, all of which may seriously complicate management and possibly inversely affect outcome through adverse effects of hypotension, hyperglycemia, and infectious complications.[25–29] Simple measures also reduce ICP, such as preventing head rotation to one side (jugular vein compression); suctioning without stimulation of the soft palate or posterior pharyngeal wall, which elicits a gag and cough reflex; and suctioning through an endotracheal tube with one passage only. Intravenous administration of lidocaine[30,31] or increasing the dose of propofol may blunt these ICP responses. Several drugs may increase ICP through an increase in cerebral blood flow by vasodilation (Table 19.5).

Hypoxemia should be aggressively managed, and after intubation, positive end-expiratory pressure (PEEP) is needed to improve gas exchange.[32] PEEP may increase intrapleural pressure and superior vena cava pressure and reduce cerebral venous outflow. ICP may become seriously elevated if PEEP values higher than 10 cm H_2O are needed, but its increase can be countered with mannitol and head elevation. PEEP may increase partial pressure of arterial CO_2 ($PaCO_2$) because of increased physiologic dead space; this effect should be anticipated and managed by increasing the minute volume of the ventilator. Conversely, the effects of hyperoxia are unclear and, when studied with microdialysis catheters, did not result in improved glucose oxidation.[33]

Systemic hypothermia (32°C–33°C) within 6 hours is not likely to be beneficial in severe head injury. Its benefit and potential complications (cardiac arrhythmias, pneumonia, coagulation problems, and increase in prothrombin time) have been investigated. There is some early indication that 35°C–35.5°C may be more optimal.[34] Certainly, fever should be aggressively treated with cooling blankets, alcohol rubbing, or, as a last re-

Box 19.1. Management of Cerebral Perfusion in Traumatic Brain Injury

Cerebral blood flow is held constant within the range of mean arterial pressure from 80 to 160 mm Hg. Outside this homeostatic range, cerebral blood flow is linearly coupled with pressure. Below the lower threshold, a decrease in CPP results in a decrease in blood flow and ischemia. Theoretically, above the upper threshold, an increase in CPP results in breakdown of the blood–brain barrier and edema, but studies suggest that high perfusion pressures are tolerated for brief periods.

Management of CPP has been advocated, but it assumes intact autoregulation, which may not be present in up to 50% of patients with severe trau-

matic head injury. Cerebral perfusion is usually aimed at 70–80 mm Hg and can be increased by increasing systolic arterial blood pressure (SABP), draining CSF pressure, and using mannitol (CPP = MAP − ICP).

These vasodilatory and vasoconstriction cascades (Fig. 19.11), have led to management of CPP irrespective of ICP.[21] Blood pressure can be increased with adrenergic receptor drugs, and normovolemia is maintained with albumin. Early results suggest good to superior outcome, but this approach (endorsed by the Brain Trauma Foundation—www. braintrauma.org) remains unproven.

sort, ice gastric lavage. These measures are certainly needed in patients with a severe sympathetic outburst, who usually have tachycardia, tachypnea, and profuse sweating, with temperature increases up to 40°C. Propofol can effectively mute shivering most of the time.

The use of prophylactic antiepileptic agents to prevent seizures has been established. Current reasonable recommendations are intravenous loading with phenytoin in patients with contusions on CT scan or depressed skull fractures.[35] Maintaining therapeutic phenytoin levels for at least 1 month, a period when seizures are most common, seems reasonable. Surgical management of extracerebral hematomas is urgently indicated. Usually, time can be allowed to evacuate the hematoma in the operating room, but in rapidly deteriorating patients without a nearby CT scanner, emergency drilling in the emergency department has been lifesaving.[36] Medical management and observation in extracerebral hematomas are considered only for patients with a maximal Glasgow coma score. Epidural hematomas with a di-

ameter less than 1.5 cm, no midline shift, and, as alluded to earlier, no lucent area inside the hematoma suggesting recent bleeding could be managed with observation.[37,38] For subdural hematomas, medical management is considered if the thickness of the hematoma is similar to the thickness of the skull. Large subdural hematomas without any shift (caused by atrophy of the brain

Table 19.5. Medications to be Avoided with Increased Intracranial Pressure

Hydralazine
Sodium nitroprusside
Halogenated inhalation anesthetics (halothane, isoflurane)
Ketamine
Calcium channel blockers (nicardipine, nimodipine)

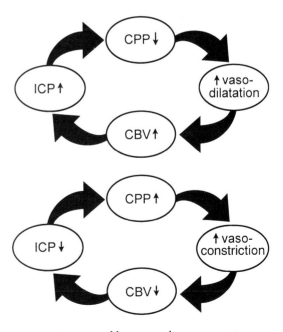

Figure 19.11 Vasodilatation and vasoconstriction cascades. CPP, cerebral perfusion pressure; ICP, intracranial pressure; CBV, cerebral blood volume.

in elderly patients or chronic alcoholics) can be surgically managed in a delayed fashion when the clinical signs are minimal. Burr hole placement after the hematoma has liquefied is preferred above a large craniotomy.

Acute chest or abdominal exploration for injury often has a priority over traumatic brain injury management due to its immediate life-threatening condition. Complicated decisions pertain to timing of fixation or instrumentation of long bone fractures. When the patient is stable for several hours, bone fixation avoids traction and its complications of prolonged immobilization but also reduces pain and possibly fat emboli.[1]

Predictors of Outcome

It is impossible to make an accurate prediction of outcome in the emergency department. Early predictors commonly have been inaccurate, proposed cut-off points in certain scales have been disproved, and successful resuscitation of a patient for systemic injuries may greatly improve the outcome. Prognosis estimates at least in the 24 hours after injury are thus unreliable.[39]

Age remains an important factor in prognosis, with 80% mortality from diffuse axonal injury in patients older than 55 years.[40] Prognosis is worse with the following factors: shock, subdural hematoma,[41] and coma in the elderly; early diffuse edema and increased ICP;[42] and failure to decrease ICP with conventional methods. In a study of MRI in 80 severely injured patients, corpus callosum lesions and dorsolateral brain stem lesions predicted an unfavorable outcome, including vegetative state.[43]

Triage

- Evacuation of any epidural or subdural hematoma if the patient has a decrease in consciousness, hemiparesis, or speech deficit.
- Evacuation of hemorrhagic contusion if mass effect occurs.
- Placement of ICP monitor and monitoring in neurologic–neurosurgical intensive care unit.

Spinal Cord Injury

Spinal cord injury may have been caused by traffic accidents in more than 50% of patients arriving at emergency departments. The demographic profile consists of men in their thirties seen most often during weekends in the summer months. Complete cord lesions have decreased in prevalence, which is tentatively explained by improved care in the field, increased use of seat belts, and, possibly, surgical care of unstable spine trauma. It is prudent to assume that spinal cord injury may have occurred in patients who have had multiple trauma, motor vehicle or sports accidents, or a documented spine fracture.[44,45]

This section is not intended to comprehensively discuss all spinal traumatic lesions and surgical management, which can be properly addressed only by experienced spine surgeons or neurosurgeons with special qualifications in the management of spine trauma. Guidelines for surgical management are outlined (Box 19.2). The field has evolved into a subspecialty in which the role of a neurologist or emergency physician is important but limited to accurate clinical description of the damage, appropriate stabilization, recognition of unstable spine fractures or dislocations, and, when necessary, early specific medical management. An overview of spine fractures can be found elsewhere.[48]

Clinical Presentation

Traumatic spinal cord injury involves the cervical cord in approximately 50% of cases, the thoracic segment in 35%, and the lumbar segment or conus in the others. Subtle signs of cervical spine injury are physical signs of an injury above the clavicle, neck pain, and tilting of the head to one side.

Tetraplegia or paraplegia is evident from the onset, but most clinical challenges involve the management of its commonly associated dysautonomia and urogenital manifestations.

In the spinal shock phase, a generalized state of hypoexcitability occurs. The marked reduction of sympathetic outflow results in peripheral vasodilatation, decreased cardiac output, bradycardia (from cardiac chronotropic activity), and venous pooling, all factors that reduce blood pressure. Blood pressure typically is less than 100 mm Hg and depends on position and volume; reduction in the sitting or upright position may result in syncope. The lower extremities may show a bluish discoloration from vasodilatation and venous pooling. Typically, pain does not produce an increase in heart rate or blood pressure. Passive

Box 19.2. Surgical Management of Spinal Cord Injury

Surgical management of spine injury in a patient with spinal cord injury is pursued to prevent further injury in incomplete lesions, to ensure stability, and to prevent deformity. Unstable cervical lesions should be expected if anterior or posterior elements are destroyed, sagittal diameter of the spinal canal is less than 13 mm, or sagittal displacement is more than 3.5 mm or 20%. A stable lesion allows for earlier mobilization and transfers. Operative stabilization has not been shown to improve recovery in complete or incomplete lesions, although one survey called for a trial based on suggestive data review.[46]

Deformity requires instrumentation and posterior fusion in many instances.[47]

engorgement of the penis (priapism) occurs as a consequence of sympathetic loss and always indicates an extensive spinal cord lesion.

Temperature may be unregulated. Shivering cannot occur below the lesion because of loss of sympathetic tone, and lack of increase in metabolism may result in hypothermia. Paradoxically, core hypothermia may be present in patients with otherwise warm extremities. The bladder is completely paralyzed, causing urinary retention and overflow. Detrusor muscle contraction only later results in spontaneous or external stimuli–induced voiding.

It is important to determine the sensory level by cutaneous innervation of the dermatomes. Pinprick sensation should be evaluated serially. It is important to memorize and document clinical markers (nipple, T4; navel, T10; midway from arm to chest, C4–T2 border). It may be difficult to determine whether the level is cervical or thoracic because the C4 and T2 levels abut each other, but examination of motor function and reflexes of the arm further helps localization.

Reflexes such as the anal wink (puckering of the anus with stimulus to the perianal region) and the bulbocavernosus reflex (traction on a Foley catheter or digital pressure on the clitoris or penis while anal sphincter contraction is monitored with a gloved finger in the rectum) should be examined. Neurologic examination should be carefully documented by use of the American Spinal Injury Association neurologic classification of spinal cord injury (Appendix 19.1). The American Spinal Injury Association Impairment Scale can also be used to monitor progress.

Interpretation of Diagnostic Tests

Neuroimaging of the spine and spinal cord has a high priority. The extent of imaging is determined by neurologic findings at presentation. Careful clinical delineation of level of involvement may tailor orientation and selection of the studies.

Neuroradiologists should have access to clinical information that may further determine certain MRI sequences. The priority in the emergency department is to diagnose unstable cervical or thoracic spine fractures or spine compression.

Spine Plain Films

Screening cervical spine radiographs for alert patients with no neck tenderness and no neurologic abnormalities have a very low yield.[49] Combined lateral, anteroposterior, and odontoid views have a high diagnostic yield and should recognize more than 90% of the lesions, although a false-negative rate of 26% was found in a study of 70 patients. The lateral cervical spine radiograph and odontoid views (Fig. 19.12) should be viewed systematically.[50,51] A common pitfall is focusing on a single fracture or misalignment while overlooking other abnormalities. The essentials of cervical spine plain film viewing are shown in Table 19.6. Evaluation is very difficult. Only the trained eye of an experienced physician can identify fractures, but even then a CT scan is often needed for confirmation. The threshold for ordering a CT scan of the cervical spine must be very low, particularly when plain films of the cervical spine give dubious information or are of marginal quality.

First, the cervical vertebral bodies should be identified, and particular attention should be paid to the lower cervical spine. Hand traction should be used to pull both arms and shoulders of the patient down. Inadequate films should prompt CT scanning of the spine. When a lateral spine film is evaluated, four lordotic curves and alignments are assessed to look for displacement (Fig. 19.12A).

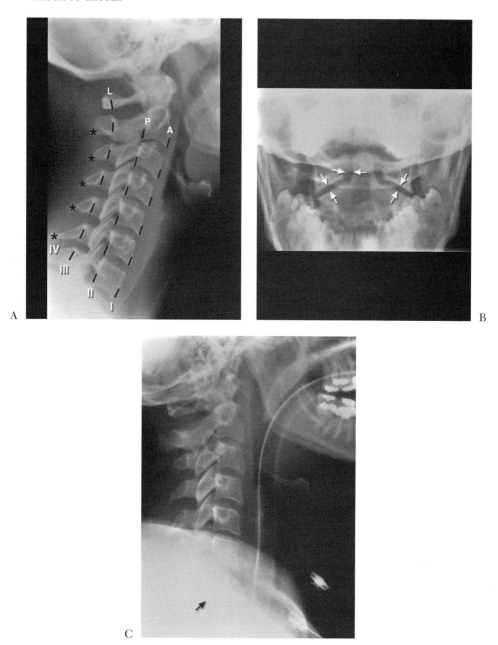

Figure 19.12 Plain spine radiographs with examination techniques to uncover fractures and dislocations. *A:* Normal alignment lines: I, normal alignment along the anterior (A) vertebral margins; II, posterior (P) vertebral margin alignment line; III, spinal laminar (L) line; IV, relation of the dorsal spinous processes. *B:* Indicators of normal odontoid interspace (*arrows*). *C:* Incomplete cervical spine examination (C7 is missing, *arrow*).

Common findings are compression of the vertebral bodies (vertebral body often several millimeters less anteriorly than posteriorly), displacement in the lateral view (more than 3 mm between adjacent vertebral bodies), and displacement of the odontoid bone (odontoid tip should be aligned with tip of clivus).

Indications of instability are displacement of a vertebral body, widening of the interspinous or interlaminar distance, widening of the facet joints

Table 19.6. Essentials of Disciplined Cervical Spine Viewing

Count the number of cervical vertebral bodies; seven cervical spine bodies and the superior end plate of T1 should be visible
Trace contour of every body to detect fractures
Evaluate the alignment lines (see Figs. 19.12, 19.13A)
  1. Anterior spinal line along the anterior longitudinal ligament
  2. Posterior spinal line along the posterior longitudinal ligament
  3. Spinolaminar line along the base of the spinous processes
  4. Line of the spinous processes
Assess soft tissue
Assess facet lines
Assess craniocervical junction
Assess space between the dens axis and lateral masses of C1

or spinal canal, disruption of the posterior spinal line, and anterolisthesis or retrolisthesis with flexion or extension (Table 19.7).[52] The odontoid bone typically lies within 13 mm of the posterior cortex of the anterior C1 arch.

Hyperflexion injuries of the cervical spine—direct trauma to the head, spine in the flexed position—can be seen in various degrees, from mild widening of the posterior intervertebral space to subluxation of the vertebra; and the inferior articular facet may become lodged on the superior facet of the vertebra below (so-called perched facet). A cord lesion is common or easily induced with further manipulation, making this a highly unstable condition.

Unilateral facet distortion can be recognized by an alteration in the laminar space, namely, the distance between the spinolaminar line and the posterior margin of the articular mass.

Table 19.7. Spine Instability

Cervical
• Widened interspinous space or facet joints
• Anterior listhesis >3.5 mm
• Narrowed or widened disk space
• Focal angulation >11 degrees
• Vertebral compression >25%
Thoracic
• Fracture dislocation
• Posttraumatic kyphosis >40 degrees
• Spine fractures associated with sternal fractures
• Concomitant rib fracture or costovertebral dislocation

Source: Imhof and Fuchsjäger.[52] By permission of Springer-Verlag.

Hyperextension injuries (sudden deceleration impact) produce fairly characteristic features, such as a hyperextension teardrop fracture (avulsion of the site of attachment of the anterior longitudinal ligament), hangman's fracture with bilateral fracture through the pars interarticularis of C2, Jefferson's fracture (fracture of the ring of C1), and odontoid fractures (tip is type I, base is type II, and extension into the body of C2 is type III). Figure 19.13 illustrates the most common unstable cervical fractures. Facial injury is more common as a result of direct impact.

Computed Tomography and Magnetic Resonance Imaging

CT scans added to a plain cervical spine film are unsurpassed in diagnostic value for demonstration of fractures. Myelography combined with CT can more clearly demonstrate the cord and nerve roots and determine whether they are compressed by the misalignment or fracture. In most instances, specific areas are scanned with axial slices 1.5–3 mm thick for the cervical spine and 3–5 mm thick for the thoracic and lumbar spines. CT scan reconstructions are very useful in imaging loose bone fragments and facet dislocation.

Intrathecal administration of contrast medium (myelography, CT scanning) is usually reserved for patients who cannot undergo MRI (presence of a pacemaker, aneurysm clips, cochlear implants, bullet fragments, and morbid obesity). It has become the second-choice imaging modality in spine injury because it is time-consuming and requires patient movement.

MRI in spine injury should first obtain sagittal T_1-weighted images, with axial images through abnormal areas.[53] A T_1-weighted image is important to rule out major abnormalities and can be followed by T_2 or gradient echo sequences (short time to acquire and sensitive for early hemorrhages in the spine). On T_1-weighted images (short TR, 300–1000 msec; TE, 10–30 msec), subacute hemorrhage is bright and CSF is dark. On T_2-weighted images (long TR, 1500–3000 msec; TE, 60–120 msec), CSF is bright, cord edema is bright, and acute hemorrhage is dark.[54] An example of cord trauma and swelling is shown in Figure 19.14.

First Priority in Management

Immediate cervical spine immobilization and endotracheal intubation are needed.

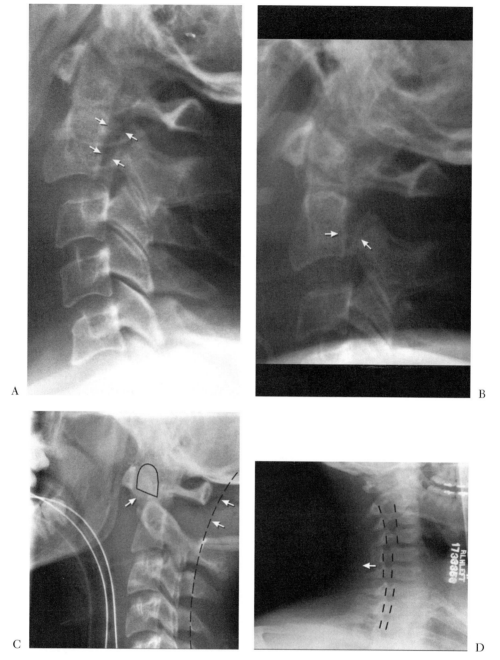

Figure 19.13 *A,B:* Two examples of hangman fracture (C2 bilateral fracture through pars articularis), common with windshield injuries. *C:* Odontoid fracture. The spinal laminar line is disrupted. Dens is outlined (*arrow*). *D:* Locked facet dislocation (*arrows*, hyperflexion injury). *E:* Jefferson C1 fracture (*arrows*).

Hypotension from unopposed parasympathetic tone is common, particularly with change in position or in the first minutes after connection to the mechanical ventilator. Volume resuscitation or an α adrenergic receptor agent, such as phenylephrine, is needed. In occasional patients, autonomic dysregulation is manifested as marked hypertensive surges, which should be treated with

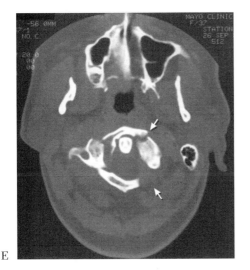

E

Figure 19.13 (*Continued*)

Table 19.8. Emergency Room Management of Traumatic Spine Injury

Intubation and mechanical ventilation with lesion at C3 or
    higher
Intubate if aspiration
Volume loading with albumin or Ringer's lactated solution
Epinephrine drip
Body warming with blanket, warming intravenous fluids
Subcutaneous heparin, 5000 U
Codeine for pain
Proton pump inhibitor (e.g., Protonix) to prevent
    gastrointestinal bleeding
Interval 0–3 hours methylprednisolone 30 mg/kg
    Infusion of methylprednisolone 5.4 mg/kg hourly for 24
        hours
Interval 3–8 hours methylprednisolone 30 mg/kg
    Infusion of methylprednisolone 5.4 mg/kg hourly for 48
        hours

labetalol. Administration of methylprednisolone has resulted in better recovery 1 year after injury (Third National Acute Spinal Cord Injury Randomized Controlled Trial).[55] Maintenance therapy depends on when therapy has been started (Table 19.8).

Catheter placement, gastric ulcer prophylaxis, correction of core hypothermia, and deep venous thrombosis prophylaxis are important before triage.

Predictors of Outcome

The degree of cord injury and the presence of head injury at presentation determine initial out-

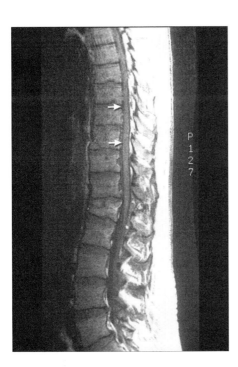

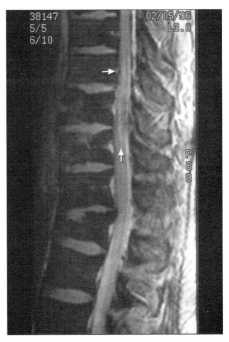

Figure 19.14 Magnetic resonance images of traumatic cord swelling (*arrows*).

come and mortality.[56–58] Patients with complete cervical transection and apnea usually do not recover. Patients are tetraplegic, depend on a mechanical ventilator, and can only operate devices for communication and locomotion (speech may be possible through a special tracheostomy). Patients with transection above the C3 level are not weaned. One study claimed weaning with an average of 80% with lower-level lesions.[56]

Complete cord lesion very rarely changes to an incomplete lesion and vice versa. Patients with incomplete lesions but no motor function and only sensory function have a 10%–30% chance of regaining some motor function. Patients with incomplete lesions but retained motor function have a 50% chance of improvement. This improvement (defined as Medical Research Council muscle grade 3 or more[57]) is then noted in half of the common muscles.

MRI abnormalities with intramedullary hematoma or contusion involving more than one segment predict a worse outcome. Central low signal intensity on T_2 images may represent central cord contusion, with poor prospects. Central high signal intensity without areas of low signal intensity with normal T_1 may represent cord edema or ischemia but no infarction. Mixtures of patterns are possible and make the use of MRI for prognosis indeterminate.

Triage

- Neurologic–neurosurgical intensive care unit for management of dysautonomia; bladder, skin, and bowel care; and planning for stabilizing spinal surgery.
- Spinal rehabilitation center if surgery is not indicated and dysautonomia is absent.

REFERENCES

1. Giannoudis PV, Veysi VT, Pape HC, et al.: When should we operate on major fractures in patients with severe head injuries? Am J Surg 183:261, 2002.
2. Marion DW, Carlier PM: Problems with initial Glasgow Coma Scale assessment caused by prehospital treatment of patients with head injuries: results of a national survey. J Trauma 36:89, 1994.
3. Partrick DA, Bensard DD, Janik JS, et al.: Is hypotension a reliable indicator of blood loss from traumatic injury in children? Am J Surg 184:555, 2002.
4. Baguley IJ, Nicholls JL, Felmingham KL, et al.: Dysautonomia after traumatic brain injury: a forgotten syndrome? J Neurol Neurosurg Psychiatry 67:39, 1999.
5. Thornbury JR, Masters SJ, Campbell JA: Imaging recommendations for head trauma: a new comprehensive strategy. AJR Am J Roentgenol 149:781, 1987.
6. Adams JH, Graham DI, Murray LS, et al.: Diffuse axonal injury due to nonmissile head injury in humans: an analysis of 45 cases. Ann Neurol 12:557, 1982.
7. Gennarelli TA, Thibault LE, Adams JH, et al.: Diffuse axonal injury and traumatic coma in the primate. Ann Neurol 12:564, 1982.
8. Blumbergs PC, Jones NR, North JB: Diffuse axonal injury in head trauma. J Neurol Neurosurg Psychiatry 52:838, 1989.
9. Piek J, Chesnut RM, Marshall LF, et al.: Extracranial complications of severe head injury. J Neurosurg 77:901, 1992.
10. Di Rocco A, Ellis SJ, Landes C: Delayed epidural hematoma. Neuroradiology 33:253, 1991.
11. Servadei F, Murray GD, Teasdale GM, et al.: Traumatic subarachnoid hemorrhage: demographic and clinical study of 750 patients from the European Brain Injury Consortium survey of head injuries. Neurosurgery 50:261, 2002.
12. Abraszko RA, Zurynski YA, Dorsch NW: The significance of traumatic intraventricular haemorrhage in severe head injury. Br J Neurosurg 9:769, 1995.
13. Lee JP, Lui TN, Chang CN: Acute post-traumatic intraventricular hemorrhage: analysis of 25 patients with emphasis on final outcome. Acta Neurol Scand 84:85, 1991.
14. Fujitsu K, Kuwabara T, Muramotoa M: Traumatic intraventricular hemorrhage: a report of twenty-six cases and consideration of the pathogenic mechanism. Neurosurgery 23:423, 1988.
15. MacPherson M, MacPherson P, Jennett B: CT evidence of intracranial contusion and haematoma in relation to the presence, site and type of skull fracture. Clin Radiol 42:321, 1990.
16. Gibson RM, Stephenson GC: Aggressive management of severe closed head trauma: time for reappraisal. Lancet 2:369, 1989.
17. Miller JD, Dearden NM, Piper IR, et al.: Control of intracranial pressure in patients with severe head injury. J Neurotrauma 9(Suppl 1):S317, 1992.
18. Bickell WH, Wall MJ Jr, Pepe PE, et al.: Immediate versus delayed fluid resuscitation for hypotensive patients with penetrating torso injuries. N Engl J Med 331:1105, 1994.
19. Mattox KL, Maningas PA, Moore EE, et al.: Prehospital hypertonic saline/dextran infusion for post-traumatic hypotension. The U.S.A. Multicenter Trial. Ann Surg 213:482, 1991.
20. Revell M, Porter K, Greaves I: Fluid resuscitation in prehospital trauma care: a consensus view. Emerg Med J 19:494, 2002.

21. Rosner MJ, Daughton S: Cerebral perfusion pressure management in head injury. *J Trauma* 30:933, 1990.

22. Kaufmann AM, Cardoso ER: Aggravation of vasogenic cerebral edema by multiple-dose mannitol. *J Neurosurg* 77:584, 1992.

23. Cruz J, Minoja G, Okuchi K: Major clinical and physiological benefits of early high doses of mannitol for intraparenchymal temporal lobe hemorrhages with abnormal pupillary widening: a randomized trial. *Neurosurgery* 51:628, 2002.

24. Kelly DF, Goodale DB, Williams J, et al.: Propofol in the treatment of moderate and severe head injury: a randomized, prospective double-blinded pilot trial. *J Neurosurg* 90:1042, 1999.

25. Bouma GJ, Muizelaar JP, Bandoh K, et al.: Blood pressure and intracranial pressure-volume dynamics in severe head injury: relationship with cerebral blood flow. *Neurosurgery* 77:15, 1992.

26. Braakman R, Schouten HJ, Blaauw-van Dishoeck M, et al.: Megadose steroids in severe head injury. Results of a prospective double-blind clinical trial. *J Neurosurg* 58:326, 1983.

27. Cottrell JE, Patel K, Turndorf H, et al.: Intracranial pressure changes induced by sodium nitroprusside in patients with intracranial mass lesions. *J Neurosurg* 48:329, 1978.

28. Rea GL, Rockswold GL: Barbiturate therapy in uncontrolled intracranial hypertension. *Neurosurgery* 12:401, 1983.

29. Ward JD, Becker DP, Miller JD, et al.: Failure of prophylactic barbiturate coma in the treatment of severe head injury. *J Neurosurg* 62:383, 1985.

30. Yano M, Nishiyama H, Yokota H, et al.: Effect of lidocaine on ICP response to endotracheal suctioning. *Anesthesiology* 64:651, 1986.

31. Evans DE, Kobrine AI: Reduction of experimental intracranial hypertension by lidocaine. *Neurosurgery* 20:542, 1987.

32. Chesnut RM, Marshall LF, Klauber MR, et al.: The role of secondary brain injury in determining outcome from severe head injury. *J Trauma* 34:216, 1993.

33. Magnoni S, Ghisoni L, Locatelli M, et al.: Lack of improvement in cerebral metabolism after hyperoxia in severe head injury: a microdialysis study. *J Neurosurg* 98:952, 2003.

34. Tokutomi T, Morimoto K, Miyagi T: Optimal temperature for the management of severe traumatic brain injury: effect of hypothermia on intracranial pressure, systemic and intracranial hemodynamics, and metabolism. *Neurosurgery* 52:102, 2003.

35. Chang BS, Lowenstein DH: Practice parameter: antiepileptic drug prophylaxis in severe traumatic brain injury. *Neurology* 60:10, 2003.

36. Mahoney BD, Rockswold GL, Ruiz E, et al.: Emergency twist drill trephination. *Neurosurgery* 8:551, 1981.

37. Hamilton M, Wallace C: Nonoperative management of acute epidural hematoma diagnosed by CT: the neuroradiologist's role. *AJNR Am J Neuroradiol* 13:853, 1992.

38. Sagher O, Ribas GC, Jane JA: Nonoperative management of acute epidural hematoma diagnosed by CT: the neuroradiologist's role. *AJNR Am J Neuroradiol* 13:860, 1992.

39. Lang EW, Pitts LH, Damron SL, et al.: Outcome after severe head injury: an analysis of prediction based upon comparison of neural network versus logistic regression analysis. *Neurol Res* 19:274, 1997.

40. Choi SC, Narayan RK, Anderson RL, et al.: Enhanced specificity of prognosis in severe head injury. *J Neurosurg* 69:381, 1988.

41. Wilberger JE Jr, Harris M, Diamond DL: Acute subdural hematoma: morbidity and mortality related to timing of operative intervention. *J Trauma* 30:733, 1990.

42. Signorini DF, Andrews PJ, Jones PA, et al.: Adding insult to injury: the prognostic value of early secondary insults for survival after traumatic brain injury. *J Neurol Neurosurg Psychiatry* 66:26, 1999.

43. Kampfl A, Schmutzhard E, Franz G, et al.: Prediction of recovery from post-traumatic vegetative state with cerebral magnetic-resonance imaging. *Lancet* 351:1763, 1998.

44. Hills MW, Deane SA: Head injury and facial injury: is there an increased risk of cervical spine injury? *J Trauma* 34:549, 1993.

45. Michael DB, Guyot DR, Darmody WR: Coincidence of head and cervical spine injury. *J Neurotrauma* 6:177, 1989.

46. Fehlings MG, Tator CH: An evidence-based review of decompressive surgery in acute spinal cord injury: rationale, indications, and timing based on experimental and clinical studies. *J Neurosurg* 91:1, 1999.

47. Donovan WH: Operative and nonoperative management of spinal cord injury. A review. *Paraplegia* 32:375, 1994.

48. Wijdicks EFM: Neurologic complications of multisystem trauma. In *Neurologic Complications of Critical Illness*. 2nd ed. New York: Oxford University Press, 2002, pp. 302–336.

49. Bachulis BL, Long WB, Hynes GD, et al.: Clinical indications for cervical spine radiographs in the traumatized patient. *Am J Surg* 153:473, 1987.

50. Kreipke DL, Gillespie KR, McCarthy MC, et al.: Reliability of indications for cervical spine films in trauma patients. *J Trauma* 29:1438, 1989.

51. Mirvis SE, Diaconis JN, Chirico PA, et al.: Protocol-driven radiologic evaluation of suspected cervical spine injury: efficacy study. *Radiology* 170:831, 1989.

52. Imhof H, Fuchsjäger M: Traumatic injuries: imaging of spinal injuries. *Eur Radiol* 12:1262, 2002.

53. Kalfas I, Wilberger J, Goldberg A, et al.: Magnetic resonance imaging in acute spinal cord trauma. *Neurosurgery* 23:295, 1988.

54. Wittenberg RH, Boetel U, Beyer HK: Magnetic resonance imaging and computer tomography of acute spinal cord trauma. *Clin Orthop* 260:176, 1990.

55. Bracken MB, Shepard MJ, Holford TR, et al.: Administration of methylprednisolone for 24 or 48 hours or tirilazad mesylate for 48 hours in the treatment of acute spinal cord injury. Results of the Third National Acute Spinal

Cord Injury Randomized Controlled Trial. *JAMA* 277: 1597, 1997.

56. Wicks AB, Menter RR: Long-term outlook in quadriplegic patients with initial ventilator dependency. *Chest* 90: 406, 1986.

57. Ditunno JF Jr, Formal CS: Spinal cord injury. In JM Gilchrist (ed), *Prognosis in Neurology*. Boston: Butterworth-Heinemann, 1998, p. 287.

58. Akmal M, Trivedi R, Sutcliffe J: Functional outcome in trauma patients with spinal injury. *Spine* 28:180, 2003.

Appendix 19.1.

American Spinal Injury Association (ASIA) Impairment Scale

ASIA

STANDARD NEUROLOGICAL CLASSIFICATION OF SPINAL CORD INJURY

MOTOR

KEY MUSCLES

R L

- C2
- C3
- C4
- C5 Elbow flexors
- C6 Wrist extensors
- C7 Elbow extensors
- C8 Finger flexors (distal phalanx of middle finger)
- T1 Finger abductors (little finger)
- T2
- T3
- T4
- T5
- T6
- T7
- T8
- T9
- T10
- T11
- T12
- L1
- L2 Hip flexors
- L3 Knee extensors
- L4 Ankle dorsiflexors
- L5 Long toe extensors
- S1 Ankle plantar flexors
- S2
- S3
- S4-5

```
0 = total paralysis
1 = palpable or visible contraction
2 = active movement,
      gravity eliminated
3 = active movement,
      against gravity
4 = active movement,
      against some resistance
5 = active movement,
      against full resistance
NT = not testable
```

Voluntary anal contraction (Yes/No)

TOTALS ☐ + ☐ = ☐ **MOTOR SCORE**
(MAXIMUM) (50) (50)   (100)

LIGHT TOUCH   PIN PRICK

R L   R L

- C2
- C3
- C4
- C5
- C6
- C7
- C8
- T1
- T2
- T3
- T4
- T5
- T6
- T7
- T8
- T9
- T10
- T11
- T12
- L1
- L2
- L3
- L4
- L5
- S1
- S2
- S3
- S4-5

TOTALS { ☐ ☐   ☐ + ☐ = ☐ **PIN PRICK SCORE** (max: 112)
(MAXIMUM) (56) (56)   (56) (56)   = ☐ **LIGHT TOUCH SCORE** (max: 112)

SENSORY

KEY SENSORY POINTS

```
0 = absent
1 = impaired
2 = normal
NT = not testable
```

Any anal sensation (Yes/No)

* Key Sensory Points

NEUROLOGICAL LEVEL The most caudal segment with normal function	COMPLETE OR INCOMPLETE? Incomplete = Any sensory or motor function in S4-S5	ZONE OF PARTIAL PRESERVATION Caudal extent of partially innervated segments
SENSORY ☐ ☐ (R L) MOTOR ☐ ☐	☐ ASIA IMPAIRMENT SCALE ☐	SENSORY ☐ ☐ (R L) MOTOR ☐ ☐

This form may be copied freely but should not be altered without permission from the American Spinal Injury Association.   2000 Rev.

Functional Independence Measure (FIM)

LEVELS		No Helper
7	Complete Independence (Timely, Safely)	No
6	Modified Independence (Device)	Helper
	Modified Dependence	
5	Supervision	
4	Minimal Assist (Subject = 75%+)	
3	Moderate Assist (Subject = 50%+)	Helper
	Complete Dependence	
2	Maximal Assist (Subject = 25%+)	
1	Total Assist (Subject = 0%+)	

ADMIT   DISCH

Self Care
A. Eating
B. Grooming
C. Bathing
D. Dressing-Upper Body
E. Dressing-Lower Body
F. Toileting

Sphincter Control
G. Bladder Management
H. Bowel Management

Mobility
Transfer:
I. Bed, Chair, Wheelchair
J. Toilet
K. Tub, Shower

Locomotion
L. Walk/Wheelchair (W/C)
M. Stairs

Communication
N. Comprehension (A/V)
O. Expression (V/N)

Social Cognition
P. Social Interaction
Q. Problem Solving
R. Memory

Total FIM

NOTE: Leave no blanks; enter 1 if patient not testable due to risk.

ASIA IMPAIRMENT SCALE

☐ **A = Complete:** No motor or sensory function is preserved in the sacral segments S4-S5.

☐ **B = Incomplete:** Sensory but not motor function is preserved below the neurological level and includes the sacral segments S4-S5.

☐ **C = Incomplete:** Motor function is preserved below the neurological level, and more than half of key muscles below the neurological level have a muscle grade less than 3.

☐ **D = Incomplete:** Motor function is preserved below the neurological level, and at least half of key muscles below the neurological level have a muscle grade of 3 or more.

☐ **E = Normal:** motor and sensory function are normal

CLINICAL SYNDROMES

☐ Central Cord
☐ Brown-Sequard
☐ Anterior Cord
☐ Conus Medullaris
☐ Cauda Equina

Chapter 20
Forensic Neurologic Injury

Nonaccidental injury to the brain is frequently encountered in the emergency department, and more so where street crime is common. Injury to the brain can be self-inflicted or due to a fight, robbery, rape, or battering. Gunshot wounds are a not-infrequent cause of death in younger individuals and adults. Because death often follows such an injury, a forensic neuropathologist typically takes responsibility for the case. Neurologists seeing patients with neurologic injury should always have nonaccidental injury in mind and, particularly, should be primed toward the possibility of spousal abuse. In some instances, crime is obvious. In others, evidence is circumstantial and these cases eventually need jurisdiction. Neurologists who evaluate patients in the emergency department may be asked to render opinions in legal proceedings. Information on neurologic injury associated with assault is difficult to obtain elsewhere; thus, including it in this monograph provides some practical value. This chapter's major focus is on the conditions that have been best characterized, but it is necessarily tentative and caveated due to lack of data in this field.

General Forensic Considerations

A detailed history may not be readily available, and the law enforcement agency involved may provide additional details about the crime scene. When the type of insult is unclear, certain clues may point toward crime. Massive fracture of the skull with comparatively little injury to the brain may be due to an immobilized head striking a wall or floor and may suggest battering. Periorbital hematomas from the use of blunt instruments or fist impacts are common in spousal abuse. Left-sided facial injuries are more frequent than right-sided injuries, reflecting the simple logic that most assailants are right-handed.[1,2] Facial fractures with dental fractures are also more common in assaults, and zygomatic complex fractures are more frequent than mandibular fractures.[2-4] In general, the combination of head, neck, and facial injury is more likely in victims of domestic violence. Other criteria, such as delay between time of injury and arrival for treatment; reluctance of the patient's companion to leave the patient during the examination; trauma to the head, face, shoulders, breasts, and abdomen; and bilateral injuries, increase the possibility of abuse.[5]

Shaken Baby Syndrome

One stunning neurologic injury is shaken baby syndrome. Shaken baby syndrome has many synonyms (shaken impact syndrome or battered babies).[6] Child abuse is a common cause of infant death but, as expected, a history suggesting neglect and foul play is commonly inconsistent or incomplete. One study on children admitted with subdural hematomas suggested that 59% had abusive injury.[7] Shaken baby syndrome is typically observed in children less than 3 years of age, with a peak incidence in the first year.[8–10] Epidemiologic studies might be complicated to interpret and less precise due to missed cases. However, a prospective epidemiologic study in pediatric units in Scotland found quite a high annual incidence of 24.6 per 100,000 children younger than 1 year. In the United States, it is common in urban regions and during autumn and winter months.[11] Risk factors for shaken baby syndrome that have been identified include younger parents, low socioeconomic status, child disability, or being premature. Fathers, boyfriends, and female babysitters most often cause the injuries; less commonly, the mother of the child is the cause. Although the clinical features are well delineated, the syndrome is still clouded in controversy and overcharged in legal proceedings.[12]

Clinical Presentation

Clinical presentation is very dramatic, and progression to brain death is common. Brain death is a consequence of sustained increased intracranial pressure that is in close proximity to the injury. A prolonged episode of lucidity between injury and the onset of symptoms is highly uncommon. On examination, the infant is comatose, is commonly mildly to moderately anemic, and may display signs of severe disseminated intravascular coagulation. Pancreatic traumatic damage may be seen, with high amylase levels, and liver injury may also be present. Femur, humerus, and rib fractures and superficial bruises should be actively sought. A fairly common finding is bilateral retinal hemorrhage (±60%), which should be specifically sought.[13] (A recent study found that more than 50% of nonophthalmologists did not visualize the retina.[14]) Presence of retinal hemorrhages together with retinal folds or detachments, which can be seen only by expert evaluation of an ophthalmologist, is much more suggestive of the diagnosis.[15]

Interpretation of Diagnostic Tests

Computed Tomography
The computed tomographic (CT) scan should include bone windows and may detect skull fractures that could be multiple and cross suture lines. The CT scan typically detects a subarachnoid

hemorrhage and subdural hematomas but may also show diffuse brain edema indistinguishable from patterns seen in anoxic-ischemic injury. The brain is hypodense, with loss of white and gray matter differentiation but with sparing of the basal ganglia and posterior fossa structures.[16] Intentional injury is more likely when the CT scan shows subdural hematoma over the convexity. In addition, subdural hematomas have a high proclivity, being located in the interhemispheric fissure. The age of the subdural hematoma may be difficult to estimate, and a magnetic resonance imaging (MRI) scan could be more useful in this determination.[17] The presence of layers of subdural hematomas of different ages is very suggestive of nonaccidental head trauma. In some infants, fractures are absent and hygromas are found.[18] Contrecoup lesions are perhaps more common and a reflection of acceleration/deceleration force.[19]

The CT scan may also include petechial or punctate hemorrhages along the gyral surfaces and the inferior surface of the frontal lobe and temporal and frontal poles (Fig. 20.1).

Eventually pathologic examination is an important adjunct in confirming the clinical diagnosis. However, the interpretation of injury is complex, and a meticulous autopsy is usually performed by experts in this field (Box 20.1).[20] Important studies have recently been published.[21,22]

Prediction of Outcome

Many neonates and children progress to brain death and may become potential organ donors. Morbidity is substantial and ranges from 15% to 40%.[23] Morbidity in survivors includes spasticity, microcephaly, and seizure disorders.[17]

Triage

- Neonatal intensive care unit.

Hanging and Strangulation

Victims of hanging, a common method of suicide, will appear in the emergency department. Attempted strangulation of an intruder or strangulation in the setting of abuse may result in a sim-

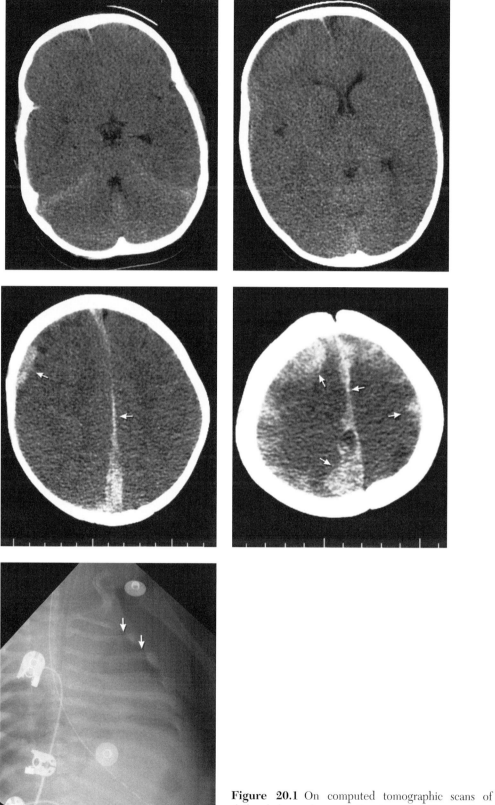

Figure 20.1 On computed tomographic scans of shaken baby syndrome, both subarachnoid hemorrhage and subdural hematomas are seen (*arrows*). On chest X-ray, note multiple rib fractures (*arrows*).

297

Box 20.1. Injury in Shaken Baby Syndrome

The term *shaken baby syndrome* suggests that impact on a flat surface is necessary to create the injury. Some evidence suggests that shaking alone may not produce the angular acceleration to create shear injuries and subdural hematoma. Small axonal size predisposes a young brain to injury, but the shell of the skull base also allows the brain to rotate more readily.[6] An "injury" should be distinguished from translational forces, such as falling down stairs. With skull fractures, skull bruises, or subgaleal hemorrhage, an impact can be assumed. Anoxic-ischemic injury seems to play a major role, which can be due to intentional suffocation as well. Other injuries include posterior rib fractures due to tight squeezing of the chest of the baby and should not be attributed to cardiopulmonary resuscitation (CPR) (none were found in 91 infants with CPR).[19] An association between subdural and retinal bleeding has been found pathologically.[21,22] Hemorrhage at the periphery (ora serrata) and posterior pole of the retina is more common.

---

ilar injury. The pathophysiologic mechanisms may be entirely due to postanoxic brain injury.

Clinical Presentation

There is a major difference between suicidal and judicial hangings. The fall from a lesser height may result in lesser prevalence of cervical spine injury (fracture or dislocation). Neck fracture occurs in fewer than 10% of hanging victims.[24] Only a fall from a major height with a sudden stop may fracture the upper cervical vertebra and detach the pons from the medulla. Drug or alcohol ingestion was present in 70% of 44 cases reported from Australia.[25]

Many patients are found pulseless, apneic, and suspended free at the scene. Marks around the neck but also subconjunctival or facial petechial hemorrhages are quite common. If severe, these may be associated with tongue hemorrhages; one study suggested that gross tongue hemorrhages were more common in strangulation.[26] Acute papilledema with hemorrhages may occur due to asphyxia. Myoclonus status epilepticus in comatose patients is observed frequently and reflects the seriousness of this injury (see Chapter 10). Brief generalized tonic-clonic seizures may occur as well. The responsible injury may be neck vein compression, carotid artery occlusion, or laryngeal injury leading to diffuse anoxic-ischemic impact.

Attempted strangulation is another condition that can produce neurologic injury, and many of the symptoms are initially nonneurologic. Patients who present to the emergency department may have petechiae of the skin of the upper eyelid and subconjunctival hemorrhages. Sore throat, hyperventilation, and uncontrollable shaking have been documented. Strangulation can cause a comatose state; then the abnormalities will involve lesions to areas that are susceptible to anoxia.

Neurologic injury associated with spousal abuse is of major concern and may be underrecognized in the emergency department.[27] Alcohol abuse, unemployment or intermittent unemployment, estranged husbands, or former boyfriends increase the risk.[28] Head, neck, and facial injuries have been found as significant markers, but there is increasing evidence of the presence of arterial dissection associated with strangulation.[29] The mechanism is thought to be compression of the carotid artery against the bony cervical vertebrae, resulting eventually in dissection of the media.[30,31] Other suggestive injuries are defensive injuries of the forearm, bruises in various stages of healing, or any poorly explained injury.[32] The time lapse between presentation may be months; thus, skin lesions may not be present.

Interpretation of Diagnostic Tests

Computed Tomography

The CT scan is rarely abnormal but may show the effects of severe anoxic-ischemic injury in the resuscitated patient.[33] In these cases, massive edema with loss of white–gray matter differentiation and sulcal architecture is common (see Chapter 9). The cerebellum may be spared.[34] Hypodensity in lentiform nuclei and thalami may be seen.[35] One report noted bilateral lobar hematomas due to massive elevated cerebral venous pressure. These could represent hemorrhagic infarcts with a mechanism comparable to cerebral venous sinus thrombosis.[36]

Magnetic Resonance Imaging

More or less specific findings have been reported on MRI, which has a much better sensitivity for lesions. Signal changes in the lentiform nuclei or the thalamus often are noted, but a rent lesion from sudden deceleration and flexion at the junction of the pons and medulla oblongata is more characteristic (Fig. 20.2). Severe anoxic injury is often combined with ischemic injury from cardiac arrest, even if brief; and, in permanently comatose patients, the cortex signal may be extremely hyperintense (Fig. 20.3).

Predictors of Outcome

The presence of a Glasgow coma score of 3, fixed dilated pupils, or cardiac arrest at the scene is associated with a grim outcome.[37] Pulmonary edema is common. Delayed anoxic encephalopathy has been reported.[39] It is very important to obtain a drug and alcohol screen in these patients, and their presence can markedly confound the assessment. Somatosensory evoked potentials (absent bilateral scalp potentials with preserved cervical cord potentials) may be considered for

prognostication. Acute dystonia and an akinetic rigid syndrome have been reported, but these findings are nonspecific and a representation of anoxic injury to basal ganglia.[40]

Triage

- Medical intensive care unit for mechanical ventilation and support.
- A mandatory law for reporting domestic violence may exist.[41]

Gunshot Wounds to the Head

The impact to the brain when penetrated by a bullet is explosive and, due to its shock wave, enormously damaging. Not only do bullets penetrate the skull, brain, and vascular structures, but the great force and high pressure in the cavity of passage also damage the surrounding structures. Details of ballistics require special expertise and are not discussed here. However, some observations seem consistent. The entrance wound often leaves unburned residues in the skin ("tattooing") and is typically smaller than the exit wound. The exit may be larger due to mushrooming of the bullet. Suicide wounds are often in the dominant temporal region or in the mouth, with an angulation

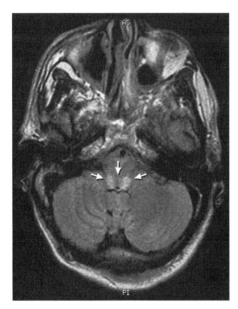 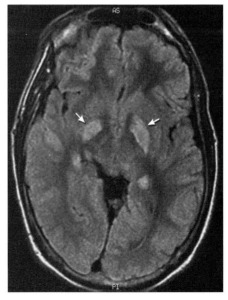

Figure 20.2 Magnetic resonance imaging (*left*) shows rent in pontomesencephalic region typical of hanging. Hyperintensities of the lenticular nucleus are also noted in globus pallidus (*right*).

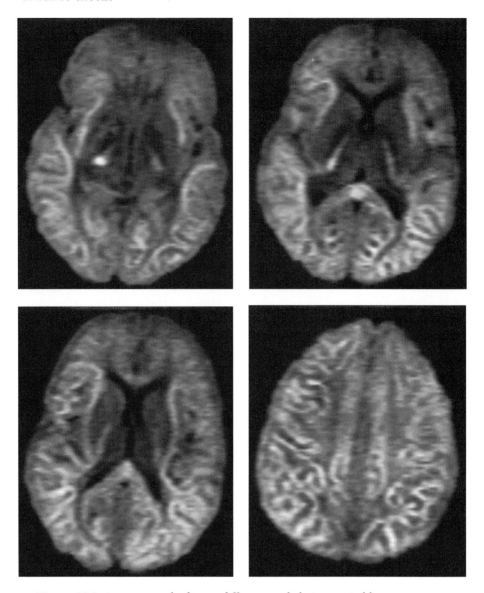

Figure 20.3 Anoxic injury leading to diffuse overwhelming cortical hyperintensities.

matching the handedness. When multiple gun-shot wounds are present, suicide is unlikely. How-ever, penetration of the head without loss of im-pairment of consciousness due to the low energy of aged ammunition may result in multiple self-inflicted wounds.[42] The brain stem and deeper structures of the brain are frequent sites of hem-orrhage, and ectopic bone fragments are seen. Guns placed in the mouth may destroy the brain stem, or bullets may lodge under the skull base, damaging the carotid artery and cranial nerve XII.[43] Gunshot wounds to the brain are complex

injuries, with skull fracture, tracks of bone, and missile fragments. Often, an associated intracere-bral hematoma determines the initial clinical con-dition. Cerebral contusions may be seen at the en-try and exit sites.

Clinical Presentation

Evaluation of patients with gunshot wounds to the head involves assessment of the Glasgow coma score, but scores are very low. Patients not un-commonly present with fixed unreactive pupils, and extensor posturing. Early deterioration may be due to enlarging intracranial hematoma or acute subdural hematoma from a fall.

Interpretation of Diagnostic Tests

Computed Tomography

CT scan images are shown in Figure 20.4. A bone window may identify small residue of metal or bone showing the track of the bullet or even lodging of a large fragment. Suicidal gunshots are often with guns placed against the temple or with the barrel inside the mouth, producing characteristic tracks. A CT scan is performed to detect parenchymal hematoma, subdural hematoma, or contrecoup lesions. The hematomas are along the tracks of the bullet in the ventricles or in the subdural space.

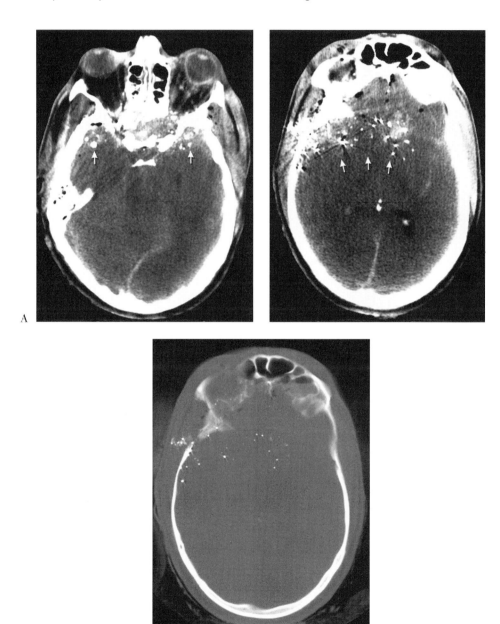

Figure 20.4 Examples of computed tomographic scans of patients with gunshot wounds. A: Gun placed on temple with bullet cutting through the brain horizontally and leaving a hemorrhage in its tracks.

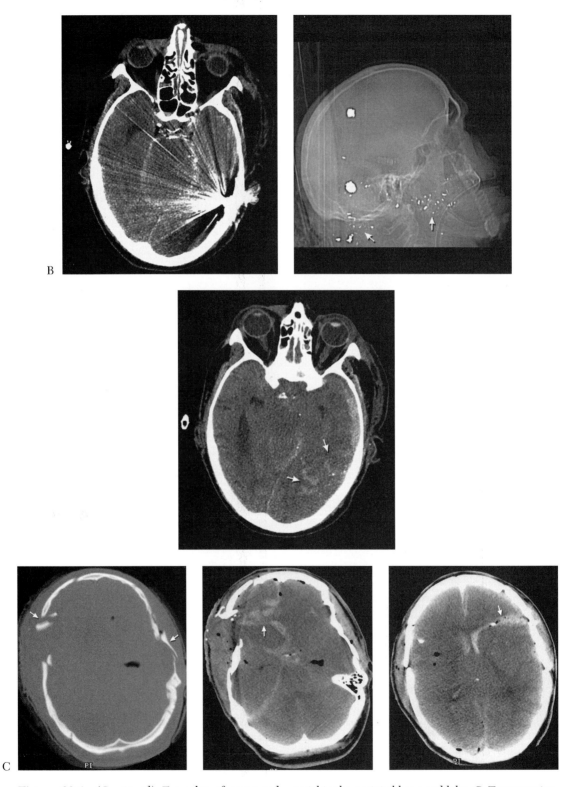

Figure 20.4 (*Continued*) Examples of computed tomographic scans of patients with gunshot wounds. *B:* Shotgun with barrel in mouth, disposing most ma-terial in the occipital bone and lobe. *C:* Transventricu-lar injury (track with intraventricular hematoma) with bone destruction (*arrows*) and intracranial air.

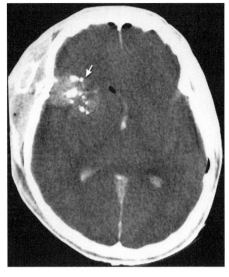

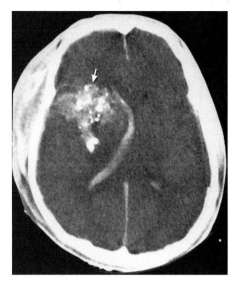

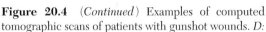

D

Figure 20.4 (*Continued*) Examples of computed tomographic scans of patients with gunshot wounds. *D:* Gunshot-induced intracranial hematoma with intraventricular hematoma. Air is visible in ventricles.

First Priority in Management

The management of gunshot wounds is similar to that of any other type of non-penetrating trauma.[44] A large intracerebral hematoma with mass effect and imminent herniation should be removed. No further therapy can be offered to patients who, after initial resuscitation, have a Glasgow coma score of 3, no operable hematoma, and no major confounder such as drug ingestion.[45] Reconstructive repair of the bone and dura should begin immediately.[38] The wound is considered contaminated, and broad-spectrum antibiotics (vancomycin with cefotaxime) should be administered early. When injury to the cerebral vasculature is anticipated, angiography can be performed, but therapeutic options other than endovascular or surgical occlusion are limited. A major problem is the early development of disseminated intravascular coagulation. Its occurrence is related to the amount of brain tissue damage; thus, it is frequent in gunshot wounds. Its appearance on laboratory tests (e.g., increased D-dimer or fibrinogen split products) denotes a poor outcome. If there is evidence of a full track throughout the brain, there appears to be very little benefit of aggressive intracranial pressure management. A bolus of mannitol, 1–2 g/kg, can be administered to determine whether improvement is possible; but if none is present, salvageability is unlikely.

Predictors of Outcome

Important factors that determine outcome relate to the size of the parenchymal hematoma, the degree of destroyed parenchymal tissue, the development of cerebral edema, infection, and mass effect.[46] The presence of contrecoup contusions could be an important additional determinant. Tension pneumocephalus may occur after penetrating injury to the frontal sinus or the anterior ethmoidal–cribriform plate area.[47–49] Gradual enlargement may occur, with clinical deterioration that requires drainage and closure of the defect (Fig. 20.5).

Poor outcome is expected in comatose patients with extensor posturing at admission, abnormal pupils, CT scan demonstrating ventricular involvement, crossing of midsagittal or midventricular horizontal planes, intraparenchymal hemorrhage, and a high volume of contused or damaged brain.[50,51] Evidence of increased intracranial pressure as noted by obliteration of the mesencephalic cisterns, presence of subarachnoid and interventricular hemorrhage, and intracranial hematoma are all associated with poor outcome, according to the National Institutes of Health Traumatic Coma Data Bank.[52,53]

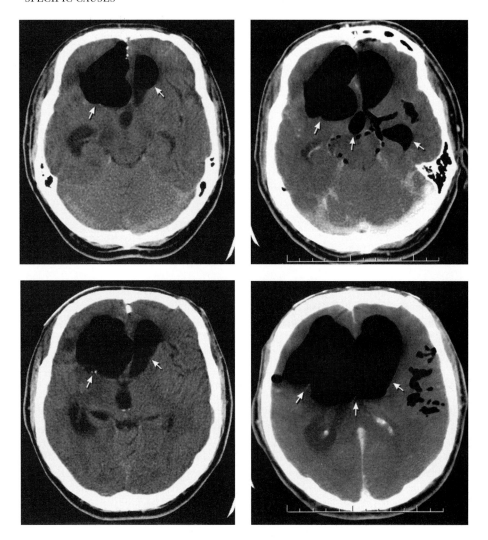

Figure 20.5 Developing tension pneumocephalus after gunshot wound.

Triage

- Surgical debridement (removal of metal and bone fragments and necrotic tissue) and evacuation of growing hematomas.
- Triage to neurosurgical intensive care unit.
- With clinical suspicion of vascular injury, consider cerebral angiogram.

REFERENCES

1. Gayford JJ: Wife-battering: a preliminary survey of 100 cases. *BMJ* 1:194, 1975.

2. Shepherd JP, Al-Kotany M, Subadan CJ, et al.: Assault and facial soft tissue injuries. *Br J Plast Surg* 40:614, 1987.

3. Perciaccante VJ, Ochs HA, Dodson TB: Head, neck, and facial injuries as markers of domestic violence in women. *J Oral Maxillofac Surg* 57:760, 1999.

4. Ochs HA, Neuenschwander MC, Dodson TB: Are head, neck and facial injuries markers of domestic violence? *J Am Dent Assoc* 127:757, 1996.

5. Flitcraft A: Physicians and domestic violence: challenges for prevention. *Health Aff (Millwood)* 12:154, 1993.

6. American Academy of Pediatrics: Committee on Child Abuse and Neglect. Shaken baby syndrome: rotational cranial injuries—technical report. *Pediatrics* 108:206, 2001.

7. Feldman KW, Bethel R, Shugerman RP: The cause of in-

fant and toddler subdural hemorrhage: a prospective study. *Pediatrics* 108:636, 2001.

8. David TJ: Shaken baby (shaken impact) syndrome: non-accidental head injury in infancy. *J R Soc Med* 92:556, 1999.

9. Duhaime AC, Christian CW, Rorke LB, et al.: Nonaccidental head injury in infants—the "shaken-baby syndrome." *N Engl J Med* 338:1822, 1998.

10. Duhaime AC, Gennarelli TA, Thibault LE, et al.: The shaken baby syndrome. *J Neurosurg* 66:409, 1987.

11. Barlow KM, Minns RA: Annual incidence of shaken impact syndrome in young children. *Lancet* 356:1571, 2000.

12. Uscinski R: Shaken baby syndrome: fundamental questions. *Br J Neurosurg* 16:217, 2002.

13. Conway EE Jr: Nonaccidental head injury in infants: "the shaken baby syndrome revisited." *Pediatr Ann* 27:677, 1998.

14. Morad Y, Kim YM, Mian M, et al. Nonophthalmologist accuracy in diagnosing retinal hemorrhages in the shaken baby syndrome. *J Pediatr* 142:431, 2003.

15. Kivlin JD, Simons KB, Lazoritz S, et al.: Shaken baby syndrome. *Ophthalmology* 107:1246, 2000.

16. Petitti N, Williams DW III: CT and MR imaging of nonaccidental pediatric head trauma. *Acad Radiol* 5:215, 1998.

17. Caffey J: The whiplash shaken infant syndrome: manual shaking by the extremities with whiplash-induced intracranial and intraocular bleedings, linked with residual permanent brain damage and mental retardation. *Pediatrics* 54:396, 1974.

18. Wells RG, Vetter C, Laud P: Intracranial hemorrhage in children younger than 3 years. *Arch Pediatr Adolesc Med* 156:252, 2002.

19. Spevak MR, Kleinman PK, Belanger PL, et al.: Cardiopulmonary resuscitation and rib fractures in infants. A postmortem radiologic–pathologic study. *JAMA* 272:617, 1994.

20. Case ME, Graham MA, Handy TC, et al.: Position paper on fatal abusive head injuries in infants and young children. *Am J Forensic Med Pathol* 22:112, 2001.

21. Geddes JF, Hackshaw AK, Vowles GH, et al.: Neuropathology of inflicted head injury in children. I. Patterns of brain damage. *Brain* 124:1290, 2001.

22. Geddes JF, Vowles GH, Hackshaw AK, et al.: Neuropathology of inflicted head injury in children. II. Microscopic brain injury in infants. *Brain* 124:1299, 2001.

23. King WJ, MacKay M, Sirnick A: Shaken baby syndrome in Canada: clinical characteristics and outcome of hospital cases. *CMAJ* 168:155, 2003.

24. Feigin G: Frequency of neck organ fractures in hanging. *Am J Forensic Med Pathol* 20:128, 1999.

25. McClane GE, Strack GB, Hawley D: A review of 300 attempted strangulation cases: part II. Clinical evaluation of the surviving victim. *J Emerg Med* 21:311, 2001.

26. Bockholdt B, Maxeiner H: Hemorrhages of the tongue in the postmortem diagnostics of strangulation. *Forensic Sci Int* 126:214, 2002.

27. Corrigan JD, Wolfe M, Mysiw WJ, et al. Early identification of mild traumatic brain injury in female victims of domestic violence. *Am J Obstet Gynecol* (Suppl) 188:S71, 2003.

28. Kyriacou DN, Anglin D, Taliaferro E, et al.: Risk factors for injury to women from domestic violence. *N Engl J Med* 341:1892, 1999.

29. Nadareishvili Z, Norris JW: Stroke from traumatic arterial dissection. *Lancet* 354:159, 1999.

30. Purvin V: Unilateral headache and ptosis in a 30-year-old woman. *Surv Ophthalmol* 42:163, 1997.

31. Malek AM, Higashida RT, Halbach VV, et al.: Patient presentation, angiographic features, and treatment of strangulation-induced bilateral dissection of the cervical internal carotid artery. *J Neurosurg* 92:481, 2000.

32. Eisenstat SA, Bancroft L: Domestic violence. *N Engl J Med* 341:886, 1999.

33. Ohkawa S, Yamadori A: CT in hanging. *Neuroradiology* 35:591, 1993.

34. Rao P, Carty H, Pierce A: The acute reversal sign: comparison of medical and non-accidental injury patients. *Clin Radiol* 54:495, 1999.

35. Ozkan U, Kemaloglu S, Ozates M, et al.: Analysis of 107 civilian craniocerebral gunshot wounds. *Neurosurg Rev* 25:231, 2002.

36. Brancatelli G, Sparacia G, Midiri M: Brain damage in hanging: a new CT finding. *Neuroradiology* 42:209, 2000.

37. Penney DJ, Stewart AHL, Parr MJA: Prognostic outcome indicators following hanging injuries. *Resuscitation* 54:27, 2002.

38. Kaki A, Crosby ET, Lui AC: Airway and respiratory management following non-lethal hanging. *Can J Anaesth* 44:445, 1997.

39. Hori A, Hirose G, Katoaka S, et al.: Delayed postanoxic encephalopathy after strangulation. Serial neuroradiological and neurochemical studies. *Arch Neurol* 48:871, 1991.

40. Kalita J, Mishra VN, Misra UK, et al.: Clinicoradiological observation in three patients with suicidal hanging. *J Neurol Sci* 198:21, 2002.

41. Feldhaus KM, Houry D, Utz A, et al.: Physician's knowledge of and attitudes toward a domestic violence mandatory reporting law. *Ann Emerg Med* 41:159, 2003.

42. Sekula-Perlman A, Tobin JG, Pretzler E, et al.: Three unusual cases of multiple suicidal gunshot wounds to the head. *Am J Forensic Med Pathol* 19:23, 1998.

43. Hagemann G, Willig V, Fitzek C, Witte OW. Gunshot-induced artery dissection with twelfth nerve palsy. *Arch Neurol* 60:280, 2003.

44. Helling TS, McNabney WK, Whittaker CK, et al.: The role of early surgical intervention in civilian gunshot wounds to the head. *J Trauma* 32:398, 1992.

45. Grahm TW, Williams FC Jr, Harrington T, et al.: Civilian gunshot wounds to the head: a prospective study. *Neurosurgery* 27:696, 1990.

46. Aldrich EF, Eisenberg HM, Saydjari C, et al.: Predictors of mortality in severely head-injured patients with civilian gunshot wounds: a report from the NIH Traumatic Coma Data Bank. *Surg Neurol* 38:418, 1992.

47. Gonul E, Baysefer A, Erdogan E, et al.: Tension pneumocephalus after frontal sinus gunshot wound. *Otolaryngol Head Neck Surg* 118:559, 1998.

48. Aferzon M, Aferzon J, Spektor Z: Endoscopic repair of tension pneumocephalus. *Otolarygol Head Neck Surg* 124:688, 2001.

49. Gardner WJ, Shannon EW: Pneumocranium from gunshot wound of brain. *JAMA* 214:2333, 1970.

50. Shaffrey ME, Polin RS, Phillips CD, et al.: Classification of civilian craniocerebral gunshot wounds: a multivariate analysis predictive of mortality. J Neurotrauma 9(Suppl 1):S279, 1992.

51. Selden BS, Goodman JM, Cordell W, et al.: Outcome of self-inflicted gunshot wounds of the brain. *Ann Emerg Med* 17:247, 1988.

52. Aarabi B, Alden TD, Chesnut RM, et al.: Neuroimaging in the management of penetrating brain injury. *J Trauma* 51(Suppl):S7, 2001.

53. Aarabi B, Alden TD, Chesnut RM, et al.: Management and prognosis of penetrating brain injury: introduction and methodology. *J Trauma* 51(Suppl):S3, 2001.

Index

Note: Page numbers followed by the letters b, f, and t denote boxes, figures, and tables, respectively